Interventional Radiology

A Survival Guide

For Elsevier
Commissioning Editor: Meghan McAteer
Project Development Manager: Hilary Hewitt
Project Manager: Anne Dickie
Illustration Manager: Mick Ruddy
Design Manager: Andy Chapman
Illustrator: Robin Dean
Marketing Manager(s) (UK/USA): Jemma Zighed/Emily McGrath-Christie

Interventional Radiology
A Survival Guide

SECOND EDITION

David Kessel, MB BS MA MRCP FRCR
Consultant Radiologist
St. James's University Hospital
Leeds, UK

Iain Robertson, MB ChB MRCP FRCR
Consultant Radiologist
Gartnavel General Hospital
Glasgow, UK

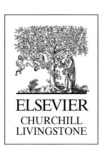

ELSEVIER
CHURCHILL
LIVINGSTONE

ELSEVIER
CHURCHILL
LIVINGSTONE

An imprint of Elsevier Limited

© 2000 Harcourt Publishers Limited
© 2005 Elsevier Limited. All rights reserved

First edition 2000
Second edition 2005

The right of David Kessel and Iain Robertson to be identified as authors of this work has been asserted by them in accordance with the Copyright, Designs and Patents Act 1988

ISBN 0 443 10044 6

British Library Cataloguing in Publication Data
A catalogue record for this book is available from the British Library

Library of Congress Cataloging in Publication Data
A catalog record for this book is available from the Library of Congress

Notice
Medical knowledge is constantly changing. Standard safety precautions must be followed, but as new research and clinical experience broaden our knowledge, changes in treatment and drug therapy may become necessary or appropriate. Readers are advised to check the most current product information provided by the manufacturer of each drug to be administered to verify the recommended dose, the method and duration of administration, and contraindications. It is the responsibility of the practitioner, relying on experience and knowledge of the patient, to determine dosages and the best treatment for each individual patient. Neither the Publisher nor the author assume any liability for any injury and/or damage to persons or property arising from this publication

The Publisher

Working together to grow
libraries in developing countries

www.elsevier.com | www.bookaid.org | www.sabre.org

ELSEVIER   **BOOK AID International**   **Sabre Foundation**

The Publisher's policy is to use **paper manufactured from sustainable forests**

Printed in China
Last digit is the print number : 9 8 7 6 5 4 3 2 1

Contents

Foreword

I am honored to write the introduction for the second edition of *Interventional Radiology – A Survival Guide* by Drs. David Kessel and Iain Roberston. When I opened the first edition in 2000, my immediate reaction was actually a horrible sinking feeling. Having recently agreed to a similar project myself, I looked through pages of concise insightful text, expertly selected and presented illustrations with comprehensive subject matter and realized that I was in trouble. This was something special. The book was the right size, the right length, easy to navigate, fun to read and truly stuffed with real-world information. It was clearly a book written by people who knew what they were doing and knew how to communicate it to others. For me, it was love at first sight.

The Survival Guide has stood up very well to the passage of the few years. As recommended reading for residents and fellows at our institution (and I am sure many others) the content remains just as valuable as when published. So why a second edition so soon – are the authors restless, sadistic, or maybe masochistic? If you look through the table of contents and the chapters, I think you will quickly see that the authors are too excited about our explosively expanding, fascinating specialty to let things be. So much has happened in just a few years, resulting in enough wonderful, new material that I guess they just couldn't help themselves. And for that the rest of us are very grateful.

Whether you are an experienced interventionalist, a fellow, a first year trainee, or a medical student, you will gain from this book. Where appropriate, the existing chapters have been revised, embellished, and strengthened. The new chapters on such topics as non-invasive vascular imaging, non-vascular intervention and fibroid embolization further the 'realness' of the book by providing the reader with the same essential and practical information required to take care of patients. The book has lost none of its character in the new edition, remaining accessible and even fun to read.

This is much more than a survival guide. This book is more akin to a fine distilled beverage, in that it concentrates the essential elements of the specialty into something that is complex, stimulating, and pleasant to ingest. Actually, after that, the analogy doesn't really hold that well; if you absorb large quantities of this book you won't just think that you are smarter and better, you will be. I raise a literary glass to Drs. Kessel and Robertson for another outstanding contribution to the specialty of interventional radiology!

John A Kaufman MD
Dotter Interventional Institute
Oregon Health & Science University
Portland, OR
19 November 2004

Preface

Second edition – how flattering, sure no problem.

Writing a second edition should be both easier and more pleasant than wrestling the text onto the page from two, sometimes disparate, minds. After all, the hard work's been done. It seemed only a limited amount of effort would be required to continue the book and perpetuate our status as authors.

We were wrong – it's been really hard work.

In the true spirit of intervention we haven't taken the quick easy route. The text has been extensively rewritten including new chapters on arterial closure, non-invasive vascular imaging and expanding the sections on GI intervention and embolization. Every chapter has been reviewed and many new figures have been added throughout the book.

Feedback from the first edition of the book has been very encouraging and we are delighted that the book has been adopted as a bench book in many departments. Indeed several departments have told us that the *Interventional Survival Guide* has now become "the book most often stolen". Certainly, there is nothing more pleasing than meeting a colleague who found the book helpful during a new or unfamiliar procedure. Well … on reflection it would be possibly even more pleasing hearing the same information from someone who had actually bought their own copy of the book!

Regardless of the ownership of this copy of the book we are sure you will find it a practical guide to surviving, and hopefully even enjoying, the rigours of interventional radiology.

Acknowledgements

We are both greatly indebted to the many people who have contributed to the delivery of this text.

Thanks to everyone who told us that they appreciated the first edition and motivated us to get typing again. We must mention the many patients who have endured and frequently entertained us during procedures and who have allowed us to use their images in the book. We are grateful to representatives from industry for providing some of the equipment that we have used to illustrate the manuscript. Lastly there are radiologists, surgeons, nurses and radiographers and nurses who have helped us practically and willingly shared their knowledge, skill and wisdom with us.

Special thanks to our families: Ben, Holly, Jamie, Ross and Anna, children who have not questioned what their dads were up to. Carrie and Debbie our much better halves who supported us throughout the writing and editing.

Abbreviations

AAA	abdominal aortic aneurysm
AV	atrioventricular
CCA	common carotid artery
CCF	congestive cardiac failure
CE-MRA	contrast-enhanced MRA
CFA	common femoral artery
CFV	common femoral vein
CIA	common iliac artery
CTA	computed tomography angiography
CVA	cerebrovascular accident
DSA	digital subtraction angiography
DVT	deep vein thrombosis
EIA	external iliac artery
ERCP	endoscopic retrograde cholangiopancreatography
FBC	full blood count
FFP	fresh frozen plasma
FNA	fine-needle aspiration
FNAC	fine-needle aspiration cytology
fps	frames per second
GTN	glyceryl trinitrate
IADSA	intra-arterial digital subtraction angiography
IJV	internal jugular vein
IM	intramuscular
IMA	inferior mesenteric artery
IV	intravenous
IVC	inferior vena cava
LAO	left anterior oblique
LGA	left gastric artery
MIP	maximum intensity projection
MPDSA	multiposition DSA
MRA	magnetic resonance angiography
MRI	magnetic resonance imaging
NSAID	non-steroidal anti-inflammatory drug
PA	popliteal artery
PE	pulmonary embolism
PFA	profunda femoris artery
PIG	peroral image-guided gastrostomy
PTC	percutaneous transhepatic cholangiography
PV	popliteal vein
PVA	polyvinyl alcohol

RAO	right anterior oblique
RAS	renal artery stenosis
RHV	right hepatic vein
RIG	radiologically inserted gastrostomy
RIJV	right internal jugular vein
RPV	right portal vein
rt-PA	recombinant tissue plasminogen activator
RVEDP	right ventricular end-diastolic pressure
SFA	superficial femoral artery
STD	sodium tetradecyl sulphate
SVCO	superior vena cava obstruction
SVT	supraventricular tachycardia
TIPS	transjugular intrahepatic portosystemic shunting
TJB	transjugular liver biopsy
TN	tibial nerve
TOS	thoracic outlet syndrome

Section One

General principles of
angiography and intervention

Chapter One

Basic principles of intervention

1

Interventional radiologists are clinicians in their own right. Along with the satisfaction of performing interventions comes the responsibility to assess the patient, explain the procedure to them and to follow up treatment outcomes. The latter is often the most rewarding aspect of clinical practice. Before rushing off to start practical procedures, stop and think, ensure that both you and your patient are properly prepared for the intervention and understand what the procedure entails. Consider the safe use of contrast, sedation and drugs. These are the cornerstones of good practice and risk management. You may be tempted to skip past here to get to the action and give this section little more than a perfunctory glance. Do so at your own peril!

Keys to successful intervention:
- Make sure that the procedure is appropriate in the clinical situation.
- Confirm that you and the patient have similar understanding of the procedure.
- Check that you have the same expectations of the likely short- and long-term technical and clinical outcomes.
- Understanding of the risks and benefits of the procedure.

Patient preparation

There are three key elements to ensure that patients are properly prepared for a procedure. Each assumes that you understand the procedure yourself.

Evaluation It is essential that patients undergoing an interventional procedure are adequately evaluated to identify any factors that may increase the risk of the procedure.

Action You must have strategies to deal with patients who are at increased risk.

Information The patient must then be given an indication of any significant risks and the likelihood of success when they are asked to give consent for the procedure.

Screening tests

Routine investigation (blood testing and electrocardiogram – ECG) of all patients is unnecessary and merely increases the cost of care. In deciding who to screen, consider the 'invasiveness' of the planned procedure and the likelihood of detecting an abnormality that would affect patient management. The guidelines below are suggestions for screening and are not absolute; if in doubt, it is better to perform a non-invasive test.

Clotting studies are indicated when the patient:
- Has clinical evidence of a coagulopathy.
- Has a disease likely to affect clotting. For instance, liver disease frequently causes deranged clotting; therefore, it is unwise to perform a liver biopsy without knowing the coagulation status as this substantially alters the risk of the procedure.
- Is taking medication that affects coagulation, e.g. heparin or warfarin.

Evaluation of renal function is indicated when the patient:
- Has a history of renal dysfunction.
- Has a disease likely to impair renal function, e.g. hypertension, especially with peripheral vascular disease.
- Is diabetic and has not had a recent evaluation of renal function.
- Has heart failure.
- Is receiving nephrotoxic drugs.

ECG is indicated when the patient:
- Has a history of cardiac disease.
- Is to undergo a procedure likely to affect cardiac output or cause arrhythmia, e.g. cardiac catheterization.

High-risk patients

Consider the risk in the context of the patient's condition. Although the risks of the procedure should be minimized, a life-saving procedure should not be delayed. From time to time you will be told that 'the patient is too unstable to bring to radiology', but remember, there is no logic saying that the patient is too ill to have a life-saving procedure! This section aims to help you keep the risk to yourself and the patient as small as possible.

This list is not comprehensive, so pause to consider before every case and never hesitate to seek advice.

The patient has a history of anaphylactic reaction to intravascular contrast   This is fully discussed in the section on contrast media (p. 11). Remember to consider alternative strategies, such as Duplex ultrasound, magnetic resonance angiography, or another contrast agent such as gadolinium or carbon dioxide (CO_2) depending on the local expertise. If angiography is essential, be prepared; if possible, get an anaesthetist, and at a minimum have the crash trolley ready and ensure the patient has venous access before starting.

The patient is anticoagulated or has a severe bleeding diathesis   The risk relates to the procedure; simple drainage and venous puncture are safer than arterial puncture or core biopsy. In the presence of mildly deranged clotting (international normalized ratio (INR) < 3), use a 3Fr catheter. If larger catheters are needed or the INR > 3, elective procedures should be postponed to allow investigation and correction of the coagulopathy. Only intervene to correct the clotting if the procedure is urgent. The risk of haematoma following angiography increases when the platelet count is 100×10^9/L. For surgery and invasive procedures the platelet count should be $= 50 \times 10^9$/L. Correction of coagulopathy is discussed in Chapter 4 (p. 27).

Tip: Abnormal clotting is relevant mainly when the time comes to obtain haemostasis. Consider using a closure device (Chapter 9). Alternatively, leave a sheath in the artery until the clotting is corrected. An arterial line may be helpful for intensive therapy unit patients.

Diabetes   Diabetic patients are at particular risk because of:
- The protean manifestations of diabetes, especially cardiovascular and renal disease.
- Potential problems with diabetic control in the periprocedural period.

Non-insulin dependent diabetics The current UK recommendation is that non-insulin dependent diabetics should stop metformin at the time of any procedure involving intra-vascular iodinated contrast, and should not restart until renal function has been checked 48 hours after the procedure. The risk of lactic acidosis is vanishingly small unless there is prior renal dysfunction. Some patients will need to take insulin to control their diabetes over this period.

Insulin-dependent diabetics should avoid prolonged fasting; they should be scheduled to have their procedure early in the morning. In this case they should take their long-acting insulin as usual but omit the short-acting insulin. If the procedure is later in the day, leave out the short-acting insulin and halve the dose of the long-acting insulin. A 5% dextrose solution should be infused to provide 5–10 g/h of glucose; this will normally maintain the blood glucose in the range 6–11 mmol/L.

Renal failure   Chronic renal impairment is relatively common in patients with peripheral vascular disease and may be exacerbated by contrast. The aetiology of contrast-induced nephropathy (a rise in creatinine of 0.5–1 mg/dL or 44–88 mmol/L) is complex. Although few patients will require dialysis, prevention is better than cure. Consider using alternative tests. The most important factor in protecting renal function is ensuring adequate hydra-tion. If iodinated contrast is essential then non-ionic iso-osmolar agents such as iodixanol (Visipaque) will minimize the risk. There is sufficient evidence suggesting a renoprotective effect of N-acetylcysteine (600 mg PO, two doses pre and post procedure) to support its use.

Tip: Remember that roughly 50% of renal function has been lost by the time the creatinine rises above the normal limit. Creatinine clearance can be estimated by the Cockcroft Gault method:

$$CrCl = [(140 - age) \times weight\ (kg)]/Cr \quad (\mu mol/L).$$
Multiply by 0.85 for female patients.

It is helpful to adopt a simple pragmatic strategy for managing patients with renal impair-ment based on the risk of developing contrast-induced nephropathy. If your centre does not have clear guidelines the following may help:
1. Is this the most appropriate investigation? (Consider MRA, Doppler, CO_2.)
2. Review medication: if possible, stop
   - NSAIDs
   - ACE-I (unless CCF)

- Metformin (stop for 48 h and restart if creatinine stable)
- Avoid loop diuretics if possible.

3. Act according to the creatinine clearance (serum creatinine if you don't have a calculator)

Minimal risk CrCl > 60 or Cr < 120

- Ensure hydration: oral fluids 1 L pre and post procedure.

Low risk CrCl 30–60 or Cr 120–180

- **Inpatient**: non-ionic contrast, IV normal saline 1 mL/kg/h 12 h pre and post procedure
- **Outpatient**: iso-osmolar contrast (iodixanol) Encourage oral fluids 1 L pre and post procedure; if possible IV normal saline started on arrival 1 L over 4 h.

Intermediate risk CrCl < 30, Cr > 180 or renal transplant

- If possible admit for procedure; iso-osmolar contrast (iodixanol) IV normal saline 1 mL/kg/h (caution if CCF) 12 h pre and post procedure; *N*-acetylcysteine 600 mg PO (two doses pre and post procedure).

High risk CrCl < 20 mL/min

- Admit for procedure; iso-osmolar contrast (iodixanol), IV normal saline 1 mL/kg/h (caution if CCF) 12 h pre and post procedure; *N*-acetylcysteine 600 mg PO (two doses pre and post procedure). Repeat Cr at 7 days.

Avoid further contrast exposure for 72 h if possible.

4. Other risk factors, e.g. diabetes mellitus, multiple myeloma, CCF, cirrhosis; consider promoting to the next level of CrCl.

Tip: Hydration – in the presence of CCF or cirrhosis with ascites use 5% dextrose instead of saline.

Hypertension   This is a common problem and is exacerbated by anxiety and pain. Hypertension increases the risk of haematoma. Review the ward charts to check the normal baseline blood pressure (BP). The Society of Cardiovascular and Interventional Radiology (SCVIR) standards define uncontrolled hypertension as a diastolic pressure >100 mmHg. Systolic hypertension is present when the systolic pressure is >180 mmHg.

Control of high blood pressure starts on the ward; the patient should take any antihypertensive medication (except diuretics) as normal. If the patient remains hypertensive in the angiography suite, he or she can be given 10 mg of nifedepine. Sedation and analgesia may also help blood pressure control. Aim to reduce the mean blood pressure by no more than 25%.

Tip: If the blood pressure cannot be controlled by these simple measures, postpone elective cases until the patient is appropriately medicated on the ward.

Heart failure   The patient's condition should be optimized before angiography. Diuretics should be avoided if possible to minimize the risk of nephrotoxicity. Limit the study to the essential details. If necessary, breathless patients can sit up slightly: this can be compensated for by craniocaudal angulation of the C-arm. Use oxygen as necessary.

Table 1.1 Fasting times prior to intervention

Oral intake	Fasting time
Solids and non-clear liquids	6–8 h
Clear liquids	2–3 h

Gastric contents It is normal to fast patients before invasive procedures, but the risk of aspiration of gastric contents is very small except in sedated patients. General guidelines are shown in Table 1.1. These are mandatory before conscious sedation or anaesthesia, and advisable before other cases.

In urgent cases, seek anaesthetic advice, avoid sedation and consider metoclopramide to promote gastric emptying, H_2 antagonists or proton pump inhibitors to increase gastric pH, and antiemetics to minimize the risk of vomiting.

Tip: Diabetic patients and those at the extremes of age should be given maintenance IV fluids to cover the periprocedural period.

Demented, anxious and agitated patients These patients may require sedation or general anaesthesia for angiography. A general anaesthetic is often the safest option for both patient and staff, and maximizes the chance of performing the procedure successfully. Consent issues are also relevant in this group of patients (see below).

Consent

Informed consent Patients have a legal (and moral) right to be given sufficient information to make informed decisions about the investigation/treatment (these terms will be used synonymously) options available to them.

Imagine what you would want to know before undergoing a procedure yourself:
- Are there alternative options?
- What are the risks or the procedures?
- What is the likelihood of the procedure being a technical success?
- Will this translate to having the clinically desired effect?
- What is the likelihood of recurrence?
- Will this treatment strategy affect their future management?

In practical terms a patient can only make a choice when they are empowered with sufficient knowledge. Your role is to provide relevant information in a way that the patient can comprehend. The laws regarding informed consent vary from country to country;

these guidelines are based on the current situation in England. The following summary outlines the key issues relating to informed consent, which are applicable in most instances.

Consent issues   The patient needs:
- Details of the diagnosis and prognosis.
- A balanced explanation of the treatment and management options along with the risks and benefits of each.
- To understand the nature and purpose of the proposed investigation or treatment, including analgesia, sedation and aftercare;
- To have realistic expectations of the outcomes of the procedure;
- Details of common and serious side effects (and their management) of the proposed intervention, especially where these may have special significance for the patient;
- To know the name of the doctor with overall responsibility for the patient, and relevant members of the doctor's team;
- To know that he/she has the right to change his/her mind or seek a second opinion at any time without prejudicing the care.

A qualified doctor who understands the risks and side effects of the procedure should be responsible for obtaining consent for treatment. Normally the doctor performing the treatment is in the best position to provide this information. If this is not practicable, the doctor may delegate to an appropriately experienced colleague.

The form of the explanation and the amount of information provided vary depending on the patient's wishes and capacity to understand, and the nature and complexity of the treatment. The patient should be allowed time to consider the information and must not be pressurized to make a decision.

Alarm: It is often considered satisfactory to mention only those complications that occur in at least 1% of patients; this is not the case! You should comment when the treatment is complex or involves significant risk for the patient's health, employment, social or personal life. Use the patient's notes to document the key elements of any explanation, and record any other wishes that the patient has in relation to the proposed treatment.

Review the patient's decision close to the time of treatment. This is mandatory when:
- Significant time has elapsed since consent was obtained.
- There have been changes that may affect the treatment.

Alarm: Compliance is not the same as consent! The patient's presence in the angiography suite does not indicate that he or she knows what the treatment entails. Checking the consent will avoid the possibility of misunderstanding later.

Special circumstances   There are instances in which it is difficult or impossible to obtain informed consent. There are some general guidelines for what is acceptable procedure. If there is any doubt, legal advice should be obtained from either the hospital administration department, your protection society or your Medical Union.

Emergencies   When consent cannot be obtained, you may only provide whatever medical treatment is necessary to save life or prevent significant deterioration in the patient's condition.

Competence to make decisions   Competence may be described as the ability to comprehend information presented in a clear way and retain it for long enough to assess it and make a decision.

Inability to comprehend   Apparently irrational decisions and refusal of treatment are not evidence of lack of competence. Take time and review whether the patient has been provided with sufficient information or has not fully understood any of the explanation. Where doubt exists, seek advice; there is guidance for the formal assessment of competence.

Fluctuating capacity   When the patient's mental state varies, consent should be obtained during periods of competence. This should be reviewed at intervals and recorded in the patient's notes. No-one can give or withhold consent to treatment on behalf of a mentally incapacitated patient. Try to establish whether the patient has previously indicated a preference, e.g. in a 'living will'. If the patient complies, you may carry out any treatment that is judged to be in the patient's best interest.

Children   At the age of 16 the patient should be treated as an adult. Below the age of 16 children have the capacity to decide whether they are able to understand the nature, purpose and consequence of the procedure or its refusal. In England, if a competent child refuses treatment, a person with parental authority or a court may give consent for any treatment in that child's best interest. Seek legal advice when there is any doubt. A person with parental authority may authorize or refuse treatment for a child who is not competent to give consent. You are not bound by parental refusal: seek legal advice. In an emergency, proceed as above.

SUGGESTIONS FOR FURTHER READING

Screening tests
Vincent GM, Brown W. Prothrombin and partial thrombin times are unnecessary before routine cardiac catheterisation. J Intervent Cardiol 1990;3:1–4.

Perioperative evaluation of patients with hematologic disorders
Fellin FM, Murphy S. Peri-operative evaluation of patients with hematologic disorders. In: Merli GJ, Weitz HH, eds. Medical management of the surgical patient. WB Saunders, 1992:84–115.
Payne CS. A primer on patient management problems in interventional radiology. AJR 1998;170:1169–1176.
A useful overview of screening for and managing high-risk patients.

High-risk patients
Aspelin P, Aubry P, Fransson S-G et al. Nephrotoxic effects in high risk patients undergoing angiography. N Engl J Med 2003;348:491–499.

Morcos SK. Prevention of contrast media nephrotoxicity – the story so far. Clin Radiol 2004;59:381–389.

Mueller C, Buerkel G, Buettner H et al. Prevention of contrast media associated nephropathy. Randomized comparison of 2 hydration regimes in 1620 patients undergoing coronary angioplasty. Arch Intern Med 2002;162:329–336.

Level 1 evidence why to use normal saline.

Rihal C, Textor S, Grill D et al. Level 1 evidence as to the advantage of iodixanol (Visipaque) over non-ionic contrast media. Incidence and prognostic importance of acute renal failure after percutaneous coronary intervention. Circulation 2002;105:2259–2264.

The true incidence of ARF and its significance in a real population: sobering reading!

Waksman R, King SB, Douglas JS et al. Predictors of groin complications after balloon and new device coronary intervention. Am J Cardiol 1995;75:886–889.

Big holes, big patients and deranged clotting.

Consent

British Medical Association/Law Society. Assessment of mental capacity: Guidance for doctors and lawyers. London: BMA Publications, BMA House, Tavistock Square, London WC1H 9JP.

General Medical Council. Seeking patients' consent: The ethical considerations. London: GMC Publications, 178 Great Portland Street, London W1N 6JE.

Up-to-date and informative booklet outlining reasonable practice in the UK. Mandatory reading.

Chapter Two

Contrast

The vast majority of angiographic procedures and many non-vascular interventions rely on contrast media to reveal the anatomy. There are many agents available, but all act by increasing differences in contrast between tissues. Contrast media can be broadly classified by their use and by their chemical structure. X-ray contrast affects tissue X-ray attenuation, ultrasound contrast affects tissue and blood reflectivity, and magnetic resonance imaging (MRI) contrast affects tissue relaxation times. Discussion in this section is confined to X-ray contrast media.

INTRAVASCULAR X-RAY CONTRAST AGENTS

The two principal categories of X-ray contrast both affect tissue X-ray attenuation. Details of the chemical and physical properties of these agents are extensively discussed in many texts, and it is important that you are familiar with the different options and their indications.

Positive contrast agents are liquids that have greater attenuation than the patient's soft tissues owing to the presence of iodine or gadolinium.

Negative contrast has lower attenuation than the patient's tissues; at present, carbon dioxide gas is the only available option.

Iodinated contrast media

These are the most frequently used agents and are derivatives of benzoic acid. In the UK, non-ionic contrast media have largely replaced the previous generation of ionic contrast agents for intravascular use. In the USA, non-ionic agents cost significantly more than ionic contrast, so the latter are frequently used. Non-ionic contrast is recommended in high-risk patients (see below).

Contrast reveals anatomy and pathology; this requires the correct strength and volume of contrast for each examination. Throughout the diagnostic angiography chapters, appropriate catheter positions, contrast volumes and flow rates are indicated.

Most diagnostic and therapeutic intervention is performed using '300 strength' contrast (300 mg/mL iodine). This density of contrast is fine for pump injections, as the contrast is effectively diluted by rapid blood flow. For selective hand injections in the vascular system, and for all non-vascular examinations, 300 strength contrast is diluted with saline to two-thirds or half strength. The aim is to opacify the vessel adequately but allow a level of grey scale that allows branches/filling defects to be seen through the contrast. Avoid high-density contrast examinations as lesions can be readily obscured.

The contrast column should opacify the entire vessel segment in the field. To achieve this, the total contrast dose and the duration of the bolus must be correct. When the blood flow is slow, it takes several seconds for the opacified blood to pass through the vessel. Hence, a long contrast bolus is necessary. This is one of the reasons for increasing the volume of contrast to image the more distal vessels. Some modern angiography equipment allows the integration of multiple images, which has the same effect as increasing the length of the bolus but can reduce image quality owing to minor degrees of patient movement between frames.

Contrast reactions with iodinated contrast media

There are two forms of contrast reaction: direct effects and idiosyncratic responses. Up to 2% of patients require treatment for adverse reactions to intravascular iodinated contrast agents. In the majority of cases only observation and minor supportive treatment are necessary, but severe reactions require prompt recognition and immediate treatment.

Direct effects   Direct effects are secondary to the osmolality and direct chemotoxicity of the contrast, and they include heat, nausea and pain. More important are the effects on organ systems.

RENAL   Chronic renal impairment is relatively common in patients with peripheral vascular disease and is exacerbated by contrast. Contrast-induced nephrotoxicity (a rise in creatinine of 0.5–1 mg/dL or 44–88 mmol/L) is common; the effect is usually transient, but may be irreversible. Patients with pre-existing renal impairment, particularly diabetics, have the greatest risk. Consider using alternative tests, iso-osmolar contrast agents (e.g. iodixanol) and non-iodinated contrast agents such as carbon dioxide.

The most important factor in protecting renal function is to avoid dehydration. There is evidence supporting the renoprotective effect of hydration with normal saline, and also the use of N-acetylcysteine (see Chapter 1). Diabetic patients treated with metformin have a risk of developing lactic acidosis if they experience renal failure. The current UK guidelines are that metformin should be discontinued on the day of the examination and for 48 hours afterwards until the creatinine has returned to the pre-examination, normal level.

CARDIAC   Cardiac problems are most likely to occur during coronary angiography and are usually manifest as arrhythmias or ischaemia. It is prudent to use non-ionic contrast in patients with ischaemic heart disease or heart failure.

HAEMATOLOGICAL   Significant haematological interactions are uncommon. Non-ionic iodinated contrast can induce clotting if mixed with blood, hence scrupulous attention to catheter flushing and the avoidance of contaminating syringes with blood are essential.

NEUROLOGICAL   Most neurological sequelae occur during carotid angiography and are related to angiographic technique. Genuine contrast-related problems are rare and are usually seen in patients with abnormalities in the blood–brain barrier.

Idiosyncratic reactions   The mechanism of these reactions is uncertain. Vasoactive agents such as histamine, serotonin, bradykinin and complement have been implicated, but a causal role has not been established. Idiosyncratic reactions are classified according to severity:

- **Minor**: Common, ~1:30, e.g. metallic taste, sensation of heat, mild nausea, sneezing; these do not require treatment.
- **Intermediate**: Common, ~1:100, e.g. urticaria; not life-threatening; respond quickly to treatment.
- **Severe**: Rare, ~1:3000, e.g. circulatory collapse, arrhythmia, bronchospasm, dyspnoea; may be life-threatening, require prompt therapy.
- **Death**: Rare, ~1:40 000, mostly caused by cardiac arrhythmia, pulmonary oedema, respiratory arrest or convulsions.

Assessing the risk   The risk of a contrast reaction varies depending on the circumstances of individual patients; however, the following are associated with an increased risk of a severe idiosyncratic reaction:

- Previous allergic reaction to iodine containing contrast and shellfish allergy – 10×
- Cardiac disease – 5×
- Asthma – 5×
- General allergic responses – 3×
- Drugs: β-blockers, IL-2 – 3×
- Age >50 years – 2× risk of death.

Reducing the risk   The vast majority of severe and fatal contrast reactions occur within 20 minutes of administration, and therefore it is vital that patients are kept under constant supervision during this period. There have been a few isolated reports of delayed hypotensive reactions hours after contrast injection.

The ideal method of reducing risk is to avoid iodine-containing contrast examinations by using other imaging modalities, such as ultrasound or MRI. When this is not possible:

- **Prepare for reaction**. Ensure that resuscitation equipment and drugs are immediately available every time contrast is injected.
- **Use non-ionic contrast agents**. Non-ionic contrast agents certainly reduce the risk of minor reactions and may reduce the risk of more significant reactions, though this has not yet been absolutely proven.
- **Reassure the patient**. Explain that contrast reactions are unlikely and that the situation is under control. In severe anxiety, short-acting anxiolytic agents may be warranted.
- **Consider steroid premedication**. There is some evidence that oral steroid premedication may reduce the risk of moderate–severe reactions, though this is hotly contested. Treatment has to be started 24 hours before contrast administration, and therefore this is only suitable for elective examinations. Intravenous hydrocortisone 200 mg has been given prior to urgent examinations, though this is of questionable value. Many departments have local guidelines on steroid administration.

In the rare patient with a documented severe reaction:

- Avoid iodinated contrast; use CO_2 or gadolinium or another imaging modality.
- If this is impossible and the examination is essential, then monitor the patient carefully.
- Ensure resuscitation personnel, equipment and drugs are immediately available. You may need expert assistance in maintaining the airway: consider enrolling anaesthetic assistance.

- Obtain secure IV access before contrast administration.
- Use non-ionic contrast.
- Consider steroid premedication; consult local guidelines.
- Reassure the patient.

Treatment of contrast reactions

Warn patients that a sense of warmth, a metallic taste and transient nausea are all common after rapid IV injection of contrast, and that these effects wear off after a few minutes.

Minor reactions

- **Nausea and vomiting**. Active treatment rarely required. Reassure and monitor patient.
- **Urticaria**. One of the commonest contrast reactions. Localized patches of urticaria do not require treatment. Simply observe and monitor the patient (pulse, BP). Generalized urticaria or localized urticaria in sensitive areas, e.g. periorbital, should be treated by chlorpheniramine 20 mg given slowly by IV injection.
- **Vasovagal syncope**. Monitor the patient's pulse, BP, oxygen saturation and ECG. Elevate the legs. Establish IV access. Give atropine 0.6–1.2 mg by IV injection for bradycardia. Volume expansion with IV fluids for persistent hypotension.

Intermediate–severe reactions

- **Bronchospasm**. Monitor the patient's pulse, BP, oxygen saturation and ECG. Give 100% O_2. Treat initially with β-agonist inhaler, e.g. salbutamol. If continuing bronchospasm, administer adrenaline (epinephrine) subcutaneously 0.3–0.5 mL of 1:1000 solution. If severely shocked, then administer adrenaline (epinephrine) 1 mL (0.1 mg) 1:10 000 by slow IV injection. IV steroids are also usually given, and in acute reactions steroids may work surprisingly quickly, though it can take a few hours for them to achieve full effect.
- **Laryngeal oedema/angioneurotic oedema**. Monitor the patient's pulse, BP, oxygen saturation and ECG. Give 100% O_2 and watch the oxygen saturation closely. Administer adrenaline subcutaneously 0.3–0.5 mL of 1:1000 solution. Chlorpheniramine 20 mg by slow IV injection should also be given. Get an anaesthetist to assess the airway. Tracheostomy may be required in severe cases.
- **Severe hypotension**. Hypotension accompanied by tachycardia may indicate vasodilation and increased capillary permeability. Monitor the patient's pulse, BP, oxygen saturation and ECG. Rapid infusion of IV fluids is essential, and several litres of fluid replacement may be necessary. Adrenaline is often of value.
- **Cimetidine**, the H_2 receptor antagonist, has been effective in severe reactions resistant to conventional therapy. The drug is given by slow intravenous infusion (cimetidine 300 mg in 20 mL saline). An H_1 receptor blocker such as chlorpheniramine should be given first.

ALTERNATIVES TO IODINATED CONTRAST

Gadolinium

Gadolinium works well as an MRI contrast agent. Its use has been described in X-ray angiography, but it is a poor X-ray contrast agent and is often difficult to see on fluoroscopy.

Gadolinium is handled in the same way as conventional contrast, and can be injected by hand or with an injection pump.

Gadolinium is nephrotoxic when doses greater than 40 mL are used: this limits its utility for most angiographic procedures. Gadolinium-based agents are much more expensive than iodinated contrast, therefore their use is reserved for patients who need a limited volume of contrast and have a good reason to avoid iodinated contrast.

Negative contrast agent – carbon dioxide

Carbon dioxide is most commonly used for the following reasons:
- History of severe reaction to iodinated contrast
- Renoprotection
- Where there is another advantage, such as the use of CO_2 for wedged hepatic venography.

Medical-grade CO_2 is an alternative to liquid contrast agents which does not cause contrast reactions or nephrotoxicity. CO_2 is only effective with digital subtraction angiography (DSA), and additional software is necessary to optimize the image. CO_2 dissolves rapidly in blood and is excreted through the lungs. Consider using CO_2 when there is a contra-indication to conventional iodinated contrast, and to opacify the portal vein during wedged hepatic venography.

Alarm: There is a risk of cerebral toxicity with CO_2, and for this reason it should never be used intra-arterially above the diaphragm, or intravenously in patients with right-to-left shunts.

Equipment
- Basic angiography set
- Medical grade CO_2 from a disposable* cylinder
- Standard bacterial filter (from a blood-giving set)
- High-pressure connector
- Three-way tap
- Lockable stopcock for each syringe
- 60 mL Luer-lock syringes.

* Reusable cylinders may be contaminated with water or rust particles, hence the need for a disposable system. The bacterial filter is a further safeguard. In an ideal world one would use disposable stainless steel cylinders: these are more expensive but cause less patient discomfort.

The circuit is set up as shown in Figure 2.1.

Alarm: The pressurized CO_2 must never be connected directly to the patient, as this risks inadvertent injection of a large volume of gas that may cause a 'vapour lock'.

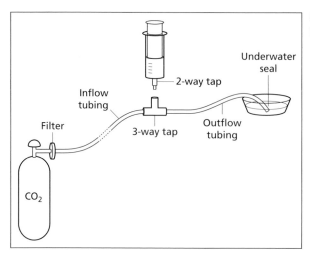

Fig. 2.1 ▓ Preparation of CO_2 for hand injection.

Injecting CO_2

You can inject by hand or via a dedicated pump. CO_2 gas has very low viscosity and so is very readily injected even through small catheters. Injecting a colourless, odourless and invisible gas is disconcerting at first. It is essential to have a foolproof system for filling the syringes to prevent inadvertent air embolization.

Filling syringes with CO_2

1. Fill a 10 mL syringe from the system; this flushes the system and purges any air from the connecting tube. Repeat this each time the gas is turned off.
2. Allow the syringe to fill 'passively' from the cylinder: this ensures that it is filling with CO_2. Stop filling when there is about 50 mL in the syringe.
3. Use the three-way tap to discard the contents three times to flush out any residual air in the syringe before finally filling.
4. Shut the lockable stopcock and disconnect the syringe from the tap.
5. The syringe will now contain CO_2 at slightly above atmospheric pressure.

 Alarm: The CO_2 in an open syringe will be replaced with air in about an hour! Always prepare CO_2 syringes just before use, and keep the stopcock closed.

The catheter is flushed with saline as normal. As the filled syringe is connected to the catheter, the stopcock is opened; this has two functions:

- Air is flushed from the catheter hub.
- The CO_2 in the syringe falls to atmospheric pressure and so the true volume of the gas is known.

The catheter is now gently flushed with CO_2; this expels the saline from the lumen. You will know when the catheter is flushed, as there is a marked fall in resistance. Close the tap and disconnect this syringe and discard its contents. Connect a fresh syringe of CO_2 and you are ready to inject. The volume and rate of injection are adjusted according to the size of the vessel. There is no dose limit as long as injections are restricted to 100 mL every 2 minutes.

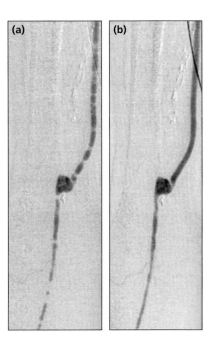

Fig. 2.2 Gas fragmentation with CO_2 angiography. (a) Image before multiple image summation. (b) After image summation.

If performing venography, always fluoroscope over the pulmonary artery to look for gas trapping.

Troubleshooting

Dependent vessels are not seen Intravascular CO_2 displaces blood rather than mixing with it like a liquid contrast. The CO_2 is buoyant and floats over the blood column, dependent branches tend not to fill, and in general there is an underestimate of vessel size. The patient should be turned to elevate the vessel of interest, e.g. side of interest up for renal angiography. C-arm angulation must be adjusted accordingly.

There is gas trapping The CO_2 collects above the blood and forms a 'vapour lock'. This reduces the surface area for the gas to dissolve. Potentially this can lead to ischaemia or thrombosis. This is most likely to happen with large (>100 mL) injections of CO_2, or in capacious vessels with anterior branches, e.g. in an aortic aneurysm. If gas trapping occurs, simply turn or tilt the patient so that the gas can disperse. If necessary, the gas can be aspirated via a catheter. **Do not elevate the patient's head!**

The gas column fragments This happens particularly in the distal vessels (Fig. 2.2). Use image summation techniques to integrate several frames on to the same image. Consider raising the leg, as this improves filling of the distal vessels.

The distal vessels cannot be seen CO_2 is a 'negative contrast' and not as good as conventional contrast media (otherwise we would use it all the time!). Sometimes bolus fragmentation and poor opacification require the use of a liquid contrast agent.

The patient experiences pain during injection Try a slower injection rate.

SUGGESTIONS FOR FURTHER READING

Complications of intravascular iodinated contrast media

Ansell G. Complications of intravascular iodinated contrast media In: Ansell G et al., eds. Complications in diagnostic imaging and interventional radiology, 3rd edn. Oxford: Blackwell Science, 1996:245–300.

An excellent summary with everything that you might ever wish to know about iodinated contrast, and more besides.

Bettmann MA, Heeren T, Greenfield A et al. Adverse events with radiographic contrast agents: Results of the SCVIR contrast registry. Radiology 1997;203:611–620.

A prospective review of adverse outcomes in over 60 000 patients. There is some study bias, but unless you are dealing with a high-risk patient, ionic contrast agents are safe.

Alternatives to iodinated contrast media

Caridi JG, Hawkins IF. CO_2 digital subtraction angiography: Potential complications and their prevention. J Vasc Intervent Radiol 1997;8:383–891.

How to work with CO_2. A useful starter.

Chapter Three

Sedation

Radiologists frequently sedate patients for prolonged or painful interventional procedures. Sedation can also be useful in anxious, confused or hypertensive patients. Unfortunately, most of us have not been trained in anaesthesia and may lack the ability to maintain a patient's airway in an emergency. Sedation may result in respiratory depression and aspiration of gastric contents; in addition, there is a small but significant mortality. Children are at particular risk.

This chapter defines conscious sedation and outlines patient selection and management in the radiology department. If you have any doubts about your ability to manage a particular patient, seek advice from an anaesthetist.

Conscious sedation

This refers to a controlled state of reduced consciousness throughout which the patient retains the ability to make purposeful, verbal responses. Protective reflexes are preserved and the airway is maintained. Drugs used in conscious sedation should have a sufficient margin of safety to make unintended loss of consciousness unlikely.

Deep sedation and anaesthesia involve a further reduction in conscious level from which the patient is not readily roused, and during which protective reflexes and the ability to maintain the airway may be lost along with the ability to respond to physical and verbal stimulation. In terms of patient management, deep sedation should be regarded as a form of general anaesthesia.

To sedate or not to sedate, that is the question

Practices differ widely between countries and cultures. Patient tolerance varies enormously: it is unnecessary to use sedation routinely. Take time to talk to patients before, during and after the procedure, and you will find that the majority are not distressed if they are actively reassured and not in pain. It is important not to equate sedation with analgesia, and if performing a painful procedure to give adequate analgesia. Remember that sedation and analgesia are synergistic, and take care. Consider sedation in the following circumstances:

- Painful procedures, e.g. transjugular intrahepatic portosystemic shunting (TIPS), biliary stenting;
- Prolonged procedures where the patient is likely to become uncomfortable;
- Patients who remain very anxious despite explanation;
- Patients who are unlikely to cooperate, e.g. children, agitated or confused patients.

By avoiding sedation, you will not expose the vast majority of your patients to the attendant risk. Try to establish whether sedation is likely to be required before starting the procedure. In this way, the patient can be properly assessed and the risks minimized.

Sedation guidelines

- Assess the requirements and risks for each patient.
- Make sure the patient has IV access and pulse, BP and O_2 monitoring.
- Remember that benzodiazepines are more potent in elderly (>60 years) patients: the dose should be reduced accordingly. Start with a small dose and increase it as necessary. A large bolus is more likely to result in hypoxia (oxygen saturation <90%) and apnoea. Most practitioners use 2.5 mg aliquots of midazolam.
- Use diazepam in patients over 70 years old (see Fig. 4.1).
- Designated personnel should be responsible for monitoring the patient and maintaining records.
- Resuscitation equipment must be readily available and staff should be familiar with its use. It helps to have a designated staff member to respond in case of emergency.

 Alarm: Do not hesitate to seek anaesthetic assistance if you have any doubts about sedation: it is much better than having to deal with a problem during a case.

Patient selection

Most serious adverse events are not predictable and can occur in 'healthy' patients. Extremes of age, pre-existing cardiorespiratory disease and severe illness contribute to and increase risk with sedation. Ask an anaesthetist to assess high-risk patients: a general anaesthetic may be safer for them than sedation. Do not forget that aspiration of gastric contents is associated with significant morbidity in patients who are not fasted.

Care and monitoring of sedated patients

Care   It is essential that there are adequate numbers of trained staff and appropriate facilities to permit constant monitoring of the patient's condition. Radiologists often take responsibility for sedation, but this is unsatisfactory during interventional procedures when your attention is focused elsewhere.

Monitoring   A named member of staff should be responsible for monitoring each patient. They must be capable of recognizing and managing important changes in the sedated patient's condition. Many of the complications caused by sedation can be avoided if the patient is closely and responsively observed during the procedure and in the recovery period. The following parameters should be monitored:

Pulse oximetry and respiratory rate Allows prompt recognition of hypoxia long before it is clinically obvious. Remember that the haemoglobin saturation is normal in anaemia despite the reduced oxygen-carrying ability. Prompt action should be taken when the oxygen saturation falls below 95%. The patient should be encouraged to take some deep breaths, and oxygen should be administered by mask or nasal cannulae. If this fails, try to establish an airway using the jaw thrust manoeuvre or a plastic airway. Seek assistance sooner rather than later.

 Tip: Give oxygen routinely to sedated patients: this saves an unseemly scuffle when the pulse oximeter alarm starts to ring.

ECG The ECG demonstrates heart rate and cardiac rhythms and detects signs of myocardial ischaemia; it is invaluable in the management of cardiac arrest and arrhythmia. **NB: Most cardiac events are late manifestations of hypoxia.**

Pulse and blood pressure These are best monitored by an automatic device. Warn the patient that this is:
(a) uncomfortable
(b) normal practice and not a sign of impending problems.

Most machines have alarms that can be set to respond to significant increases or falls in blood pressure. Record the pressure every 5 minutes and make additional recordings during procedures likely to affect the blood pressure. **NB: Tachycardia and hypertension are usually the response to pain, but may also reflect hypercapnoea.**

 Alarm: Clinical observation is vital during conscious sedation; machines do not detect responsiveness. Maintain verbal and tactile contact with the patient, and assess his or her mental state and alertness.

Aftercare

Remember that sedated patients require close observation until they are alert and oriented and able to drink. Inpatients may return to the ward as soon as they are stable enough to be cared for on the ward, but this varies considerably with the type of ward. Baseline observations should be stable for at least 1 hour before discharge. Outpatients should not drive or operate machinery for 24 hours, and must be accompanied by a responsible adult. Clear instructions should be provided for the carer, detailing what to expect in the postprocedural period. State clearly who should be contacted (and how to contact them) in case of problems.

SUGGESTIONS FOR FURTHER READING

Royal College of Radiologists and the Royal College of Anaesthetists. Sedation and anaesthesia in radiology: report of a joint working party. London: Royal College of Radiologists and the Royal College of Anaesthetists, 1992.
A good overview, compiled jointly by anaesthetists and radiologists.
Scholer SG, Schafer DF, Potter JF. The effect of age on the relative potency of midazolam and diazepam for sedation in upper gastrointestinal endoscopy. J Clin Gastroenterol 1990;12:145–147.

Chapter Four

Drugs used in interventional radiology

This chapter provides a brief guide to the use of some of the drugs frequently used in interventional radiology, broadly grouped according to their actions. Familiar drugs in common general usage will not be discussed in detail. The list is not comprehensive and we do not address pharmacological interactions. For other drugs and paediatric dose schedules, consult conventional texts and local guidelines.

Anaesthetics, analgesics and sedatives

Local anaesthetics

Local anaesthesia is the first stage in almost every interventional procedure. Warn the patient that the injection may sting for a few seconds before the anaesthetic takes effect. Remember to wait before making that first incision! Local anaesthetics are remarkably free from adverse reactions. The majority of 'reactions' are psychogenic or the result of systemic toxicity, usually owing to inadvertent intravascular injection, overdose or rapid absorption. True anaphylactoid and anaphylactic reactions to lidocaine occur very rarely (about 1 per year in the UK) and represent only 1% of reported adverse reactions. Skin testing may be useful to establish cases of true type I hypersensitivity. In true allergy, prilocaine should be used. Systemic effects on the central nervous system include dizziness, confusion, paraesthesia and convulsions with bradycardia, and cardiovascular effects (e.g. arrhythmia and hypotension).

Lidocaine hydrochloride (xylocaine, lignocaine)
- **Action** Stabilizes nerve membrane, preventing generation and transmission of impulses.
- **Indication** Local anaesthesia. NB: Lignocaine is also a class I antiarrhythmic agent.
- **Dose** 1% lignocaine (10 mg/mL) is sufficient for local anaesthesia; the total dose should not usually exceed 20 mL (200 mg).
- **Cautions** Allergic reactions.
- **Monitor** Pulse, BP and oxygen saturation.
- **Reversal** None. Oxygen helps prevent and treat systemic effects; give circulatory support and maintain airway.

Prilocaine hydrochloride
- **Indication** Allergy to lignocaine; adverse reactions are commoner with prilocaine, but there is little cross-reactivity.
- **Dose** 1% prilocaine (10 mg/mL). Maximum dose 400 mg.

Bupivacaine hydrochloride (marcain)   Bupivacaine is a long-acting local anaesthetic and is sometimes useful for prolonged procedures or when a device is left in situ. It is not used to induce anaesthesia, as it takes up to 30 minutes to reach full effect.

- **Indication** Prolonged local anaesthesia.
- **Dose** 0.25% bupivacaine (2.5 mg/mL). Maximum dose 150 mg (60 mL).

Analgesics

Prolonged and painful interventional procedures are often very uncomfortable for the patient. Even the most stoic will become restless after a time, and if they are also in pain their confidence in you will be lost. Analgesia should be given before this stage is reached. This is not the time for paracetamol: **opiate analgesics** are the order of the day. Use a preparation that you are familiar with; pethidine and morphine are commonly used.

- **Cautions** Start with a low dose and increase as necessary. Elderly patients are often very sensitive. Opiates and sedatives have a synergistic effect.
- **Monitor** Pulse, BP and oxygen saturation.
- **Reversal** Naloxone 100–200 mg (1.5–3 mg/kg) by IV injection. If response is inadequate, give increments of 100 mg every 2 minutes. Repeat as necessary.

Sedatives

The use of sedation increases the risk of any procedure, but sedatives should be considered in anxious and restless patients. Remember that in confused and agitated patients there is often a narrow divide between sedation and anaesthesia. Start with a small dose and titrate it to individual requirements. If the patient has cardiorespiratory disease, it is prudent to seek anaesthetic advice (see p. 4). Benzodiazepines are the most commonly used sedatives as their dose requirement decreases with increasing age.

Midazolam

- **Action** Short-acting benzodiazepine with a half-life of 2 hours.
- **Indication** Conscious sedation.
- **Dose** 2.5–10 mg, IV or IM; IM injection gives slower absorption in elderly patients. The potency of midazolam increases in patients over 60, and for this reason diazepam is recommended in elderly patients, especially those over 70 years old (Fig. 4.1).
- **Cautions** Reduce dose in elderly patients, respiratory depression, aspiration.
- **Monitor** Pulse, BP and oxygen saturation. Give oxygen by nasal prongs or by mask.
- **Reversal** Flumazenil (Annexate) by IV injection, initial dose 200 mg over 15 seconds, then 100 mg at 60-second intervals to a maximum dose of 1 mg. Flumazenil is short acting and an infusion of 100–400 mg/h can be instituted in the presence of long-acting benzodiazepines.

Diazepam

- **Action** Benzodiazepine with a long half-life and active metabolites.
- **Indication** Sedation of elderly patients. Compared with midazolam, the relative potency of diazepam changes little with age, giving it a wider margin of safety.
- **Dose** 2–10 mg by slow IV injection into a large vein.
- **Cautions** Thrombophlebitis common.

Monitoring and reversal are as for midazolam.

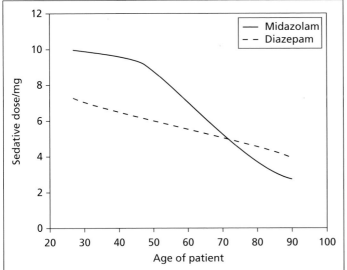

Fig. 4.1 ■ Age-related changes in the sedative dose of diazepam and midazolam. (Modified from Scholer SG et al. J Clin Gastroenterol 1990;12:145–147.)

Vasoactive drugs

Vasodilators

Vasodilator drugs are used in angiography to prevent and relieve vascular spasm (prevention, as always, is better than cure) and to augment flow during measurement of intra-arterial pressure gradients. Several drugs are in common use and are discussed below. Typically use glyceryl trinitrate (GTN) to prevent spasm, and tolazoline and papaverine to augment flow and reverse spasm. Nifedipine (an antihypertensive) can also be given prophylactically in situations where spasm is anticipated.

Tolazoline
- **Action** α-Adrenoreceptor blockade.
- **Dose** 20–50 mg by slow intra-arterial injection.
- **Cautions** Palpitations, angina and nausea are common side effects.
- **Monitor** Pulse, BP and ECG.

Papaverine
- **Action** Direct smooth muscle relaxant.
- **Dose** 20–60 mg by slow, selective intra-arterial injection. May be followed by infusion of 30–60 mg/h.
- **Cautions** Hypotension.
- **Monitor** Pulse, BP and ECG.

Glyceryl trinitrate
- **Action** Complex, mixed venous and arterial vasodilator.
- **Dose** 100–200 mg boluses by selective intra-arterial injection. May be infused at 15–20 mg/min and increased as necessary if the blood pressure allows.

- **Cautions** Hypotension.
- **Monitor** Pulse, BP and ECG.

Tip: GTN typically comes in a solution of 1 mg/mL; to measure small doses accurately, draw up the desired dose in a 1 mL syringe and dilute to 1 mL with saline.

Vasoconstrictors

Vasopressin is the only vasoconstrictor in common use.
- **Action** Synthetic, antidiuretic hormone that has direct vasoconstrictor effects.
- **Indication** Used to control variceal and gastrointestinal haemorrhage.
- **Dose** Selective intra-arterial infusion 0.1–0.4 units/min. May be given IV for variceal bleeding 0.2–0.8 units/min.
- **Cautions** Ischaemic heart disease and peripheral vascular disease.
- **Monitor** Pulse, BP and ECG.
- **Reversal** The half-life is only 10 minutes.

Antihypertensive agents

Hypertension is a common problem and is exacerbated by anxiety and pain. Hypertension increases the risk of haematoma. When faced with a hypertensive patient, review the ward charts to check the normal baseline blood pressure and to ensure that the patient has taken any antihypertensive medication as normal. Blood pressure reduction is indicated if the diastolic pressure rises above 100 mmHg before or during an interventional procedure. Sedation and analgesia may also help blood pressure control. If the patient remains hypertensive in the angiography suite, aim to reduce the mean blood pressure by no more than 25%.

Nifedipine
- **Action** Calcium channel blocker.
- **Dose** 10 mg; this can be repeated at 20-minute intervals up to a dose of 30 mg.
- **Monitor** Pulse, BP and ECG.

Tip: To speed up the effect, the capsule should be chewed and the contents swallowed. The effect begins in 5–10 minutes, peaks at 40 minutes and lasts 6 hours.

Labetalol
- **Action** Mixed α- and β-adrenoreceptor blockade.
- **Indication** Patients with phaeochromocytoma, hypertensive crisis.
- **Dose** Usually 100 mg orally, twice daily. In emergency, slow IV injection of 50 mg repeated at 2-minute intervals up to a maximum of 200 mg.

- **Cautions** Asthma and heart block. Postural hypotension for up to 3 hours.
- **Monitor** Pulse, BP and ECG.

Drugs affecting coagulation

Heparin
- **Indication** Prevention of vascular and pericatheter thrombosis during endovascular procedures.
- **Dose** 50–100 units/kg (3000 u for a small woman, 5000 u for a large man). The half-life is about 60 minutes. Give a further 1000 units every hour in prolonged procedures.
- **Cautions** Heparin infusions should be stopped 3 hours before the procedure and the activated clotting time (ACT) checked on arrival in the catheter laboratory.
- **Monitor** ACT, check baseline level, aim for a 2.5× increase for effective anticoagulation. Sheaths can be removed when the ACT has returned to near baseline and is below 200 s.
- **Reversal** Protamine given by slow IV injection to a maximum single dose of 50 mg.

Tip: As a general rule, 1 mg of protamine will neutralize 100 units of heparin. The dose should be halved every 30 minutes after heparin administration.

Correcting coagulopathy – when and how

The risk of bleeding relates to the procedure: clearly, simple drainage and venous puncture are safer than arterial puncture or core biopsy. Elective procedures should be postponed to allow investigation and correction of the coagulopathy. Only intervene to correct the clotting if the procedure is urgent.

Reversing heparin Protamine, see above.

Reversing warfarin Warfarin has a half-life of about 2½ days and is generally stopped 3 days before an elective procedure. When continuous anticoagulation is necessary, the patient should be heparinized to cover the periprocedural period. Warfarin can be reversed with fresh frozen plasma (FFP) or vitamin K_1.

Fresh frozen plasma A unit of FFP has clotting factors equivalent to 1 unit of fresh blood. At least 2 units are normally required. The effect only lasts about 6 hours, so the FFP is usually given at the time of the procedure.

Tip: FFP is used when immediate correction of coagulopathy or temporary reversal of anticoagulation is necessary.

Table 4.1 Correction of coagulation with vitamin K

INR	Dose of vitamin K_1
6–10	0.5–1 mg
10–20	3–5 mg
>20	10 mg

Vitamin K_1 is given a few hours before the procedure by slow IV injection (1 mg/min.). The dose depends on the INR and the condition of the patient (Table 4.1).

 Alarm: Following vitamin K_1, it may take 2–3 weeks to re-establish anticoagulation with warfarin. Do not use vitamin K_1 when continued anticoagulation is desired!

Thrombocytopenia The risk of haematoma following angiography increases when the platelet count is $<100 \times 10^9$/L. For surgery and invasive procedures, the platelet count should be $>50 \times 10^9$/L. Below this level, platelet transfusion is advisable. Each unit of platelets contains the same number of platelets found in 1 unit of fresh blood. One unit of platelets raises the platelet count by approximately 5×10^9/L; transfusions of 4–6 units are usually sufficient to cover the procedure.

Antiplatelet agents

Platelet activation has a central role in thrombus formation and can be inhibited by many agents. Different drugs have different modes of action to inhibit platelets.

Aspirin
- **Action** Aspirin irreversibly inhibits platelet cyclooxygenase.
- **Indication** All patients with peripheral vascular disease should take low-dose aspirin.
- **Dose** 75 mg daily.
- **Caution** Active peptic ulceration, children under 16 years of age, bleeding diathesis.

Clopidogrel
- **Action** Clopidogrel is a thienopyridine and inhibits binding of adenosine diphosphate.
- **Indication** Carotid artery stenting.
- **Dose** 75 mg daily. Ideally clopidogrel should be started 1 week before the procedure and continued for 1 month afterwards. If the case is more acute then give 200 mg 24 hours before the procedure and continue with 75 mg daily.
- **Caution** Active bleeding, planned surgery within 7 days, ischaemic stroke within past 7 days.

Thrombolytic agents

Blood clot comprises platelets and blood cells in a mesh of fibrin polymer. Thrombolytic drugs activate plasmin to break down fibrin and factors V and VIII. Fresh clot has less cross-linked fibrin and is more likely to respond to thrombolysis. Several drugs are available for thrombolysis; all cause a systemic lytic state. The most widely used are recombinant tissue plasminogen activator (rt-PA) and urokinase. Streptokinase is cheaper but is associated with more side effects. rt-PA and urokinase are probably safer and more effective than strepto-kinase. rt-PA has become the favoured drug in the UK and urokinase in the USA.

The indications for thrombolysis and the techniques and dose regimens are discussed in detail in Chapter 12. All of the drugs cause a systemic lytic state, which can result in haemorrhagic complications that should be reversed with FFP.

Recombinant tissue plasminogen activator
- **Action** rt-PA is activated by the presence of fibrin and is only weakly active in the circulation.
- **Dose** Bolus 5 mg, to a maximum of 20 mg. Infusion 0.5–4 mg/h. Total dose should be kept to 40 mg.

Urokinase
- **Action** Urokinase acts directly on circulating plasminogen to form plasmin.
- **Dose** Bolus 30 000–60 000 units. Infusion 60 000–240 000 units/h.

Streptokinase
- **Action** Binds to circulating plasminogen; this complex converts free plasminogen to plasmin.
- **Dose** Bolus 50 000 units; infusion 2500–5000 units/h.
- **Cautions** Causes fever (33%) and allergic responses (20%). Circulating antibodies can completely neutralize its action up to 5 years after exposure.

Newer thrombolytic agents are being developed, but there is no evidence that they are any more effective than those currently in use.

Drugs causing thrombosis

Thrombin
- **Indication** Injection of false aneurysm.
- **Dose** Variable according to clinical response. Usually given in aliquots of 100 IU in 0.1 mL of saline, repeated until thrombosis achieved.
- **Caution** Thrombin is not licensed for intravascular use in the UK but is widely used to treat false aneurysms. Some haematology departments will generate autologous thrombin from a specimen of the patient's blood. Otherwise there are formulations of human and bovine thrombin available. Bovine thrombin is immunogenic, and repeated exposure carries a risk of anaphylactic reaction and coagulopathy due to cross-reactivity with human clotting factors.

Drugs reducing peristalsis

Antispasmodic drugs are used to abolish bowel peristalsis during digital subtraction angiography (DSA) and are essential for any serious abdominal and pelvic angiography.

Hyoscine butylbromide (Buscopan)
- **Action** Antimuscarinic cholinergic blockade.
- **Dose** 40 mg by intra-arterial injection. Maximum total dose 160 mg.
- **Cautions** Heart failure and tachycardia.
- **Monitor** Pulse, BP and ECG.

Tip: There is no point in asking patients whether they suffer from glaucoma. If they do they will be on treatment, and the others will not know!

Glucagon
- **Action** Polypeptide with direct smooth muscle relaxant mediated by c-AMP.
- **Dose** 1 mg intra-arterial injection.
- **Cautions** Insulinoma and phaeochromocytoma; may produce hypoglycaemic and hypertensive crises.

ANTIBIOTICS

Local policy will often dictate the choice of antibiotics and govern their use. We use antibiotics when puncturing synthetic vascular grafts, implanting permanent devices and performing biliary manipulation in obstructed biliary or urinary systems. Choose antibiotics targeted at likely causative organisms.

ANTIEMETICS

Nausea is not an uncommon problem, especially during embolization procedures.

Metoclopramide is a dopamine antagonist with central antiemetic action. It also increases gastrointestinal motility and gastric emptying. **Prochlorperazine** is a phenothiazine with a central antiemetic action. Both these drugs can cause dystonic reactions, especially in the young and the very old.
- **Reversal** Procyclidine 5–10 mg by IV injection rapidly relieves the dystonic reaction.

Drugs to prevent and treat contrast reactions

A crash trolley should be immediately available for the interventional suite. In addition to the standard drugs found on the resuscitation trolley, the following are essential:

Chlorpheniramine (Piriton)   Used in the treatment of generalized urticaria post contrast, and in the emergency treatment of anaphylactic contrast reactions.
- **Action** Blocks the H_1 receptor-mediated actions of histamine.
- **Dose** 10–20 mg by slow IV injection over 1 minute.
- **Cautions** Will cause drowsiness; rapid injection may cause hypotension.

Hydrocortisone sodium succinate   Used in the treatment and prevention of severe contrast reactions. The mechanism of action is usually too slow to be of immediate benefit in acute reactions, and steroids are used in addition to more immediate treatment such as adrenaline.
- **Action** Multiple effects inhibiting release of a variety of inflammatory mediators.
- **Dose** 200 mg by slow IV injection, repeated at 4-hourly intervals during procedure.

Prednisolone   Used in prophylaxis against contrast reactions in high-risk patients.
- **Dose** 50 mg orally 13, 7 and 1 hour(s) before contrast administration.
- **Cautions** Active peptic ulceration.

Epinephrine (adrenaline)   A cornerstone of the treatment of severe contrast reactions, epinephrine is used for anaphylactic shock, laryngeal oedema and severe bronchospasm.
- **Action** Multiple actions – cardiac stimulant, vasoconstriction of peripheral vessels and bronchodilation.
- **Dose** The route of administration is determined by the clinical status of the patient. If the patient remains well perfused, then the subcutaneous route is safest. 0.3–0.5 mL of 1:1000 solution is given to a maximum of 2 mL in 5 minutes. In severe shock with peripheral shutdown, IV adrenaline is required: 1 mL of 1:10 000 solution (0.1 mg) is given by slow IV injection.
- **Cautions** Ventricular arrhythmias, hypertension and cerebral haemorrhage have all been described. Clearly, the drug carries considerable risks for patients with pre-existing myocardial ischaemia and should only be used in an extreme situation.

Atropine   Used in the treatment of bradycardia.
- **Action** Competitive inhibitor for acetylcholine.
- **Dose** 0.6–1.2 mg by IV injection. Maximum dose is 3 mg.
- **Cautions** Dose-related anticholinergic effects – dry mouth, urinary retention, blurred vision. Contraindicated in closed angle glaucoma.

Cimetidine   A second-line treatment for severe contrast reactions resistant to epinephrine.
- **Dose** 300 mg dissolved in 20 mL saline as a slow IV infusion.
- **Cautions** Patients should receive an H_1 blocking agent before cimetidine. Rapid infusion may cause cardiac effects.

Antiarrhythmics   Most of these drugs are best administered by a physician skilled at interpreting the electrocardiogram and managing cardiac arhythmia. If the patient has SVT it is usually safe to try adenosine.

Adenosine

- **Indication** This is the treatment of choice for supraventricular tachycardia. It has a short duration of action, with a half-life of about 10 seconds.
- **Dose** 3 mg IV over 2 seconds. This may be followed with 6 mg after 1–2 minutes, and 12 mg after a further 1–2 minutes.
- **Contraindications** Second- or third-degree atrioventricular (AV) block. Patients with heart transplant or taking dipyridamole should receive a reduced dose, e.g. 0.5–1 mg.

SUGGESTIONS FOR FURTHER READING

Drugs used in the imaging department

McConnell CA. Drugs used in the imaging department. In: Ansell G et al., eds. Complications in diagnostic imaging and interventional radiology, 3rd edn. Oxford: Blackwell Science, 1996: 27–46.
A comprehensive overview.

McDermot V, Schuster M, Smith T. Antibiotic prophylaxis in vascular and interventional radiology. AJR 1997;169:31–38.

Section Two

Vascular intervention

Chapter Five

Non-invasive vascular imaging

Traditionally, vascular imaging has involved some form of assault on the patient with a needle and catheter to obtain a diagnostic angiogram. Although the quality of DSA images has improved considerably, so have other imaging modalities for assessing the circulation. Diagnostic angiography exposes the patient to the risks of arterial puncture, ionizing radiation and iodinated contrast agents, and requires at least a few hours' stay in hospital. The rivals can be performed without a hospital stay and are no more invasive than an intravenous injection of contrast. MRA and ultrasound do not involve ionizing radiation, and MR contrast agents such as gadolinium are relatively innocuous. In addition, these modalities have the ability to give far more information than a DSA. IADSA will probably retain an important role as arbitrator and where imaging of small distal vessels is necessary, but in the not too distant future most diagnostic angiography is likely to become sidelined by these non-invasive techniques. This book is no place for a treatise in vascular imaging, but we will try to give you a flavour of what can be achieved with contemporary equipment, and a guide to prioritizing patients.

Vascular ultrasound

Modern vascular ultrasound imaging is incomparably better than even 5 years ago. Ultrasound can show the vessel wall, the flowing lumen and surrounding structures, and can image in any plane. Doppler gives physiological information that is not available on an angiogram.

Basic principles

Ultrasound has several potential advantages over DSA: it demonstrates the vessel wall, the flowing lumen, flow direction and abnormal flow patterns. Ultrasound will only succeed if you choose the correct equipment and settings.

Probe   Linear array (5–9 MHz) for peripheral and 7–12 MHz for carotid artery imaging. It is essential to use a linear array as the colour and spectral Doppler can be steered to allow an appropriate angle of insonation of the vessel. Curvilinear array for general renal imaging: the linear array is often still best if the main renal artery is to be interrogated.

Settings   Most modern machines have a range of presets; these optimize the greyscale and Doppler parameters for a given type of study. This does not mean that you can rely exclusively on them, and a key to success is making adjustments as you scan.
- **Depth and focus** These are easily forgotten in all the excitement.
- **Colour velocity scale** This must be appropriate to the flow in the vessel. If the scale is too low then aliasing will be seen with normal flow; too high and sensitivity will be compromised.

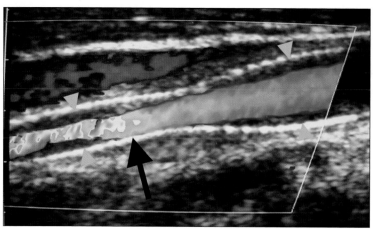

Fig. 5.1 ▦ This shows most of the features you need to recognize on colour flow imaging. Neointimal hyperplasia (turquoise arrows) within a carotid artery stent. The flow changes from uniform velocity to turbulent flow, with aliasing in the proximal internal carotid artery (black arrow).

- **Colour gain** Should be set to close to the maximum that does not result in colour extending beyond the vessel wall or flow in stationary tissues.
- **Doppler cursor** Should be in the centre of the target vessel and set at an appropriate angle (40–60° is optimal). The cursor width should encompass the centre of the lumen.

What to look for With the ultrasound image optimized you are set to find the abnormalities.
- **Greyscale imaging** Plaque morphology and reflectivity may be of some use in the assessment of carotid artery disease, but in the main you will be looking for calcification (Fig. 5.1).
- **Colour flow** Narrowing of the lumen, abnormally high velocities. The colour becomes lighter as velocity increases. Aliasing is present if the colour changes from red to blue passing through white as it exceeds the range of the velocity scale (Fig. 5.1). This must be discriminated from flow reversal, which is indicated by colour changing from red to blue through black (black = zero velocity), and turbulence (chaotic colour). In peripheral arterial disease visible collaterals usually indicate an impending stenosis or occlusion.
- **Doppler spectrum** Changes in peak systolic velocity are usually most important, with a doubling corresponding to approximately 50% diameter narrowing. The velocities are usually measured on either side of a stenosis, as well as at the point of maximal luminal narrowing. Turbulent flow is indicated by infilling of the Doppler spectral trace, representing a wider than normal range of velocities. The morphology of the waveform may also change, but this varies according to the artery being studied.

Principal uses

Ultrasound guided intervention The principles of ultrasound guidance are set out in Chapter 19. Current guidelines recommend the use of ultrasound guidance for all central venous punctures. It is essential to use ultrasound when performing thrombin injection of deep or superficial false aneurysms, and when puncturing the portal and hepatic veins. Ultrasound is invaluable for simplifying vascular access when there is complicated anatomy, e.g. in the presence of a femorofemoral crossover graft, and in patients in need of last-ditch venous access.

Assessment of abdominal aortic aneurysm (AAA) This goes without saying. However, remember that there is a tendency for ultrasound to underestimate the diameter of AAA.

Assessment of patients with peripheral vascular disease Think practically here. It is easiest to scan the femoropopliteal segments. If these are diffusely diseased the patient will need surgery and should have MRA or IADSA. If there is focal disease they will probably be suitable for angioplasty, but should have a formal diagnostic angiogram at the time of the procedure.

Assessment of patients with renal arterial disease Ultrasound is used in the first instance as it will give information on renal size, parenchyma and upper tract dilatation.

Assessment of patients with carotid artery disease This is extensively covered in many other sources and will not be considered here.

Follow-up of vascular intervention This is to be recommended, as seeing patients you have treated is very informative, rewarding, and often gives sobering insight into the outcomes of your intervention.

Most carotid artery Doppler and assessment is performed by sonographers, and so this chapter will be limited to the consideration of peripheral and renal arterial Doppler.

Peripheral vascular Doppler

In the peripheral arteries normal flow has a triphasic waveform. As the extent of arterial disease increases, the flow becomes first biphasic and then monophasic. When there is severe disease the patient will be maximally vasodilated and peripheral resistance is low; antegrade flow may be seen throughout systole and diastole. With any artery, trace it in entirety from proximal to distal, noting the velocities as you go (the machine will normally remember them for you and issue a report if you can find someone to show you how).

 Alarm: A triphasic common femoral artery waveform will be found in about 10% of patients with significant iliac arterial stenosis.

Iliac vascular ultrasound This is quite challenging because the arteries lie deep in the pelvis, often concealed beneath bowel gas and blubber. Applying the general principle that there is no vessel that cannot be reached with a good strong right arm and an appropriate ultrasound probe (modified from *The House of God* by Samuel Shem), most iliac arteries can be seen with a bit of determination. Start imaging in the transverse plane around the umbilicus and identify the aorta; as you scan caudally the iliac bifurcation will be seen. Unfortunately this is usually not the best view for a Doppler study. Place the probe in the iliac fossa of interest and angle medially and cranially until the common iliac artery (CIA) springs into view. There will normally be a favourable angle of insonation. Trace the CIA distally; the deepest point in the pelvis is usually the transition between CIA and the external iliac artery (EIA). If you are lucky you can confirm this by demonstrating the internal iliac artery origin (most often detected with no steering on the colour box). The EIA will now course generally upwards towards the groin.

Tip: In the 'less than lean' patient you will need to press hard. Suddenly pressing very hard always results in the patient tensing the abdominal muscles; instead, engage the patient in conversation and gradually press more and more firmly until the vessel comes into range.

Femoropopliteal segment This is the region most commonly scanned: the vessel is relatively superficial and there is no bowel in the way. Things are generally straightforward until you reach the adductor canal, where the superficial femoral artery (SFA) plunges deeper. Stay calm and adjust the depth, focus and colour flow gain until you find it again. The artery will eventually be too deep to see. Note how far above the upper pole of the patella you are. Ask the patient to turn on to their left side and to flex the contralateral knee. Find the popliteal artery behind the knee and trace it proximally. This is so simple that you will wonder why you persevered so long from the front. Trace it caudally in the traditional fashion.

Calf vessels This is time-consuming and difficult, but the good news is that some form of angiographic assessment is usually required to fully assess the crural vessels, so you can give up relatively early with your pride intact. Scanning may be difficult from proximal to distal: if you are having difficulty, work backwards. Start by checking the posterior tibial artery behind the ankle (right where you would feel the pulse) and the anterior tibial artery in front of it. If there is a good multiphasic waveform there is unlikely to be too much wrong proximally. If you cannot see the arteries look for the paired calf veins that accompany them. Remember to adjust the machine: you will usually need to reduce the colour flow scale. In general, to scan the posterior tibial artery scan from the medial aspect of the calf, the peroneal from the posterolateral aspect, and the anterior tibial from anterolateral.

Common pitfalls in peripheral vascular ultrasound

- **Artery obscured by bowel gas** Try pressing even more firmly to displace the bowel, or try an alternative view.
- **Calcification in the vessel wall obscures detail** Try another view, but usually not much can be done about this. Fortunately, if there is a significant stenosis there will usually be evidence of turbulence, altered waveform, and increased velocity downstream.
- **Unfavourable angle of insonation** As angles increase the velocities become less reliable. Try adjusting the view and angling the transducer to optimize the angle. It may be impossible to assess the native renal arteries even with a linear array.
- **Pressing too hard on an artery** This is surprisingly easy to do, and not uncommon in the distal external iliac and common femoral arteries. The effect is to compress the artery and mimic a stenosis.
- **Incorrect velocity settings** Too high and it will be difficult to demonstrate flow, too low and there will be aliasing everywhere.

Renal vascular ultrasound

It is very difficult to demonstrate the entire renal artery and almost impossible to demonstrate accessory vessels. It is even harder to insonate the artery at a suitable angle for velocity measurements. This has led to the adoption of indirect measures to investigate

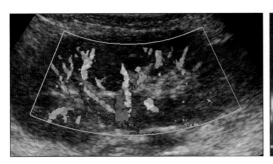
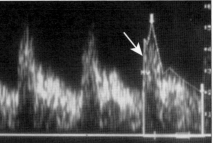

Fig. 5.2 ▦ Intrarenal blood flow on contemporary ultrasound. The Doppler trace has a sharp systolic upstroke with an acceleration time less than 0.07 seconds (large arrow).

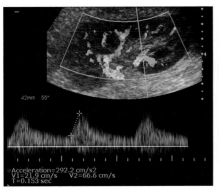
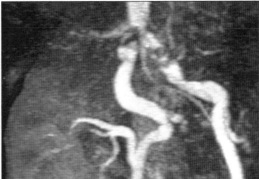

Fig. 5.3 ▦ Parvus tardus waveform in a renal transplant interlobar artery secondary to iliac artery stenosis, clearly shown on the accompanying MRA scan.

renal artery stenosis. Start with the simplest thing to do: measure the kidneys. If they are shrunken with relatively normal cortical echogenicity, or there is >2 cm difference in size, this raises the possibility of renal artery stenosis. Next switch on the colour: arterial and venous flow should be readily demonstrated throughout the kidney (Fig. 5.2). Interrogate the waveform of the interlobar arteries in the upper and lower poles and the interpolar region of each kidney. The normal renal artery trace has a very steep systolic upstroke, an early systolic peak, and flow throughout diastole. Severe renal artery stenosis is associated with a parvus tardus waveform and a slowly rising systolic upstroke. In between there is a spectrum of changes in the slope of the systolic upstroke, and loss of the early systolic peak. A systolic acceleration time of <0.07 s is normal.

The most helpful results of renal Doppler are a parvus tardus waveform (Fig. 5.3), indicating a definite problem in the main renal artery or inflow, or a completely normal study. Anything else will require further imaging.

Tip: When there is a bilateral parvus tardus waveform this may indicate a coarctation of the aorta. Scan the femoral and brachial arteries as well, and look for abnormal femoral and normal brachial waveforms to confirm the diagnosis.

Renal transplant Doppler

The same principles apply to renal transplant Doppler as to study of the native kidneys, except that it should be possible to study the entire renal artery. As always, it is essential to know the anatomy. Be aware that there are alternative causes of transplant renal artery stenosis to look out for:

- Anastomotic stricture
- Clamp injury (NB: only in live related donors: clamping should not be required in a cadaveric kidney)
- Kinking of the renal artery
- Inflow iliac arterial disease (Fig. 5.3).

Only meticulous attention to detail will suffice. If you cannot see the entire renal artery then you should proceed to MRA. Remember, if there is an abnormal waveform and you don't identify a stenosis, look for inflow disease.

Magnetic resonance angiography (MRA)

At present MRA is a relatively limited resource, mainly because MR scanners are clogged up by musculoskeletal and neurological cases. It is easy to understand how this has come about, but not so simple to change. One of the best arguments must be on the risk–benefit basis of non-invasive versus invasive procedures. No-one would dream of returning to conventional myelography; similarly, we should protest against the need to subject patients to catheter angiography. If you intend to perform peripheral MRA, make sure your new scanner has a stepping table and a dedicated peripheral coil.

What you need to know about MR physics Basically, the scanner is best regarded as a 'black box' capable of producing beautiful angiographic images. For most applications you are interested in traditional time of flight, and phase contrast studies are either irrelevant or have been replaced by the much faster contrast-enhanced MRA (CE-MRA). This is basically an angiographic study showing the flowing lumen of the vessel and little else.

The scanning sequences used in CE-MRA:

- **Rely on giving contrast** Gadolinium reduces the T_1 of blood.
- **Are fast**, enabling data acquisition during breath-holding and large areas to be scanned in a single study.
- **Are flow independent**, enabling scanning to be performed in any plane.
- **Suppress the background tissues** High flip angles and very short pulse repetition times lead to increased signal-to-noise ratios.
- **Are relatively free of artefact** There is still a tendency to overestimate stenoses, but this is nowhere near as marked as in time-of-flight imaging.

CE-MRA keys to success

- **Timing data acquisition to correspond to the arterial peak level of gadolinium** This is usually achieved by looking at the time of maximal signal following a test dose of

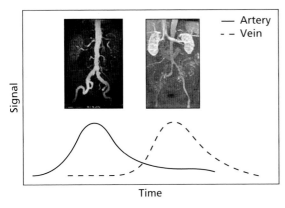

Signal

Time

— Artery
- - Vein

Fig. 5.4 ▪ Figure variation of arterial and venous signal following intravenous gadolinium. Scanning at the peak of arterial enhancement gives optimal angiographic imaging with peak signal to noise ratio. Scanning too late reduces the signal to noise ratio and results in venous contamination.

gadolinium. This results in the highest signal from the artery and optimal image quality. Scan too early and there is no contrast there; too late and there is venous filling (Fig. 5.4). Venous contamination can be particularly troublesome in the calf, where it obscures the arterial signal.

- **Scanning in the coronal and sagittal planes** This improves resolution, increases the field of view, reduces the number of slices required to cover the area of interest and reduces 'wrap' artefact. Typically the coronal plane is used for peripheral, renal, arch and carotid MRA, and the sagittal plane for mesenteric MRA.

- **Restricting the volume scanned** This shortens the time to acquire data and allows thinner slices to increase spatial resolution. The key to volume restriction is to set up the scan carefully by performing localizer sequences that clearly show the position of the target arteries. This is where you might become involved. The volume of interest will change for the different stations in MRA of the peripheral arteries, much as it does in conventional angiography. For example, when scanning the renal arteries you would choose a volume starting just anterior to the aorta and extending no further back than the posterior aspect of the kidneys.

- **Image review** Don't rely on MIP images: go to the console and review the source images when there is any doubt!

- **Understand the artefacts and limitations of the technique** Image quality may be degraded by venous contamination, especially in views of the calf in patients with critical limb ischaemia. New sequences are reducing this, and scanning just the calf and foot on the affected side in the sagittal plane may help. Interference from metallic objects, stainless steel stents and embolization coils will completely obliterate the signal from the vessel (Fig. 5.5).

Areas in which CE-MRA is accepted

- Patients with a documented history of severe contrast reaction.
- Patients with severe renal dysfunction.
- Peripheral arterial imaging: **priority** should be given to those patients.
  - with no femoral access in whom the arm approach would carry a risk of CVA.
  - in whom ultrasound has indicated a pattern of disease unsuitable for endovascular intervention. Intra-arterial DSA can then be reserved for those patients in whom you are likely to proceed to intervention.

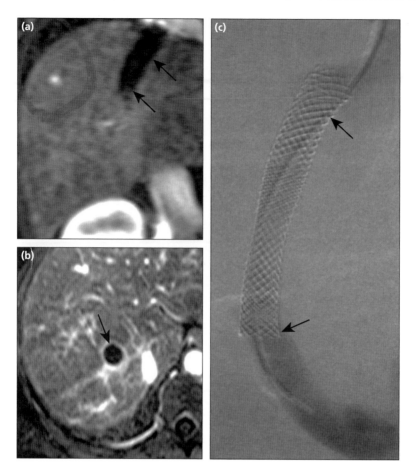

Fig. 5.5 ▦ (a) and (b) Contrast-enhanced MR scans of a patient with a TIPS. Apparent occlusion of the TIPS tract (arrows) due to signal loss caused by the ferromagnetic Wallstent. (c) Subsequent normal TIPS venogram as part of routine follow-up.

- in whom ultrasound and IADSA have failed to show the distal circulation.
- who indicate a preference for non-invasive imaging during informed consent.
- Carotid artery imaging for carotid arterial stenosis and dissection: intra-arterial DSA should only be performed when there is a contraindication to MRA, or when MR and ultrasound are discordant.
- Renal artery imaging: CE-MRA has become the modality of choice for:
  - investigation of atheromatous renal artery stenosis.
  - assessing the anatomy of potential live renal donors.
  - imaging transplant renal arteries. Remember to check the surgical anatomy, cadaveric transplant vs live related donor.

The use of MRA to investigate young patients with possible fibromuscular dysplasia is less well established and the disease may be distal and subtle. However, in a young patient with hypertension MR can still be justified, as it allows simultaneous assessment of the adrenal glands. There should be an understanding that if the MR scan is negative the patient should proceed to IADSA.

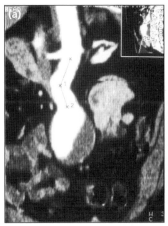 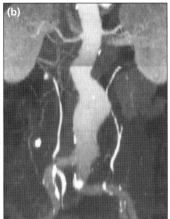 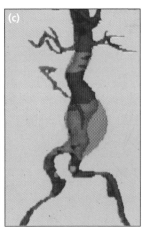

Fig. 5.6 ■ CT reformats of a patient with AAA. (a) Multiplanar reformat in coronal oblique plane shows all tissues in the reformatted volume. (b) Maximum-intensity projection – near angiographic image, but also shows calcification and areas of high attenuation, e.g. kidneys and ureters. Need to subtract the spine. (c) Shaded surface rendering – regions of interest created to show both the lumen and the thrombus.

Computed tomography angiography (CTA)

CTA has been available since the 1990s, but is improving fast with the advent of multislice CT scanners. As CT involves high doses of iodinated contrast and ionizing radiation, the only advantage it has to offer is that it is non-invasive. At present CTA remains second choice to MRA and ultrasound, but it may be that it will become more widely used in patients who have a contraindication to MRA. It will probably help hasten the demise of diagnostic arteriography. Images are generally produced as MIPS akin to MRA (Fig. 5.6). Volume rendering, three-dimensional shaded surface renderings, curved and multiplanar reformats will also be helpful, especially in dealing with aneurysmal disease (Fig. 5.6). Much will depend on the type of scanner and software locally available. The keys to successful CTA are similar to those for MRA: scans must be acquired at the peak of arterial enhancement, and oral contrast should not be used. A test bolus is normally required to achieve optimal timing. Doses and infusion rates vary, but usually 100–150 mL of contrast are needed.

 Summary: Non-invasive vascular imaging is set to replace most of conventional angiography: if you don't want to be left behind, get involved. Think about the most appropriate test and tailor it for each patient.

Chapter Six

Angiography – getting the picture

This chapter briefly reviews the key areas in image acquisition and manipulation. A successful angiogram depends on cooperation between the patient, the radiographer and the radiologist. A little understanding of the basic principles of angiography can vastly improve the standard of the final study!

Fluoroscopy

Fluoroscopy or screening This is used to provide real-time imaging during catheter and guidewire manipulation. Continuous fluoroscopy is used when optimal image quality is required, e.g. selective catheterization; it is the only option on many machines. Pulsed fluoroscopy is used when less detail is required, e.g. positioning a pigtail catheter, or when screening over sensitive organs, e.g. during uterine fibroid embolization. Radiation dose is reduced as the production of X-rays is intermittent; the image from each pulse is saved on the monitor to give an impression of continuity. At fewer than seven pulses per second the image is rather jerky and only suitable for crude catheter positioning, e.g. positioning a pigtail catheter. Whenever possible use fluoroscopy rather than DSA runs, as this keeps the dose to a minimum.

Last image hold The fluoroscopic image is automatically stored on the monitor. In systems with two monitors, this image can be transferred to the reference monitor and used for guidance.

Guide to good fluoroscopy Aim to keep everyone's radiation exposure to a minimum. You are the person most at risk!
- Keep the image intensifier close to the patient.
- Centre over the area of interest.
- Use collimation.
- Use pulsed fluoroscopy if available – there is little dose reduction at >7 frames/s (FPS).
- Keep your hands out of the field – you may need your fingers in years to come.
- Use runs to sort out anatomy and pathology – do not perform repeated fluoroscopic injections.
- Keep your foot off the pedal unless you have a reason to screen!

Catheter guidance

Roadmap (subtracted fluoroscopy) In this mode a subtracted fluoroscopic image is obtained after a few seconds of fluoroscopy. Contrast is injected to opacify the vessels and

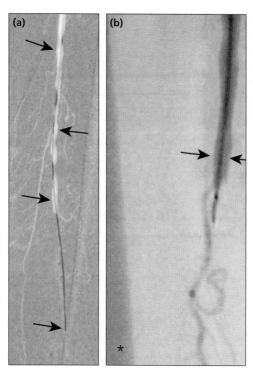

Fig. 6.1 ▪ The principal techniques for guiding catheters and guidewires. (a) Roadmap: the guidewire (arrow) can be seen with an image of the vessel (arrows) on a subtracted background. (b) Fluoroscopy fade: an image of the vessel (arrows) is superimposed on the standard fluoroscopic image (*, bone edge).

fluoroscopy stopped. The next time screening is activated, the catheter and guidewire will be seen on the subtracted image of the blood vessels (Fig. 6.1a). This is used particularly to navigate past strictures and avoid branch vessels.

 Tip: Roadmapping is not effective in the chest and abdomen, as respiration and peristalsis interfere with the subtraction and degrade the image.

Roadmap (non-subtracted fluoroscopy) An image from a DSA is superimposed on the normal fluoroscopic image (Fig. 6.1b). The density of the superimposed image can be adjusted to suit the application. It is particularly useful in the chest and abdomen, as the superimposed image does not move with respiration. Confusingly, this is called by a different name by each of the manufacturers, e.g. on a Seimens machine it is called fluoroscopy fade.

Digital subtraction angiography: basic principles

The vast majority of angiography is now performed using a DSA technique. DSA uses a computer to subtract an image without contrast (mask) from each subsequent image acquired in exactly the same position after contrast injection. The resultant images show only the opacified blood vessels; the underlying bone or soft tissue is not displayed. Movement between the mask image and the contrast image will result in image degradation because of visible bone edges. Most DSA examinations are performed with positive (iodinated) contrast media; however, negative (CO_2 gas) contrast can be used.

Digital subtraction angiography techniques Multiposition DSA (MPDSA)
Angiography is performed in discrete sections, each with its own contrast injection.
In peripheral angiography this usually gives the best results at the expense of an increase
in radiation dose.

Stepping-table DSA Only used in peripheral angiography. The table or C-arm moves
in a series of overlapping steps. Five positions are usually needed to cover from the
abdominal aorta to the feet. Mask images are obtained in each position. A bolus of
contrast is injected and the table advanced when the vessels in that position are opacified.
The technique only works well with an experienced radiographer and a patient with
broadly symmetrical disease. Additional runs are frequently necessary, particularly of the
crural vessels.

Tip: Stepping-table DSA gives best results when the blood flow is the same
in each limb. Use MPDSA if symptoms or pulses are markedly asymmetric.

Bolus-chasing DSA Only used in peripheral angiography. The technique resembles
stepping-table DSA. Mask images are obtained at multiple levels (approximately every
5 cm); the table is then panned to keep up with the contrast bolus.

Rotational angiography This is a variation on MPDSA. The C-arm is rotated in an arc
around the patient while masks are acquired. The rotation is repeated during the injection
of contrast. The mask is matched with the image acquired at the same obliquity. Rotational
angiography is most useful when multiple oblique projections are required, e.g. renal transplant angiography.

Hard copy

The best study in the world can be sabotaged by careless and inadequate hard copy.

Angiography is unique in that we discard much of the study almost immediately after
acquisition. The hard copy represents only the edited highlights of the angiogram. Vital
information may be lost irretrievably if we fail to convey to radiographic staff the essential
objectives of the study. In particular, complex or unfamiliar studies should be reviewed at
the console with the radiographer and images for hard copy identified.

Suboptimal imaging is most often due to elementary errors. Try to apply the following basic
guidelines:
- Image all phases of the run: arterial, capillary and venous.
- Optimal image density is a grey which allows overlying vessels to be discriminated from
  each other. Set window levels accordingly. Too black an image will obscure pathology
  (Fig. 6.2).
- Include non-subtracted images to show landmarks.
- Annotate views with relevant information, e.g. tube angulation when it has been difficult
  to obtain a suitable oblique projection.

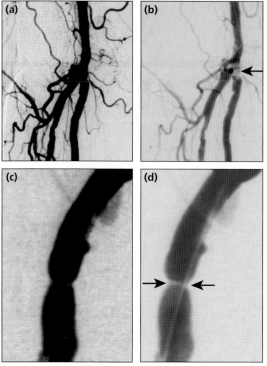

Fig. 6.2 ■ Effect of incorrect window settings. (a and b) Profunda oblique view: the large posterior plaque (arrow) is obscured by narrow windows. (c and d) Subtle 'weblike' stenosis (arrows) in a vein graft is only appreciated on correct settings.

Tip: Although it is always worth trying to blame the radiographer, no amount of radiographer ingenuity can make up for images that were never there: always review the study on the console before removing the catheter.

Pixel shifting If there is no movement between the mask and the run, then a single mask image will suffice. In reality most patients do not keep completely still, especially if a large volume of contrast has been injected. If there has only been slight movement, then the resultant image can often be markedly improved by pixel shifting (Fig. 6.3). This entails realigning the chosen mask with the image to allow effective subtraction. Pixel shifting is not as helpful when there is considerable movement, such as respiration, or when there is rotation.

Masking Some patients are unable to stop breathing for the duration of image acquisition, especially if a long sequence is involved. In this case, the solution is multimasking. Multiple masks are made over several respiratory cycles before injecting contrast. Normal respiration is continued throughout the run. Images from the run can then be matched with a mask in the same phase of respiration, allowing subtraction.

Tip: Multimasking is essential in most patients during prolonged runs in the chest and abdomen. No amount of pixel shifting and remasking can compensate for bowel peristalsis. Paralyse the bowel with buscopan or glucagon.

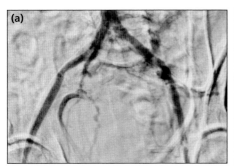
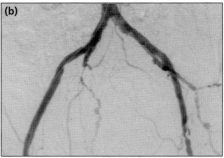

Fig. 6.3 ■ Severely degraded image (a) is salvaged (b) by choosing an appropriate mask and pixel shifting.

Pump injectors

Even the strongest angiographer cannot hand-inject rapidly enough for aortic runs. Pump injectors are used to deliver a controlled bolus of contrast while you stand back and reduce your radiation dose. The settings may seem confusing at first, but there are only six parameters to consider:

- **Volume** This is the total volume of contrast that will be delivered.
- **Injection rate** The flow rate in mL/s. Volume/injection rate determines the duration of the bolus.
- **Maximum pressure (PSI)** The peak pressure the pump will generate during injection.
- **Pressure rate rise** The time to peak pressure. In practice, it seems permanently set at 0.4 seconds.
- **Inject delay** Delays the injection of contrast to allow mask images to be acquired. This is necessary when contrast will reach the target vessel immediately after injection, e.g. imaging the aortoiliac segment.
- **X-ray delay** Delays the X-ray exposure. This avoids unnecessary images prior to the contrast arriving at the area of interest, e.g. injecting in the aorta and imaging the feet.

Tip: Parameters 2–4 are limited by the catheter. Details of the maximum permissible pressure are displayed on the catheter hub and information about flow rates is on the catheter packaging. The maximum flow rate is only achievable at the maximum PSI.

Chapter Seven

Equipment for angiography

Catheters come in a wide range of shapes and sizes, and simple rules govern their choice. Most angiographers rely on a relatively small selection of catheters to perform almost all cases.

Catheters

There are three important factors concerning catheter size:
- Outer diameter (French size)
- Length in centimetres (obvious really)
- Inner diameter – relates to the diameter of guidewire that will pass through the catheter.

The length of the catheter refers to the usable length from the hub to the tip. Helpfully, it is to be found on the packaging, and also on the catheter hub. Make a mental note of it and you will be able to select an appropriate length guidewire.

Catheter diameters are based on the French (Fr) system, which is the outer circumference of the catheter shaft in millimetres. For easy reference, the diameter in mm is approximately the French size divided by 3, e.g. 6Fr = 2 mm. The majority of catheters in current use are 5Fr or smaller. Small-calibre catheters may be less traumatic in terms of the size of the puncture site, but the cost is often reduced turning ability or *catheter torque*. Catheter torque is also affected by many other factors, including catheter material, catheter length and vessel tortuosity. Most non-selective angiograms can be performed with 3Fr catheters, but selective catheterization, particularly if tortuous vessels are involved, usually requires 4Fr catheters or larger.

Tip: French sizes
Catheter size = outer circumference
Guide catheter size = outer circumference
Sheath size = inner circumference

Flow rates   Maximum flow rates vary between catheters, depending on the internal diameter and length and the number of sideholes. Typical maximum flow rates for pigtail catheters are:

3Fr 6–8 mL/s
4Fr 16–18 mL/s
5Fr 20–25 mL/s

The maximum flow rate and injection rate (PSI) are usually on the catheter packaging or catheter hub – check them before giving everyone a contrast shower.

To avoid catheter recoil, pump-injected selective angiograms should be performed with an appropriate rate rise (the time for the pressure to reach its peak value). Typically 0.4 seconds is used.

Catheter flushing   It is essential that catheters are flushed at regular intervals to prevent occlusion or thrombus formation at the tip. Outside the cerebral circulation, a single flush technique is appropriate. A syringe containing saline is attached to the catheter hub and held vertically; aspirate until a small bead of blood enters the syringe. Any air bubbles aspirated will rise to lie against the syringe plunger and will therefore not be introduced when the saline is injected.

In the cerebral circulation, because the injection of even a small thrombus or air bubble could be disastrous, a double-flush technique is used. A syringe with saline is attached to the hub of the catheter and aspiration applied until blood flows freely into the syringe. This syringe is discarded and the catheter is then flushed with a syringe containing clean saline, meticulously prepared to exclude air bubbles.

Tip: Multiple-sidehole catheters should be flushed vigorously to ensure adequate flow through both the tip and the sideholes.

Essential catheters

Catheters divide into two distinct groups: non-selective (flush) and selective. Non-selective catheters are used to inject contrast in large to medium-sized vessels and have multiple sideholes to increase the injection rate. Selective catheters are shaped to a wide variety of angles to allow catheterization of branch vessels.

Non-selective catheters

Pigtail catheter   This is the workhorse of diagnostic angiography. The catheter has an end-hole and multiple sideholes extending down on to the distal 1–2 cm of the shaft. The pigtail usually forms when the guidewire is withdrawn, but if it does not, simply push the catheter forward while twisting. The pigtail shape minimizes inadvertent catheterization of small branch vessels, and the distribution of sideholes produces a homogeneous contrast bolus.

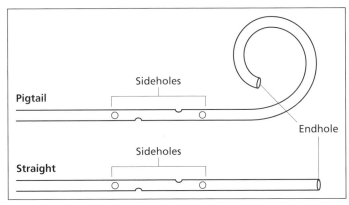

Fig. 7.1 ▨ Pigtail and straight multi-sidehole catheters. Unless the catheter is flushed briskly the flush exits via the proximal sideholes and will not flush the catheter tip, with resultant clot formation.

In practice, the endhole of the catheter is larger than the sideholes and therefore has greater flow. It is essential that a test injection of contrast is made to verify that the endhole is not in a small branch before the rapid injection of a contrast bolus. As the pigtail loop measures approximately 15 mm across, this catheter should not be used in vessels smaller than this diameter.

Straight catheter Endhole and multiple sideholes on a straight shaft (Fig. 7.1). This catheter is used in vessels too small to form a pigtail, but with reasonably rapid flow, e.g. the iliac arteries.

Tip: To locate the catheter tip, pull the J wire back until a catch is felt as it begins to straighten on the catheter.

Selective catheters

Endhole vs sideholes Selective catheters come in two main designs: endhole only, and end- and sidehole.

Endhole catheters are used for hand-injected, diagnostic angiograms and embolization procedures. Pump injections are potentially hazardous with endhole-only catheters, as the high-flow jet coming out of the single endhole is likely to displace the catheter and may dislodge plaque or cause dissection.

End- and sidehole catheters are used for pump-injected runs (e.g. superior mesenteric artery angiograms), as the multiple sideholes deliver a rapid, safe bolus of contrast; however, sidehole catheters should not be used for embolotherapy, as coils may become trapped in the sideholes and particulate matter may escape to non-target territory via the sideholes.

Tip: Endhole catheters will not aspirate if the catheter tip rests against the vessel wall. Rotate the catheter and try again.

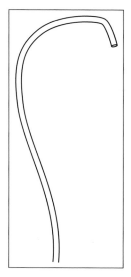

Fig. 7.2 ▧ Cobra catheter.

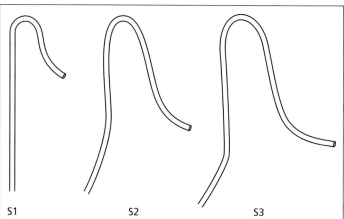

Fig. 7.3 ▧ Sidewinder catheter.

S1　　　　S2　　　　S3

Top five selective catheters

Cobra An invaluable catheter for visceral and peripheral selective arteriography (Fig. 7.2). The catheter is pulled down to engage a vessel, but is pushed forward over a guidewire to allow deeper catheterization. Cobra catheters come in three curves, C1–C3; in practice, simply use a C2.

Sidewinder Very useful for visceral angiography. The Sidewinder reverse curve comes in three sizes, S1–S3, with progressively larger curves and longer limbs (Fig. 7.3). Reforming the reverse curve can be difficult for the uninitiated. There are a variety of techniques, but the simplest is the 'quick aortic turn'. As the catheter is formed in the aortic arch there is a small risk of causing a stroke.

Forming the Sidewinder: quick aortic turn (Fig. 7.4):
1. Advance the catheter until its knee is across the apex of the aortic arch.

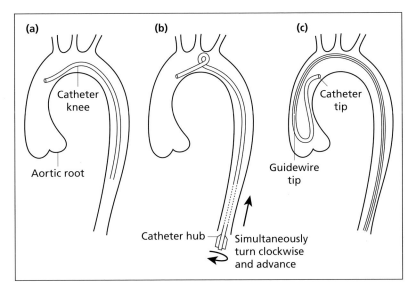

Fig. 7.4 ▓ Reforming the Sidewinder catheter.

2. Simultaneously push the catheter forwards and rotate clockwise to reform the reverse curve.
3. Under continuous fluoroscopy, pull the catheter down into the aorta. The catheter may occasionally engage vessels on the way down. Remember to push the catheter in to disengage, then withdraw, rotating it slightly.

The aortic turn manoeuvre can be difficult in the unfolded aortic arch, so insert a guidewire to the level of the knee of the catheter and try again. Alternatively, carefully advance the catheter into the left subclavian artery as far as the apex of the catheter, then push and rotate clockwise. In elderly patients or those with cerebrovascular disease an alternative is to form the reverse curve over the iliac bifurcation. To do this, another catheter (Cobra or Renal double curve) is used to catheterize the contralateral iliac artery. A guidewire is passed down at least as far as the common femoral artery, and then the catheter is exchanged for the Sidewinder. The Sidewinder catheter is now introduced over the wire until the apex of the loop is over the bifurcation. The wire is now pulled back to the apex, and the catheter and wire are advanced together.

The catheter is positioned above the target vessel and then pulled down and steered by gently rotating the shaft towards the target vessel (Fig. 7.5). Once the knee of the catheter has reached the vessel ostium, further traction will pull the tip back! At this stage, deeper catheterization can be achieved by advancing the catheter over a guidewire. This is easiest with an S3, possible for the gifted with an S2, and only for the divine with an S1.

The Sos Omni catheter is simply a Sidewinder shape with a small curve and a short limb. It has the advantage that it can be formed in the abdominal aorta. It is simple to engage an artery with the Sos Omni, but almost impossible to advance it further into a vessel.

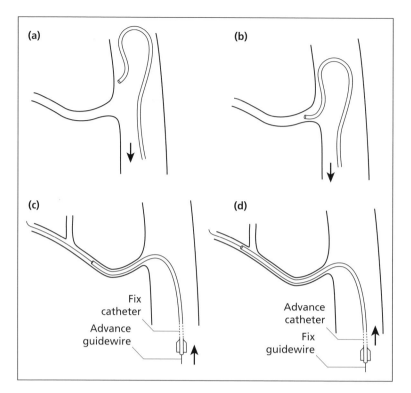

Fig. 7.5 ▪ Using the Sidewinder. (a) Pull back to engage catheter tip in the vessel ostium. (b) The catheter is advanced further by pulling back until it is in as far as the knee. (c) For deeper catheterization, advance a guidewire into the vessel. (d) Push the catheter over the fixed wire.

Tip: If the catheter loop is too large for the aorta, the tip of the catheter is held away from the aortic wall and will not engage branch vessels. Try introducing a guidewire around the apex of the catheter curve to straighten out the limb; if this fails, choose a smaller curve.

Berenstein Endhole only (Fig. 7.6); the tip is angled and therefore at its best when catheterizing forward-facing vessels such as the aortic arch vessels.

Renal double curve (RDC) As the name suggests, this is designed for selective renal work (Fig. 7.7). The tip points downwards, and therefore it is very useful for getting across the aortic bifurcation. At least one of the authors thinks this is a useful catheter for inferior mesenteric artery catheterization.

Headhunter This catheter has a forward-facing primary curve and is available with and without sideholes (Fig. 7.8). It is used primarily to catheterize the head and neck vessels.

Tip: Cobra, Sidewinder and straight catheters are available with hydrophilic coatings. These catheters when used in combination with a hydrophilic wire can be advanced into small vessels of the distal arterial bed.

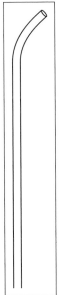

Fig. 7.6 ▦ Berenstein catheter.

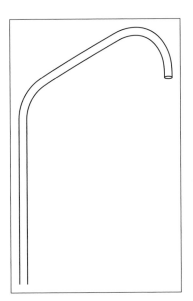

Fig. 7.7 ▦ Renal double curve catheter.

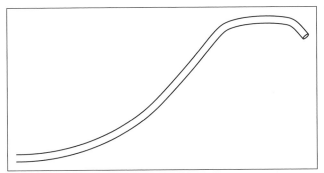

Fig. 7.8 ▦ Headhunter catheter.

Selective catheterization

Choosing your weapon   The most important factor in catheter choice is the angle at which the target vessel arises from the parent vessel. Review the diagnostic runs, then choose logically; if the vessel points downwards, then even the most skilled angiographer will struggle with a forward-facing catheter such as the Berenstein. Use Figure 7.9 to aid your choice.

Keys to success

- Always obtain a high-quality diagnostic angiogram. This allows you to be sure where the target is and to make a logical choice of selective catheter.

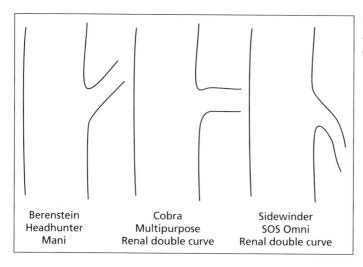

Fig. 7.9 ▪ Choose an appropriately shaped catheter for the target vessel.

Berenstein	Cobra	Sidewinder
Headhunter	Multipurpose	SOS Omni
Mani	Renal double curve	Renal double curve

- Use roadmapping when possible.
- Keep the catheter shaft straight – this allows the catheter maximum opportunity to rotate. Turn the catheter gently towards the target. If the catheter does not turn readily, then either it is catching on aortic plaque or most of the torque is being taken up in tortuous iliac vessels. To improve torque, either increase the catheter size, e.g. go from 4Fr to 7Fr, or better still insert a long sheath or guide-catheter.
- Check to see if the catheter tip is facing forwards or backwards. Turn the catheter towards you:
  - If the tip turns towards you, the catheter faces forwards.
  - If the tip turns away from you, the tip faces backwards.
- Using fluoroscopy, rotate and advance the guidewire smoothly and gently. If the wire starts to buckle or push the catheter back, STOP. Do not try to force it. Retract the wire, then try advancing at a different angle.
- Get a reasonable length of guidewire into the target vessel – a catheter will not advance across the floppy section of the guidewire.
- Keep the guidewire absolutely fixed and under tension when advancing the catheter.
- Advance the catheter smoothly and gently into the target vessel under fluoroscopy. If the catheter starts to buckle, STOP. The catheter and wire will spring out of the vessel. Try again, this time with more wire to increase stability, or exchange for a different catheter.

Microcatheters

Microcatheters are coaxial catheters, only 2–3Fr in size, that allow catheterization of even the smallest and most tortuous of vessels (Fig. 7.10). They were initially developed for cerebral catheterization, but are being increasingly used for superselective hepatic, visceral and peripheral catheterization. A conventional catheter is initially used to selectively catheterize a branch of the proximal circulation. The coaxial catheter is then

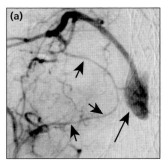 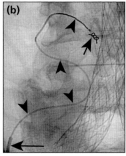

Fig. 7.10 ■ Microcatheters will negotiate the most tortuous vessels. (a) Tiny iliolumbar collaterals (short arrows) causing type II endoleak (long arrow) following endovascular aortic aneurysm repair. (b) Microcatheter (arrowheads) delivering embolization coils (small arrow) into the lumbar artery. 5Fr guide-catheter in the iliolumbar branch of the internal iliac artery (large arrow).

advanced through the conventional catheter using a Tuohy–Borst adapter to maintain haemostasis.

Microcatheters come in a variety of lengths; it is essential to choose a catheter long enough to pass through the conventional catheter and out to the target site. Microcatheters have improved enormously over the past few years. There are now hydrophilic catheters with integral guidewires (e.g. Progreat, Terumo). There are additional auxillary guidewires available that offer greater and lesser degrees of support and steerability.

Tip: Always advance the coaxial catheter over a guidewire. The small-calibre microcatheter does not have enough rigidity to advance by itself.

Guide-catheters

Guide-catheters are large-calibre catheters, most frequently 7–9Fr, which are used to provide a safe and stable conduit from the arterial puncture site to the target vessel. They come in a variety of lengths, from ~50 to 100 cm, and shapes include straight, hockey stick and RDC. The guide-catheter is designed to be introduced to the vessel ostium; conventional catheters and guidewires should be used for more distal catheterization.

Guide-catheters are most frequently used during stenting procedures, when the extra rigidity and increased bail-out options are a reasonable trade-off against the increased puncture site size. Occasionally, a guide-catheter can be very useful to take up the torque from tortuous iliac vessels and thus allow selective visceral catheterization. When selecting a guide-catheter make sure you choose an appropriate length: too long and your catheter will not pass through it, and too short and it will not reach the target vessel.

Tip: Guide-catheters are sized by their outside circumference. Therefore, a 7Fr guide-catheter will fit through a 7Fr sheath but will not allow a 7Fr catheter through it.

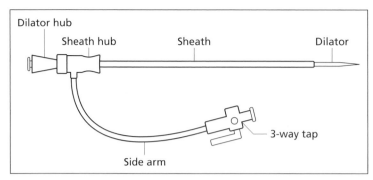

Fig. 7.11 ■ Vascular sheath with side-arm for flushing.

Vascular sheaths

Vascular sheaths provide an atraumatic arterial or venous access route. The sheath consists of a hollow plastic tube connected to a haemostatic valve with a side-arm for flushing (Fig. 7.11).

Sheaths are invaluable for any case that is likely to use more than one catheter, and are essential for angioplasty cases as they prevent the wings of the balloon creating an irregular arteriotomy. The sheath is sized by the calibre of catheter it will accept, e.g. a 5Fr sheath takes a 5Fr catheter, but actually has an approximately 6Fr outer diameter.

Most sheaths are thin-walled and will kink if they enter the vessel at a steep angle – typically an antegrade puncture in an obese patient. Try to puncture at a shallow angle to prevent this, or if a steep puncture is essential, then consider using a reinforced sheath such as the Arrowflex.

Troubleshooting

The sheath will not aspirate　Try to remember to flush the sheath regularly and after every catheter exchange – but it is too late for that now! Adhere to the following guidelines:

- Do not be tempted to clear the sheath with a 'gentle' injection.
- Use fluoroscopy to check whether the sheath is kinked.
- Try to aspirate with an empty 50 mL syringe, as this will generate the maximum amount of vacuum.
- If this fails and there is still a guidewire through the sheath, then the simplest action is to exchange the sheath for a new one.
- If there is no guidewire through the sheath, then apply suction with a 50 mL syringe to the side-arm and insert a straight wire and exchange for a new sheath. This carries a very small risk of distal embolization and should be used cautiously, particularly for patients with diseased runoff.

Alternatively, the more economical can reuse the same sheath. Put the sheath dilator back on the guidewire. Aspirate on the sheath and remove it as above. Compress the puncture site. Get your assistant to flush the sheath to clear the thrombus, and then replace the introducer and insert the sheath as normal.

The sheath kinks This usually occurs during antegrade puncture in 'the larger patient'. It is almost unavoidable if the abdominal fold was retracted during arterial puncture. This is one indication for choosing the contralateral CFA for access.

- Try straightening out the sheath by flattening it against the abdomen.
- If this fails, advance a guidewire into the sheath until it stops. Carefully reinsert the dilator to the point of obstruction, then apply traction to straighten the sheath; the guidewire will generally advance.
- If this fails, then remove the sheath and repuncture.

Tip: If the puncture has to be at a steep angle you may need a reinforced sheath to prevent recurrence. Reinforced sheaths have an external diameter 1–2Fr greater than a standard sheath.

GUIDEWIRES

Guidewires are a key element to successful catheterization as they support and steer the catheter to the target vessel. The choice of the correct wire can seem baffling when confronted with a rack full of wires, but there are some simple rules.

Basic properties

Guidewires divide into two groups: non-steerable guidewires simply allow the catheter to be positioned but are not designed to negotiate stenoses or select branch vessels; steerable guidewires are designed with shaped tips and good torque control, and some have special hydrophilic coatings which will cross even the tightest stenosis if used properly.

Hydrophilic wires must be kept wet. Wet the wire before initial use and do not let it dry out. Dry wires are very sticky; catheters do not slide, and the wire may stick to your gloves and be accidentally pulled out. For complex procedures have a bowl full of saline to keep catheters and wires clean and moist.

Length Length is important! The length of the wire becomes critical when trying to exchange catheters, especially if in a hard fought-for selective position. A standard-length wire is 140 cm and is fine for most uses; however, longer wires of 180 and 260 cm may be needed when:

- working in the upper limb from the groin;
- working in the visceral/renal/hepatic circulation and needing to exchange catheters;
- working with 90 cm+ guide-catheters or angioplasty balloons.

Tip: The minimum length of guidewire necessary to allow catheter exchange = the length of the catheter + the length of the guidewire in the patient. Having too short a wire is very frustrating!

Some guidewires, such as the TAD II, can have extensions added to increase their length, e.g. for catheter exchange, or when using guide-catheters. The extensions are always very expensive, so do not use them if they are not necessary.

Wire tip   The length of the 'floppy tip' is variable and can be very important. As a general rule choose a wire with a long floppy tip unless there is little wire purchase (space in the target vessel to position the wire tip) in the target vessel and additional support is needed, e.g. Amplatz wires come with a 6 cm floppy tip as standard, but a wire with a 1 cm floppy tip is also available and is useful for carotid artery and hepatic vein intervention. A key to successfully advancing a catheter over the wire is to ensure that the transition between the floppy tip and the main body of the wire is within the target vessel.

Stiffness   Guidewires vary enormously in their stiffness – if you use a very stiff wire to negotiate a tortuous diseased vessel, you are sure to dissect! Pick the right tool.

STIFFNESS RATINGS OF GUIDELINES

- **Floppy** Bentson, movable core.
- **Normal** Hydrophilic guidewire, standard 0.035 = J or straight guidewire.
- **More supportive** Heavy-duty J or straight guidewire, stiff hydrophilic guidewire.
- **Stiff** TAD wires, Flexfinder, Amplatz super and extra-stiff wires.
- **Unreasonable force** Lunderquist wires. These are coat hangers with a floppy tip; they should only be used in extreme circumstances, e.g. to straighten vessels during stent-grafting (Fig. 7.12).

Alarm: Stiff guidewires should be introduced through a catheter that has been placed over a conventional guidewire. Do not attempt to steer a very stiff wire through even mild curves.

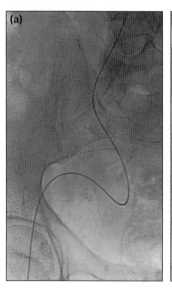
(a)

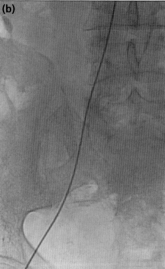
(b)

Fig. 7.12 ▇ (a) An extremely tortuous iliac artery with an Amplatz super-stiff guidewire in situ. (b) Following exchange for a Lunderquist guidewire, the artery has straightened markedly.

Diameters Guidewires come in a range of diameters from 0.014 to 0.038 inches. Small-calibre wires of 0.014–0.018 inches are used with microcatheters and for small vessel work, but do not have the same strength as larger wires.

0.035 inch guidewires are used for the majority of cases and will fit through a 4Fr or larger catheter. 0.038 inch wires were used a lot in the past, and some 4/5Fr catheters, most commonly the Terumo glidecatheters, will accommodate this size of wire.

Non-steerable guidewires

3 mm J guidewire This is the most frequently used wire. The 3 mm refers to the radius of the curve; also available in 5, 10 and 15 mm curves. The J tip does not dig up plaques and misses small branch vessels – ideal for retrograde femoral catheterization. The larger curves are used to avoid branch vessels, e.g. the 15 mm J will avoid the profunda femoris artery during antegrade puncture (Fig. 7.13).

Straight wire Length of the flexible tip varies from 1 to 6 cm, depending on particular wire type. Take care when passing plaques and branch vessels.

Bentson wire This wire has a very floppy, atraumatic 5 cm distal tip. If the end of the wire engages a branch vessel, then often gently continuing to advance the wire under fluoroscopy forms an atraumatic loop within the main vessel which pushes the wire tip out of the branch. It is particularly useful in combination with steerable catheters to negotiate stenoses and occlusions, as it does not readily dissect.

'Heavy-duty' guidewires have a stronger inner core than standard wires and therefore provide extra support.

Rosen wire comes as straight or 1.5 mm J. It provides extra support for advancing a catheter.

Amplatz super-stiff Supportive enough for introducing stents, stent-grafts and other devices. Treat with respect. This wire is strong and should never be used for selective catheterization! Amplatz wires normally have 6 cm floppy tips, which can be too long for some situations. They can also be obtained with a 1 cm floppy tip. Choose the correct length depending on the length of target vessel available as an anchor.

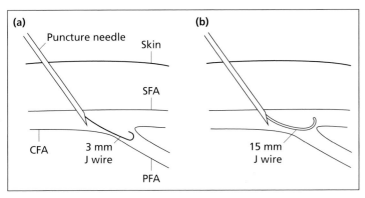

Fig. 7.13 ▦ (a) During antegrade puncture of the common femoral artery (CFA) the 3 mm J wire will often enter the profunda femoris artery (PFA). (b) The increased radius of curve of the 15 mm J wire usually will pass directly down the superficial femoral artery (SFA).

Steerable guidewires

Hydrophilic guidewires, e.g. Terumo, Road-runner. The coating on these wires makes them remarkably slippy and frictionless, allowing them to cross the narrowest of stenoses. The wire retains good torque control, though you will need a pin-vice to achieve this. The Terumo wire also comes in a 'stiff' supportive version, most frequently used for non-vascular intervention. Membership of the 'whoops Terumo' club is easily obtained by letting the wire slip through your fingers and on to your shoe. Take care when using hydrophilic wires and avoid using them for catheter exchange until you are proficient. A recent addition to the fold is the Sensor wire (Boston Scientific). This has a hydrophilic tip and supportive shaft and can be useful for extraluminal angioplasty.

Platinum-plus A 0.018 inch wire on a supportive stainless steel shaft with a 4 cm shapeable atraumatic floppy tip. The tip is highly visible.

TAD A graduated guidewire extending from a 0.018 inch 4 cm long floppy tip to an 0.035 inch stiff shaft. An excellent wire, particularly useful for renal angioplasty.

A steerable wire needs some space to work. If only a few millimetres extend beyond the catheter, then the wire will not torque correctly; back the catheter off until you achieve the desired effect. The tip of the guidewire can be shaped by placing it over some forceps and pulling it back between the forceps and your thumb.

Guidewires: a step-by-step guide

1. Advance the wire smoothly and carefully under fluoroscopic guidance. STOP if you feel any resistance; withdraw the wire a few centimetres, then carefully advance again. Use fluoroscopy to see what is wrong.
2. Insert a good length of wire before trying to introduce or exchange a catheter through the skin. You are less likely to lose position and you will have some wire to withdraw if it buckles.
3. Never let the wire move forwards when trying to introduce the catheter into the skin. It will buckle at the catheter tip and make the job much harder. Hold the wire out straight under slight tension.
4. Steerable guidewires have improved torque control; rotating the shaft will steer the tip in the same direction. Use this in combination with roadmapping to pass branch vessels and enter target vessels. You can use a pin-vice to help torque a steerable guidewire.
5. Do not be fooled by an assistant giving you the wrong end of the straight wire. Always check the flexibility of the end of the wire.

Tip: Always assume that your assistant is determined to pull the guidewire out during catheter exchanges. Get a grip!

OTHER ESSENTIAL EQUIPMENT

There are a few miscellaneous pieces of equipment whose existence greatly simplifies yours!

High-pressure connectors   These are non-compliant tubes used to connect the catheter to the injection pump. Most incorporate a two-way tap. Connectors should also be used during hand-injection to reduce your radiation exposure. Remember the inverse square law: even a small increase in distance causes a significant dose reduction.

Taps   There are many commercially available taps, and not all have been designed to allow high-pressure injection. Check before you treat everyone to a contrast shower. Only two types of tap are of importance angiographically:
- **Two-way taps** These have two positions, on and off, and come in two styles. The standard tap has a rotating valve and is almost ubiquitous. The other variety of tap functions using a 'sliding switch', so that it can be turned on and off very quickly; it is useful for CO_2 angiography.
- **Three-way taps** These taps have a sideport which allows air bubbles to be flushed out when a syringe is connected. It also permits two syringes to be attached together. This allows one to be used as a reservoir, e.g. during thrombolysis. Three-way taps are also used in pressure measurement circuits to allow the system to be calibrated to atmospheric pressure.

Pin-vice   This device is used to grip and steer guidewires and is particularly helpful when using hydrophilic and 0.018 inch wires. Remember to check that the device you use is the correct size for your wire: a standard pin-vice will not grip an 0.018 inch wire.

Vascular snares   Snares are used to retrieve foreign bodies and to capture guidewires for pull-through procedures. The best-known and most popular snare is the Amplatz Gooseneck (Fig. 7.14). This is made of Nitinol and comes in a range of sizes from 2 to 25 mm, which should be matched to the target vessel. The snare is supplied with its own 6Fr catheter, which has a radio-opaque end marker. This catheter can be shaped if necessary to increase manoeuvrability. Gooseneck snares are like lassoes and can be rotated, advanced and withdrawn, as well as tightened. The snare is placed around the target object and then the catheter is advanced, shortening the loop and gripping the target. The snare and its prey can now be pulled back to the access site and removed.

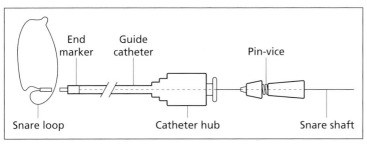

Fig. 7.14 ■ Amplatz 'gooseneck' snare.

End marker   Guide catheter   Pin-vice

Snare loop   Catheter hub   Snare shaft

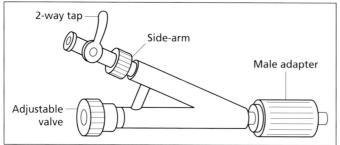

Fig. 7.15 ■ Tuohy–Borst adapter.

Alternative snares are also available. The EnSnare (Hatch Medical) has a trilobed configuration which can simplify capture in some circumstances (see Fig. 18.2).

Tuohy–Borst adapter   This invaluable but slightly fiddly Y-shaped device allows a haemostatic seal to be formed around guidewires that are smaller than the catheter lumen (Fig. 7.15). In addition to preventing a puddle of blood on the floor, it allows contrast or drugs to be injected through the side-arm of the adapter around the wire. Tuohy–Borst adapters are available in sizes that will seal around devices from 0.014 inch to 9Fr (approximately 3 mm). Probably the most frequent use of this device is to permit a 0.018 inch guidewire to be used with a standard catheter without leakage.

Learning to flush the device properly will place you ahead of many of your colleagues. Connect a two-way tap to the side-arm. Attach a syringe containing heparinized saline to the tap, then attach the Tuohy–Borst to the catheter and hold the system vertical. Start with the adapter valve open and allow flush to come out through it along with any residual air within the device. Now close the valve and flush the catheter. The catheter is now passed over the guidewire, which will stop at the valve. Loosen the valve sufficiently to allow the wire to exit, and then tighten it so that it forms a snug fit but allows the catheter to slide on the wire.

Chapter Eight

Vascular access

Vascular access is the starting point for all diagnostic and interventional angiography. Several basic principles apply, and similar problems are encountered at any access site. Choice of puncture site is dictated by the planned procedure; think what you need to achieve, consider the site of the lesion, and the size of sheath and catheter required.

The basic technique, first described by Seldinger, has three components:
- Vessel puncture.
- Passage of the guidewire.
- Introduction of the catheter.

The following section describes arterial access; venous access is discussed at the end of the chapter.

Arterial puncture

Puncture sites are points where the artery is relatively fixed and is compressible over bone to obtain haemostasis. The most commonly used site is the right common femoral artery (CFA). However, many factors, such as the strength of the pulse and the site of the disease, will influence the decision. The shortest, straightest route is nearly always best.

Arterial puncture: a step-by-step guide

1. Choose the optimal puncture site, take time to find the pulse, clean and drape the area.
2. Palpate the pulse and gently tension the skin. Infiltrate from skin to artery with 1% lidocaine. Leave the needle in situ to mark where to make the skin incision.
3. Make a skin incision appropriate to catheter/sheath size.
4. Place gauze swabs to absorb blood.
5. Insert the needle at 45° to the skin, aiming towards the pulse. A change in resistance is felt at the arterial wall and on entry to vessel lumen.
6. Free pulsatile backflow indicates that the needle tip is intraluminal. Poor flow is seen when using a 21G needle, or below a high-grade stenosis or occlusion.
7. The needle position is usually quite stable: it does not need to be held with a vice-like grip.

If the arterial pulse is not palpable, puncture can be attempted using the normal anatomical landmarks. Fluoroscopy may also demonstrate vascular calcification. If this is unsuccessful, use a form of guidance, either ultrasound or a roadmap image from another catheter. If you cannot obtain access at your preferred site, use an alternative approach. Remember to include the original access site in the subsequent angiogram to clarify the situation.

Consent issue: The main complications of arterial puncture can be readily remembered as the three Bs: Bruising, Bleeding and Blockage of the vessel. Less than 1% of patients should need either a blood transfusion or an operation to put things right.

Passage of the guidewire

The 3 mm J wire is the most frequently used guidewire. Arterial sheaths often come with guidewires with straight and J tips; the straight end is useful in small vessels. Use the introducer to advance the wire into the needle. If the introducer is not immediately available – which usually means it has migrated to the floor – it is possible to straighten the J wire by applying tension to the inner mandril (Fig. 8.1). The wire should advance smoothly and without resistance when held loosely between finger and thumb. Use fluoroscopic guidance to ensure that the wire follows the expected path without buckling or deforming (Fig. 8.2). It is better to put plenty of wire in the vessel rather than too little!

Alarm: Never use force on a guidewire: something is wrong. STOP and CHECK. Use fluoroscopy to check wire passage. Force is never necessary and always harmful.

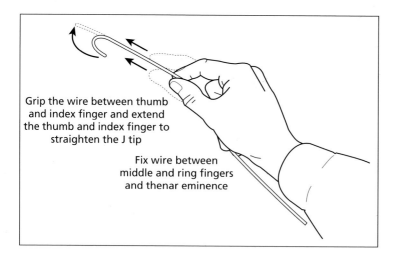

Grip the wire between thumb and index finger and extend the thumb and index finger to straighten the J tip

Fix wire between middle and ring fingers and thenar eminence

Fig. 8.1 ▦ Straightening the J wire. Fix the wire between the middle and ring fingers and the thenar eminence. Grip the wire between thumb and index finger and extend the thumb and index finger to straighten the J tip.

Troubleshooting

The wire will not advance beyond the needle tip

- It is not intraluminal. Usually the needle has been advanced too far and is in the far wall of the vessel. Remove the wire and verify pulsatile backflow; reposition as necessary.
- The needle tip is abutting plaque. Alter the angle of the needle: flattening towards the skin is often helpful. Try straightening the wire tip and redirecting (Fig. 8.3).

Use a test injection of contrast via the puncture needle to confirm intraluminal position. A roadmap may help guide the wire. Use tight collimation; keep your fingers out of the main beam (you may need them in years to come).

- Try another wire: many sheath wires have both a J and a straight tip. The straight end will often pass when the J tip will not advance. The Bentson wire often finds its way past plaque (Fig. 8.4) that the J wire will not negotiate. Never use a Terumo wire because the hydrophilic coating may shear off in the cutting bevel of the needle.
- If you have no success, obtain haemostasis and try again, or consider another approach.

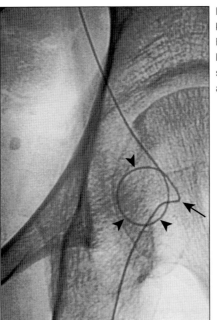

Fig. 8.2 ▦ A 0.018 inch guidewire has kinked at the end of the catheter (arrow). Further pressure has caused a subcutaneous loop to form. The wire was pulled back and straightened to allow the catheter to be advanced.

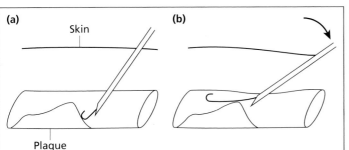

Fig. 8.3 ▦ Flattening the needle against the skin will often allow the wire to negotiate plaque adjacent to the puncture site.

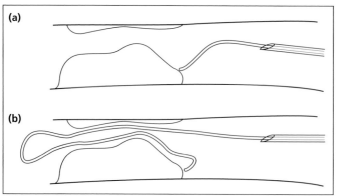

Fig. 8.4 ■ The very floppy tip of the Bentson wire will negotiate plaque with minimal risk of dissection.

The wire stops after a short distance
- Confirm that the wire is taking the expected route and is not in a branch vessel. Redirect as necessary.
- Introduce a 4Fr dilator over the wire and then try again; consider using an angled hydrophilic wire.
- Use a roadmap and a steerable wire to negotiate diseased and tortuous vessels.

Introduction of the catheter

The choice of catheter depends on the procedure. If the guidewire is held straight under slight tension, the catheter should slide smoothly along it. In a scarred groin it often pays to use a dilator and consider changing for a stiff guidewire. Use the following basic rules:
- Always insert plenty of guidewire.
- The guidewire should be held out straight and under slight tension.
- Hold the catheter close to its tip, within 1–2 cm of skin.
- Push and twist the catheter to advance it.
- Feel the catheter slide freely along the wire.

 Alarm: If the catheter seems to stick and pulls on the wire, the wire has kinked. Stop. Use fluoroscopy to show the problem (Fig. 8.5).

Pull back the catheter until the kink is outside the skin. Then, applying tension to the wire, try to advance the catheter again.

 Tip: This was why you put in lots of wire! Pull back the catheter and wire until the kink is outside the skin. Try again using a 4Fr dilator, and then change the wire that has been damaged.

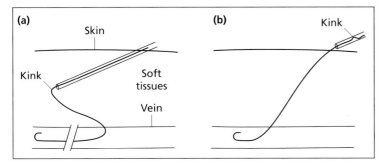

Fig. 8.5 ■ (a) If the catheter is difficult to advance through the skin, the wire may have kinked. (b) Pull back the catheter until the kink is outside the skin. Then, applying tension to the wire, try to advance the catheter again.

The catheter tip is often difficult to see, especially when using 3Fr catheters in obese patients. Pull back the guidewire until it takes the shape of the catheter tip; J wires can be felt to engage the catheter tip. The position is now readily seen on fluoroscopy. Use a test injection of contrast to confirm intraluminal position before flushing the catheter or performing a run. If the catheter is extraluminal, an extensive dissection will be avoided!

Commonly used arterial puncture sites

 Consent issue: An additional risk of the arm approach is causing a stroke as the catheter passes across the great vessels of the arch. Patients should be reassured that the risk is low (1%), but even that will be too high for some. Consider using non-invasive arterial imaging if the femoral approach is contraindicated.

Common femoral artery The CFA runs over the medial half of the femoral head. When the pulse is weak (Fig. 8.6) it is worth checking your position on fluoroscopy. Always aim to puncture the artery at the level of the midpoint of the femoral head, whether for retrograde or antegrade puncture. This is usually the point where the pulse is most readily palpated.

 Alarm: Puncturing too high – above the inguinal ligament – increases the risk of bleeding. Puncturing too low, i.e. superficial femoral artery puncture, increases the risk of false aneurysm and arteriovenous fistula (Fig. 8.7).

The wire generally does not need any steering to enter the external iliac artery; however, occasionally a plaque may deflect the wire into the deep circumflex iliac artery, which comes off the common femoral artery at approximately 10 o'clock. This is usually easily

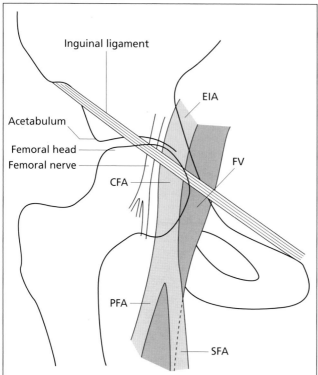

Fig. 8.6 ▇ The femoral anatomy. Note that the femoral vein lies medial to the artery in the groin, but then passes deep to the superficial femoral artery (SFA). CFA, common femoral artery; EIA, external iliac artery; FV, femoral vein; PFA, profunda femoris artery.

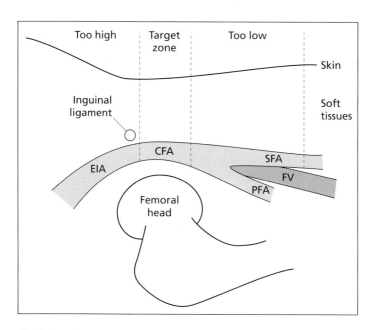

Fig. 8.7 ▇ Target puncture zone in the common femoral artery. Puncture at sites too low or high cannot be effectively compressed. CFA, common femoral artery; EIA, external iliac artery; FV, femoral vein; PFA, profunda femoris artery; SFA, superficial femoral artery.

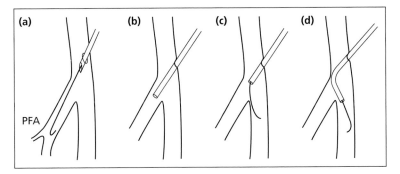

Fig. 8.8 ▮ Antegrade common femoral artery. (a) Wire repeatedly enters the profunda femoris artery (PFA). Insert a 4Fr dilator. (b) Perform an angiogram in the profunda oblique to confirm puncture is proximal to the superficial femoral artery. (c) Carefully pull back the dilator to the common femoral artery and try to direct an angled hydrophilic wire down the SFA. (d) If still unsuccessful, exchange for a Cobra catheter and use this to direct the wire into the SFA.

appreciated on fluoroscopy. Take care in this vessel, as it is prone to severe spasm that will retain the wire in a vice-like grip. It usually responds to vasodilation with nitrates and the passage of time.

Antegrade puncture (Fig. 8.8) Antegrade puncture is more difficult and carries an increased risk, as dissection flaps tend to occlude the vessel lumen. The point of skin puncture is always higher than you expect. Aim to hit the artery at the level of the midpoint of the femoral head. In obese patients it may help if an assistant holds back the abdominal folds. The profunda femoris artery (PFA) arises posterolaterally. This is in line with the needle, and so the guidewire tends to pass preferentially into it. To catheterize the superficial femoral artery (SFA) under these circumstances:

- Flatten the needle and point it towards the SFA. If the wire still passes into the PFA, try steering by straightening the wire tip.
- Put a 4Fr dilator into the PFA. Withdraw it slowly into the proximal PFA, injecting contrast to show catheter position.
- Obtain a roadmap image in the profunda oblique projection (ipsilateral anterior oblique 25°). Inject hard enough that contrast refluxes into the CFA and then opacifies the SFA. Ensure that the puncture site is proximal to the SFA origin. If it is not, start again.
- Try using an angled hydrophilic wire or a 15 mm J wire to select the SFA. Do not exchange over a hydrophilic wire: put the dilator into the SFA and change to a safer wire.
- No luck? Put the guidewire deep into the PFA and exchange for either a 4Fr Cobra or an RDC. The catheter is pulled back into the CFA and the wire is directed into the SFA.

Brachial artery (Fig. 8.9) This is used when the femoral approach is precluded; it is often the best route for upper limb angioplasty, stenting and fistulography. For diagnostic angiography, the left brachial artery is the preferred approach as it is usually the non-dominant arm and this route crosses the fewest cerebral vessels. The brachial artery is a small muscular artery and is prone to spasm. To prevent spasm, use a straight wire and administer prophylactic intra-arterial GTN. Consider a surgical cutdown for sheaths larger than 7Fr.

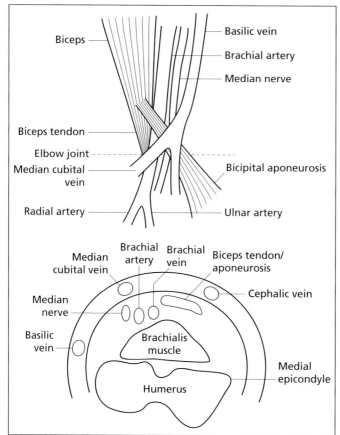

Fig. 8.9 ■ Anatomy of the antecubital fossa. The artery is punctured in the antecubital fossa above the elbow joint; it lies medial to the biceps tendon.

Tip: From the arm, the guidewire tends to pass into the ascending aorta. Use the left anterior oblique (LAO) 30° projection, advance the wire to open out the curve of the pigtail catheter and direct the wire into the descending aorta. If this fails, use an RDC catheter.

Radial artery This is an alternative route for diagnostic angiography. It is fiddlier than other approaches but has advantages for haemostasis. Bedrest is not necessary, so it is well suited to an outpatient procedure. Use a micropuncture set, a 4Fr sheath and prophylactic GTN. A 120 cm-long catheter is needed, which restricts flow rates to 6 mL/s. Long-term rates of thrombosis are not known.

Tip: Perform Allen's test to confirm the ulnar arterial supply to the hand. Alternatively, place a pulse oximeter on the middle finger. Compress the radial and ulnar arteries: desaturation will occur. Release the ulnar artery; resaturation confirms dual blood supply to the hand.

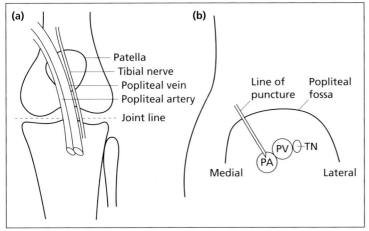

Fig. 8.10 ■ The popliteal fossa. (a) The popliteal vein (PV) lies superficial and lateral to the popliteal artery (PA). (b) Puncture at the level of the patella, medial to the popliteal vein and tibial nerve (TN).

Popliteal artery (Fig. 8.10) Occasionally used to access the SFA and CFA when angioplasty via the CFA has failed. SFA occlusions may be easier to traverse from below, especially in the presence of collaterals. Balloons up to 6 mm can be used through a 4Fr sheath. With the patient prone, use ultrasound to puncture the artery at the level of the patella.

Axillary artery Not the best initial choice. Puncturing the mobile axillary artery is difficult, and haemostasis no easier. There is a significant risk of brachial plexus injury secondary to haematoma. This approach is less safe than brachial puncture and is seldom used nowadays.

Translumbar aortogram Historical interest only (if that). From the days when radiologists were picadors, before haemostasis became fashionable.

Venous puncture

The principles of venous access are similar to those for arterial access, but remember that veins are thinner walled, compressible and prone to spasm. Venous spasm is readily provoked by injudicious catheter and wire manipulation. This can be a real catheter-gripping affair. Do not be tempted to start a tug-of-war – completely avulsing part of the venous system is seldom a satisfactory outcome. STOP and let the vein settle down for at least 5 minutes. If this does not work, try either GTN via the catheter or oral nifedipine. Blood pressure monitoring is advisable. Veins are more fragile and prone to dissection than a correspondingly sized artery, but fortunately bleeding is less severe.

Venous puncture: a step-by-step guide

1. Choose the optimal site depending on the planned procedure; clean and drape the area. Infiltrate the skin with 1% lignocaine. Leave the needle in situ to mark where to make the skin incision.
2. Make a skin incision appropriate to the catheter/sheath size.

3. Attach a 5 mL syringe to the puncture needle. Advance the needle at 45° to the skin, aspirating as you go – a change in resistance may be felt on entry to the vessel lumen.

4. Confirm intraluminal position by aspirating blood. If the tip is not in the vein, aspirate as the needle is slowly withdrawn. Flush the needle between attempts.

5. Guidewire passage and catheterization are the same as for arterial puncture.

Tip: Use ultrasound if available – even just one failed entry to the venous system is usually enough to cause a haematoma that will compress the vein and make subsequent puncture difficult.

Occasionally it may be helpful to use Valsalva or Trendelenburg manoeuvres to distend the vein.

Commonly used venous access sites

The approach chosen depends on the objective of the procedure.

Common femoral vein (CFV) The CFV lies medial to the CFA. Palpate the CFA and infiltrate local anaesthetic 1–2 cm medial to it. Aim to puncture the vein at the level of the midpoint of the femoral head. The right femoral vein is preferred to the left as it has a much straighter course to the inferior vena cava (IVC). Use ultrasound guidance if there is any difficulty, or when there is a contraindication to arterial puncture, e.g. pre-thrombolysis.

Tip: Remember, veins are easily compressed. Do not palpate over the vein during puncture because this just flattens the vein. Always aspirate as the needle is withdrawn, as sometimes a compressed vein has been transfixed during puncture and will open as the needle is pulled back.

Internal jugular vein (IJV) The IJV is one of the most important venous access points; it is used for central venous catheterization, hepatic venous intervention and IVC filter insertion. The right IJV provides a straight path to the right atrium and IVC. The left IJV detours via the (left) brachiocephalic vein; this angled course limits its utility for interventional procedures. The vein is punctured 1–5 cm above the clavicle, either using traditional anatomical landmarks or guided by ultrasound. Guidance makes the procedure simpler, safer and quicker.

Ultrasound-guided jugular vein puncture A 5–7.5 MHz ultrasound probe offers the best combination of resolution and depth for guidance. Turn the patient's head away from the side to be punctured and scan the neck to identify the vein lateral to the carotid artery, and infiltrate local anaesthetic. It is usually easiest to position the probe transversely unless it has a very small footprint. Position the transducer 1–2 cm below the skin puncture site and line up the vein with the midpoint of the probe head. Slowly advance the needle into the scan plane and on to the anterior vein wall. The vein is easily compressed and should be punctured with a quick stab: free aspiration of blood confirms intraluminal position.

'Blind' jugular vein puncture Many practitioners puncture the IJV blind, but few will be able to claim that they have never punctured the carotid artery or caused a pneumothorax. With the patient's head turned away, palpate the carotid artery midway between the mandible and the clavicle. Infiltrate local anaesthesia between the two heads of sterno-mastoid. The puncture needle is advanced at 45° to the skin and directed towards the ipsilateral nipple. If jugular venous pulsation is visible, direct towards it. If the carotid artery is punctured, gently compress it for 5–10 minutes to obtain haemostasis. A haematoma will compress the adjacent vein and make subsequent puncture more difficult.

Subclavian and axillary veins The subclavian vein is frequently used for central venous catheterization. It is a poor first choice for venous access. Besides the obvious risk of pneumo-thorax (1–2%), the vein is impalpable and cannot be compressed to secure haemostasis. In the long term it is prone to symptomatic stenosis and thrombosis. The axillary vein shares similar problems, though haemostasis can be secured by compression.

Subclavian vein puncture Infiltrate local anaesthesia at a point two-thirds of the way along the clavicle and 1 cm inferior to its inferior margin. The puncture needle is advanced just deep to the clavicle, aiming towards the head of the clavicle. Fluoroscopy can be helpful and, if in difficulty, a venogram from a peripheral injection may be used to guide puncture.

Axillary vein puncture The axillary vein is usually punctured under ultrasound guidance at a point just lateral to the first rib. The axillary vein and artery run closely parallel. Make sure the target vessel is compressible, to avoid inadvertent arterial puncture.

Median cubital vein This is the medial superficial vein in the antecubital fossa; it drains into the basilic vein and is the best arm vein for obtaining central venous access for IV DSA. The cephalic vein can also be used, but it may be difficult to negotiate from it into the subclavian vein. A hydrophilic guidewire and catheter are indispensable in this situation.

 Tip: In the absence of superficial veins at the elbow, inject contrast into a hand vein (preferably on the ulnar border) to opacify the basilic vein. It can then be punctured under fluoroscopic guidance.

Esoteric venous access sites

These sites are not used in daily practice but may be useful for some forms of intervention, and also in cases where there are no options left.

Inferior vena cava The IVC can be used for long-term central venous access. It is punctured under fluoroscopic guidance using a posterior approach to the right of the spine. If possible, place a pigtail catheter in the IVC below the renal vein; this provides a target to aim at and also helps to hold the vein open during puncture.

Hepatic vein The hepatic veins are another approach for long-term venous access and may also be used for intervention in Budd–Chiari syndrome. The target vein is punctured peripherally under ultrasound guidance. It is helpful to have colour Doppler to clarify that the vein is patent, and that it is not a portal vein radical. The mini-access set is very useful in these circumstances. The initial puncture uses a 21G needle, which is relatively atraumatic.

Collateral veins As a last resort, the central venous system can be accessed via collateral veins. These are usually identified and punctured using ultrasound guidance; alternatively, try a peripheral contrast injection and use fluoroscopy to target the vessel. Even using hydrophilic catheters and wires, it can be very difficult to navigate these small tortuous vessels.

SUGGESTIONS FOR FURTHER READING

Kaufman JA, Kazanjian SA, Rivitz SM et al. Long-term central venous catheterization in patients with limited access: A pictorial essay. AJR 1996;167:1327–1333.
Spies JB, Berlin L. Complications of femoral artery puncture. AJR 1998;170:9–11.
Trerotola SO. Management of hemorrhagic complications. J Vasc Intervent Radiol 1996;7:92–94.
What to do when the wheels come off, or how to keep your head while all around are losing theirs.

Chapter Nine

Haemostasis

Even if you enjoy talking to your patients, obtaining haemostasis after a diagnostic or therapeutic angiogram is tedious. Hence the art of staunching the flow is often neglected, or delegated to the most junior member of staff in the vicinity. Don't adopt this approach: it results in haematoma or haemorrhage. Stopping the bleeding is usually straightforward unless:

- The patient is severely hypertensive.
- The patient is obese.
- The patient is excessively anticoagulated or has a bleeding diathesis.
- You didn't puncture the artery in the correct place.
- You made a bigger hole than normal, i.e. >7Fr.
- Or, as is often the case, all the above.

Tip: If you are anticipating problems call for help before you remove the sheath. Consider using an arterial closure device. If necessary leave the sheath in situ, keep the patient heparinized, and have it removed surgically. Less than 1% of patients should require transfusion or emergency surgery.

How to prevent haemorrhage and haematoma (Fig. 9.1)

If you have only recently given 5000 units of heparin, stop and have a cup of tea before taking out the sheath. When both you and the patient are ready and have emptied your bladders you can start.

Remember that the puncture site is higher than the skin entry. In overweight patients it may be considerably higher.

- Place a finger on either side of the catheter, proximal and distal to the hole in the artery. You should be able to feel the pulse: this confirms that it is the correct place to press.
- Press firmly down until the pulse reduces; if increasing the pressure abolishes the pulse you are in control.
- Look at a clock and check the time.
- Remove the sheath and continue pressing, feeling the pulse, and watching the puncture site.
- After 5 minutes slowly reduce the pressure and check the puncture site.

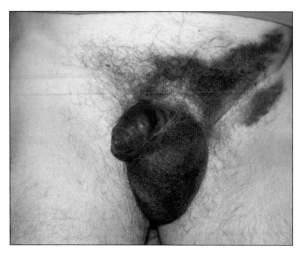

Fig. 9.1 ■ Large haematoma in left groin, penis and scrotum following bilateral iliac stenting. Note that the right groin puncture site is free of bruising. No transfusion required, but moderate discomfort persisted for several weeks.

- Still pulsatile bleeding? Press for at least another 10 minutes before you check again.
- Gentle ooze? Then press for another 5 minutes before checking.
- If the bleeding has stopped, get someone else who understands the principles of haemostasis to press for a further 5 minutes just to be on the safe side.
- When the bleeding has completely stopped the puncture site will remain dry. Place a swab over it, place the patient's hand on the pulse, check that they can feel it. Instruct them to keep pressing until they get back to the ward, and to remember to press if they cough, sneeze etc.

Bed rest post angiography There is no scientific formula and precious little evidence to tell us what is the optimum period of rest before mobilizing. For uncomplicated 3 and 4 Fr punctures it is probably reasonable to sit up after 30 minutes and to get out of bed after about an hour. For larger punctures a period of 4 hours' bed rest is probably prudent. Make sure that you advise patients to rest as much as possible for the remainder of the day. Day cases and outpatients should be given clear instructions what to do and who to contact if bleeding starts again after discharge.

Troubleshooting

The bleeding doesn't stop Stay calm and reassure the patient. If your fingers are numb ask someone to help you and prepare your contingency plan, i.e. notify the vascular surgeon that it may be necessary to repair the artery. Usually this act of contrition is sufficient to stem the flow, but if the bleeding is continuing after an hour it is usually better to put a suture in the artery. At least you mentioned this eventuality to the patient at the time of consent.

A large haematoma develops Stay calm and reassure the patient. Make frequent observations of the pulse and blood pressure. Try to find the pulse and continue compression. If you cannot do this, get an ultrasound machine and use colour Doppler to check for continuing bleeding or false aneurysms. Use the ultrasound probe to direct compression. A large haematoma will be painful, so give strong analgesics as necessary. Inform the vascular surgeon and assess the patient.

The patient has signs of bleeding   These may be overt haemodynamic instability, or subtler signs such as yawning, sweating or confusion. Resuscitate the patient with colloids infused rapidly, and call for help. Look for haematoma in the pelvis: this usually displaces the bladder and is readily shown on ultrasound and fluoroscopy if there is contrast in the bladder.

Remember, if bleeding will not stop you can always tamponade the puncture site by placing an angioplasty balloon from another access point. This will stop the bleeding and allow the patient to be stabilized, and everyone else to compose themselves and work out the best solution.

Arterial closure devices

These will not help you once the above problems have set in, but they can help prevent them occurring. Closure devices are relatively expensive and are not without their own problems; they are not a panacea. The devices and the techniques for deploying them are evolving and improving, making them more reliable; the following description is a general overview and is not a substitute for hands-on training. Each system has its own idiosyncrasies, which require familiarity, but there are a few basic principles which, if followed, will generally result in haemostasis. There are no precise rules regarding mobilizing the patient after using a closure device. It makes sense to encourage them to rest as much as possible, as for conventional haemostasis. Usually it is safe for the patient to get up after 1–2 hours, but they must be given clear instructions what to do if bleeding restarts. If the patient is being discharged home it is prudent to ask them to perform a test walk before they leave the department.

There are two basic types of closure device.

Suture-mediated closure devices, typified by the Perclose device (Abbott Laboratories). This comes in 6Fr and 8Fr sizes, depending on the sheath size being used. With a suture device there is immediate haemostasis and the artery may be punctured again immediately afterwards.

The design of the Perclose is quite complex. In essence, it passes two needles through the vessel wall adjacent to the puncture site; these retrieve a suture loop. Pulling the button out of the handle pulls the suture through and out of the skin. A slipknot is formed, and as this is tightened it closes the hole in the artery. The current device has the knot already tied within it. Sounds easy? Using the Perclose is not actually difficult, but there are quite a few elements to remember and carry out in the correct order.

The device needs a minimum of a 5 mm vessel to allow the footplate to open properly. The manufacturer recommends an angiogram of the puncture site in the oblique plane to be certain that the vessel is a suitable size, and the puncture is through the CFA.

Basic steps in using the Perclose

Phase 1 Introducing the catheter

1. Introduce the monorail suture device over a standard 0.035 inch guidewire up to the wire exit channel. Do not use a hydrophilic wire, as the catheter also has a hydrophilic coating and is quite slippery. The metal handle is not.

2. Remove the guidewire.
3. Continue introducing the device; when the transition point between flexible plastic and rigid metal is reached it usually helps to change the angle of approach from about 45° to a shallower angle. When pulsatile blood flow is seen from the clear plastic sidearm the device is far enough into the artery.

Phase 2 Catching the suture (Fig. 9.2)

1. Lift up the lever on the front of the device to open the footplate.
2. Hold the device at approximately 45° to the skin and gently pull it back until resistance is felt. This apposes the footplate to the inner wall of the artery.
3. Firmly depress the button on the end of the device until it stops.
4. Pull the button right back out of the handle; the two needles will appear. Hopefully only one will have a green suture attached.
5. Cut the suture close to the needle.
6. Push down the lever on the front of the device to retract the footplate.
7. Pull the device back until the guidewire channel is visible and replace the guidewire – this is useful if the device fails.

Phase 3 Tying the knot

1. The knot and sutures will now be visible.
2. Harvest the sutures from the device window. Don't pull hard on either of them until you know which is which.
3. Irrigate the sutures with a syringe full of saline; this makes it easier for the knot to slide and easier to see the colours.
4. The green suture (the longer one) is the rail suture, i.e. the knot slides down this suture.
5. The white suture is the locking suture; place it carefully to one side.

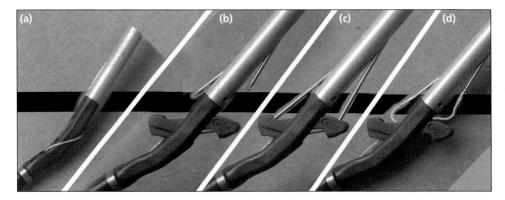

Fig. 9.2 ■ How the Percloser works. (a) The device is inserted into the artery and held at an angle of 45°. (b) The footplate is opened and the needles advanced. (c) The needles pass through the wall and 'dock' in the footplate. (d) The needles are retracted, bringing the sutures back through the artery wall with them.

DO NOT PULL THE WHITE SUTURE!!

Phase 4 Advancing the knot

1. Attach the knot pusher to the rail suture above the knot.
2. Keep tension on the **rail** suture while pulling the delivery catheter out. The suture should slide progressively further into the puncture site as you do this. If the bleeding stops, maintain tension on the rail suture and remove the guidewire.
3. Advance the knot pusher along the rail suture to deliver the knot against the arterial wall. It is usually possible to feel the knot against the wall.
4. Relax the pressure and inspect.
5. No bleeding? Ask the patient to cough; if still no bleeding, proceed to cut the suture.
6. If there is still some bleeding try steps 3 and 4 again.
7. Now is the moment to pull on the **WHITE** suture: this locks the knot tight.

Phase 5 The final cut

1. Advance the knot pusher down on to the knot; press the red lever and a tiny blade will cut the suture – above the knot, not through it. Honest!
2. If there is no bleeding after 10 minutes then sit the patient up.

Tip: On the current Perclose device the manufacturer has helpfully put a number 1 on the footplate lever, a number 2 on the end button and a 3 to indicate suture withdrawal – how much easier can it be?

Troubleshooting

Only one suture end is captured   Well, we warned that it was not perfect. Replace the guidewire and consider using an Angioseal, or compressing as normal. Sometimes rotating the angle of fire of the needles will be successful with a second Perclose.

Alarm: Remember, with the latest version of Perclose only the longer 'rail' suture emerges with the needle – look to see if the knot is tied; if it is, both sutures were captured.

The suture won't slip   Wet it and try again. Unfortunately, this is usually a prelude to the suture snapping and failure. Did you leave the wire in place?

The suture snaps   See above.

Bleeding continues despite your best efforts   If the wire is still in try an Angioseal if the puncture site is 8Fr or smaller; if not, press on (literally).

Tip: The Perclose can be used for larger sheaths by deploying the suture in advance of placing the larger sheath. If you are going to do this, keep each end of the suture in moist gauze. By using two sutures this technique can be used to close holes up to 18 Fr. Hardly surprisingly, the manufacturer does not recommend this.

Collagen plug and anchor Typified by the Angioseal (St Jude Medical). The Angioseal comes in 6 and 8Fr sizes. This system resembles that used to attach plastic price tags to clothing. A collagen footplate is deployed in the artery lumen using a version of a pusher system. The anchor is attached to a thread with collagen 'wadding' on it. The wadding is tamped down the thread with a pusher to form a plug at the puncture site. Haemostasis is rapid. The collagen footplate dissolves over about 10 weeks and the artery should not be punctured again within 3 months, as there is a risk of dislodging the anchor plate; this subsequently forms an effective embolus.

Tip: If you do need to access the artery again the plug can be identified with ultrasound and a puncture made as far away from it as possible.

Using the Angioseal is not actually difficult: there are just a few elements to remember and carry out in the correct order.

Basic steps in using the Angioseal

Phase 1 Assembling the delivery catheter

1. Open the packaging and you will find: a green dilator, a delivery catheter which has Angioseal written on it with the letters conveniently spaced 1 cm apart, a guidewire, and a sealed foil packet. This contains the seal itself; open it as well.
2. The catheter is basically like a sheath. Pass the green dilator into the catheter until it engages.
3. Note that there is a hole in the side of the catheter just beyond the distal end of the sheath, and another proximal to the sheath.

Phase 2 Inserting the delivery catheter

1. Keep the side with the writing facing up. The catheter is introduced just like a conventional sheath over a guidewire.
2. Continue to introduce until pulsatile flow is seen from the proximal sidehole.
3. Pull the catheter back until pulsatile flow stops; this indicates that the distal end lies just outside the artery. Note which letter of ANGIOSEAL is at the skin surface (usually G, unless the patient is large).

4. Advance the catheter in by 1 cm (to the next letter) – pulsatile flow should start again.

5. Fix the delivery catheter firmly in place and remove the wire and dilator.

Phase 3 Deploying the 'footplate' (Fig. 9.3)

1. Take the component containing the seal and introduce it into the sheath until the two components positively engage with a click. Do this quickly for the first few centimetres, or the collagen plug gets wet and won't advance. The footplate is now dangling freely in the artery lumen.

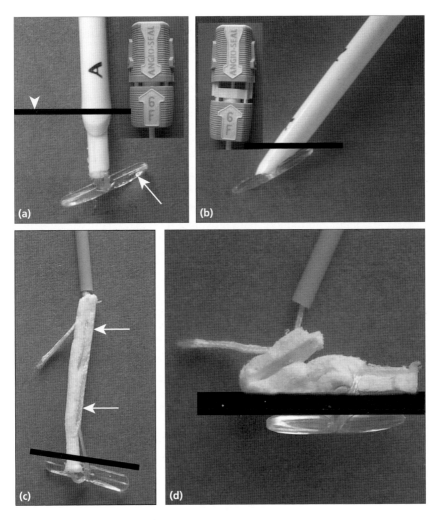

Fig. 9.3 ▓ Angioseal – the basics. (a) The footplate (white arrow) is released in the artery. Black line (arrowhead) represents the artery wall. Insert shows the delivery mechanism. (b) The footplate is retracted to the end of the delivery catheter (insert shows the delivery mechanism). (c) The catheter is withdrawn to leave the footplate in the artery and the collagen 'wadding' (white arrows) outside it. (d) The wadding is tamped down to effect a seal.

2. Keeping the delivery catheter still, disengage the two components you just clicked together. Pull back the second catheter about 5 mm – it usually makes two clicks as you do this. The footplate is held taut sitting across the end of the delivery catheter.

Phase 4 Deployment of the device
1. Press gently over the puncture site as if to obtain haemostasis.
2. Pull back the delivery catheter and second catheter together until they stop. A firm steady pull is usually required. A thread will be seen coming out of the puncture site. The collagen sponge can be seen on this, and behind it a green plastic pusher.
3. Keeping the thread taut, use the pusher to tamp down the collagen sponge until bleeding stops or a black transition is seen on the thread; this indicates that the plug is packed firmly enough.
4. Check the femoral pulse.

Phase 5 The final cut
1. Place a clip on the thread just behind the green plastic. This will keep the plug in place, which is probably unnecessary but will remind everyone to be careful of the puncture site.
2. Transfer the patient to the recovery area.
3. If there is no bleeding, tension the suture and cut it close to the skin.
4. Wait a few more minutes and sit the patient up.
5. Tell them that the artery should not be punctured for 3 months, and give them the patient information sheet provided. It does no harm to place the same information in their case notes!

Troubleshooting

Bleeding persists   The device may have been suboptimally deployed. There is only one thing to do – press on it.

The femoral pulse is weak or absent   This is much more worrying and implies that either the plug and the footplate are intra-arterial or the footplate has embolized. Perform an ultrasound to verify the situation and contact a vascular surgeon. It is likely that the patient will need an arteriotomy.

The patient's leg becomes ischaemic despite a good femoral pulse   This implies embolization of the endplate. If ultrasound does not give the answer you may need an angiogram to find it. Once you have located it consider snaring the footplate, but you have probably already caused enough trouble for one day.

Chapter Ten

Complications of angiography and vascular intervention

Puncturing arteries and blowing up balloons in them can and does occasionally cause problems, but they never seem so bad if you know what to expect and what to do. Basically, most mishaps can be categorized into immediate and delayed and, with hindsight, predictable and unpredictable. Immediate and unpredictable complications are often more spectacular, and the delayed are more sinister.

 Tip: Try to avoid predictable complications! What seems unpredictable to you may well be commonplace: consult others when trying something new. Whenever you experience a complication, review the case and make sure that you learn from your mistakes.

Remember the central tenets of crisis management:
- Stay calm.
- Stop and think what is likely to be the problem.
- Plan your action.
- Get help.
- Action your plan.

Immediate complications

Whenever a complication occurs, stay calm and try to think logically. A downward spiral of disaster can easily set in, so ask for help sooner rather than later. Document the episode carefully in the patient's notes and explain what has happened to the patient or the patient's relatives. Many misunderstandings occur because of poor communication, and patients frequently complain about not being told what was happening. Immediate complications can be grouped according to the site affected:
- Puncture site
- Intervention site
- Remote.

Puncture site complications

These are the commonest and most predictable.

Haematoma (see Fig. 9.1 of haematoma.) Some bruising is inevitable, but significant haematomas requiring either transfusion or surgery are rare (<1%). The risks increase with increasing catheter size, increasing patient size, hypertension, anticoagulation and low platelet levels. Think carefully before you delegate the removal of an 8Fr sheath in an obese, hypertensive patient who has just been heparinized!

Bleeding Haemorrhage at the puncture site almost always occurs during haemostasis. A large haematoma can accumulate very quickly and will alert you to the problem. More sinister is occult bleeding into the pelvis. This happens when the arterial puncture is above the inguinal ligament. Be alert for signs of blood loss, yawning, confusion, agitation, faintness, tachycardia and hypotension. Act quickly as soon as you suspect a problem.

Basic survival strategy:
- Do not struggle alone – call for assistance.
- Lie the patient down and elevate the legs if necessary.
- Attempt to control the bleeding, try to find the pulse and apply local pressure.
- Resuscitate the patient, put in a large drip and take blood for cross-match and clotting studies. Start a rapid infusion of a plasma substitute or saline, and give oxygen by mask.
- Closely monitor the patient's pulse, BP, oxygen saturation and ECG.
- Correct any clotting abnormality, e.g. protamine to reverse heparin (p. 27).
- By the time the surgeon arrives, the situation is normally under control. If not, don't hesitate – the patient should have an urgent arterial repair, usually requiring just one or two sutures.
- If you have time, get an ultrasound machine and document the site of the bleeding and the extent of any haematoma. Ultrasound-guided compression can be very effective when there is a large haematoma. If the bleeding has been occult, look in the pelvis for haematomas displacing the bladder.

False aneurysm This is more likely to occur with low puncture in the SFA where the artery cannot be compressed against the femoral head. If a pulsatile swelling develops, perform an ultrasound to differentiate between simple haematoma and a false aneurysm: the latter typically has 'in and out' flow. It is usually possible to identify a jet of flow arising from the hole in the artery.

Management of puncture-site false aneurysms

False aneurysm occurs when there has been inadequate haemostasis. Fortunately, this complication is usually caused by someone else (frequently a cardiologist). There are reasons for this, principally the vigorous use of anticoagulation, antiplatelet drugs, large sheaths, early mobilization of patients and low puncture. Whatever the aetiology, it frequently falls to us to treat it.

Options include ultrasound-guided compression, thrombin injection and surgical repair.

Ultrasound-guided compression was very popular when first introduced, as it was the only alternative to surgery. It is recognized that it works best for acute false aneurysms,

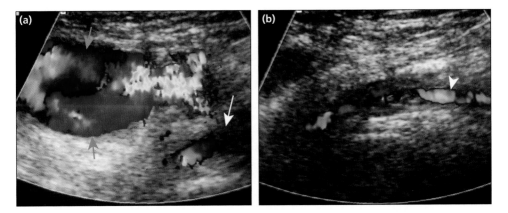

Fig. 10.1 ▪ Ultrasound-guided compression of a femoral false aneurysm. (a) Large false aneurysm (turquoise arrows) 24 hours after removal of a 9Fr femoral sheath. Note the characteristic flow pattern: turbulent jet adjacent to the neck (white arrow) and 'in and out' flow within the false aneurysm itself. (b) During compression, flow is maintained within the femoral artery but there is no flow in the false aneurysm.

with the chance of success diminishing after a few days. It is a simple technique: scan the puncture site and use colour flow Doppler to look for the jet of flow in and out of the false aneurysm. Keep the colour on and use the probe to compress over this point. The aim is to press hard enough to occlude the flow in the false aneurysm while preserving flow in the main artery. In simple cases this is just like obtaining haemostasis, and the aneurysm will thrombose after a few minutes. If you do succeed, bring the patient back for a follow-up scan after 24 hours to ensure that the aneurysm has not recurred.

Commonly the patient will have a large and tender haematoma and find the whole procedure very uncomfortable. Some patients will either not tolerate this or only manage a few minutes despite analgesia/sedation. Both you and the patient will be very uncomfortable if you need to press hard for more than about 15 minutes. If this is the case then consider the other options (Fig. 10.1).

Tip: You are much less likely to succeed if the patient is anticoagulated. Reverse this where possible before attempting compression.

Thrombin injection This technique has been widely adopted as it is quick and easy, but it is not cheap, and complications have been reported, including anaphylactic reactions to the thrombin (especially the bovine preparation) and thrombosis of the donor artery. Pass a 23G needle into the false aneurysm under ultrasound guidance. Attach a 1 mL tuberculin syringe containing 1000 IU of thrombin (DO NOT ASPIRATE, or you will need to start again from scratch!!). Aim towards the inflow defect and inject in 0.1 mL aliquots, keeping the colour flow on throughout. Thrombosis usually occurs very rapidly, and further injection will risk thrombus – or, worse, thrombin being injected into the artery, with potentially calamitous results.

Troubleshooting

If thrombosis does not occur

- Check that the needle is in the false aneurysm by injecting saline and looking for turbulence. Reposition as necessary and try again.
- Check that it is thrombin, not just saline in the syringe.
- Consider placing an angioplasty balloon across the defect from an alternative access point. Inflate the balloon to cover the hole and inject a small volume of thrombin. Slowly deflate the balloon and check for thrombosis. Do not overinject the false aneurysm sac or you will simply inject a bolus of thrombin into the artery when the balloon is deflated.
- Check the clotting and reverse coagulopathy if necessary.
- If it still won't thrombose, it's back to surgery.

The false aneurysm thromboses but a tongue of thrombus is seen in the artery

If this is a small amount and there is no problem with limb ischaemia, accept this and stop. Consider heparinizing the patient. Rescan after 24 hours.

The artery thromboses   This is usually the time to call the vascular surgeon and explain what has happened.

Arteriovenous fistula This is very uncommon with a CFA puncture and is much more likely if the SFA is punctured, as the femoral vein lies deep to it.

Thrombosis This normally occurs if the artery is severely diseased at the puncture site, or if there has been arterial dissection during antegrade puncture. Check the condition of the limb: if there is acute ischaemia, then urgent surgical revascularization is required. If you have vascular access, get an angiogram to demonstrate the extent of the problem. If the situation is less urgent, thrombolysis may be appropriate; fresh thrombus is particularly likely to lyse. If the patient is asymptomatic, consider terminating the procedure and reviewing their clinical progress.

Nerve damage This is very uncommon and may result from direct injury, ischaemia, local anaesthetic and compression by haematoma.

Intervention site complications

It is hardly surprising that occasional arterial injuries occur when you consider what we are doing inside these structures with catheters, guidewires and balloons.

Arterial dissection As angioplasty works by stretching and tearing the vessel lining, some dissection is to be expected. It is important if it is flow limiting, and it most commonly happens with antegrade approaches; retrograde dissections are usually self-limiting. If a dissection flap is causing significant obstruction, make sure that the patient is heparinized. There are four treatment options:

- Do nothing: only a consideration if the problem is unlikely to lead to a clinical deterioration.
- Perform a prolonged (5–10 min) low-pressure balloon inflation: try to stick the dissection flap back to the wall (Fig. 10.2).
- Stent the dissection: this provides an immediate and durable solution, but is not advisable if the dissection involves a point of arterial flexion.
- Call your friend the vascular surgeon again.

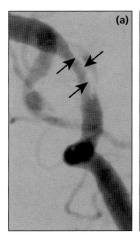 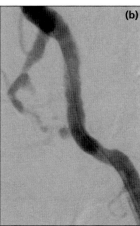

Fig. 10.2 ■ (a) External iliac artery showing extensive postangioplasty dissection (arrows) with residual 30 mmHg pressure gradient. (b) Abolition of pressure gradient and improved angiographic appearance after prolonged low-pressure inflation.

Arterial occlusion This is not uncommon when treating severely diseased vessels and may be of little clinical significance, e.g. when a severely narrowed artery becomes occluded. Occlusion is important if it:

- Results in an acute decrease in perfusion, such as when important collaterals are blocked. In this case, a bail-out procedure such as stenting, thrombolysis or surgery is indicated.
- Modifies the treatment options for the patient, e.g. when the length of an occlusion is increased, thereby affecting the type of surgery required.

Heparinize the patient and consider the treatment options, stenting and surgery.

Arterial rupture Minimize the chances of this occurring by using a correctly sized balloon and asking the patient to let you know if discomfort is experienced during inflation. Mild discomfort is normal but marked pain is not; do not be surprised if the vessel splits if you stretch the adventitia much more. Arterial rupture is an emergency and can lead to rapid destabilization of the patient's clinical condition (Fig. 10.3). Apply the basic survival strategy as above. Whatever you do, keep control of the bleeding by gently inflating an angioplasty balloon across or proximal to the injury. If you have a correctly sized stent-graft, now is the time to use it.

Venous filling A little filling of the venae comitantes is nothing to worry about, but if there is a brisk arteriovenous shunt, stop and think. This is unlikely to happen, as rupture is much more common.

Remote problems

This means that the problems are not at the sites above, not that they are remote from you.

Distal macroembolization Thrombus or atheroma may break off from the wall of a diseased vessel and will migrate distally until it occludes a vessel of a suitable diameter, usually at a bifurcation. Once again, the treatment should be based on the clinical scenario. If a

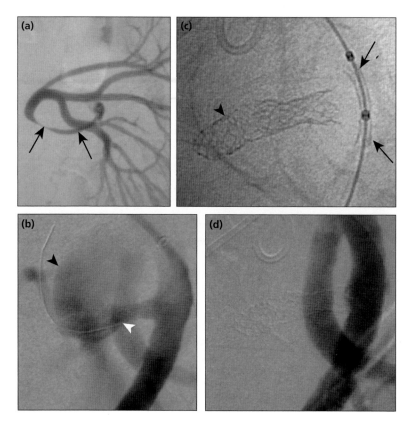

Fig. 10.3 ▓ Rupture of a renal transplant artery. (a) An unusual 5 cm long high-grade stricture (black arrows) in an acutely non-functioning transplant. (b) Arterial rupture (white arrowhead) following placement of three stents, extensive extravasation (black arrowhead). (c) Site of the rupture (black arrowhead). Unfortunately, it was impossible to place a stent graft in the ruptured artery. A covered stent is being deployed over the origin of the transplant artery (black arrows). (d) Completion angiogram showing complete occlusion of the artery.

small and unimportant vessel is affected, do nothing. If the limb has become ischaemic or a vital vessel has been blocked, then some action is necessary:

- Heparinize the patient.
- Attempt to aspirate the embolus (Fig. 10.4) (thrombosuction, p. 188).
- Stent over the embolus.
- Call 0800 Fogarty.

Distal microembolization Microembolization can affect any organ system, and cholesterol, thrombus and atheroma can all cause severe problems. Catheter manipulation in the diseased aorta is the most common cause, with the resultant microemboli causing occlusion of the distal vascular bed. If the patient experiences sudden severe back or abdominal pain during the procedure, this indicates massive embolization and has a poor prognosis. More commonly, there will be cutaneous manifestations (livido reticularis), which come on after a few hours. Renal dysfunction is common; this may be abrupt in onset or manifest by a

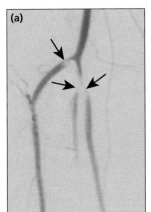 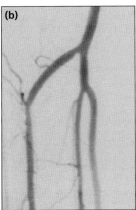

Fig. 10.4 ▓ (a) Distal embolization of atheroma into the crural vessels post angioplasty. (b) Flow is restored after thrombosuction with a 5Fr catheter.

progressive, often irreversible, loss in renal function starting days after the procedure. 'Trash foot' is a serious outcome frequently requiring amputation, and it presents classically as distal tissue necrosis in the presence of palpable pulses.

Cardiorespiratory failure This can result from fluid overload, bronchospasm, drugs, sedation and contrast reaction. A vicious cycle is set up, with hypoxia and myocardial ischaemia. The patient should be given oxygen and vigorously resuscitated.

Chapter Eleven

Diagnostic angiography

Obtaining good-quality diagnostic angiograms is the first step to any successful intervention. This chapter discusses the indications, equipment, procedural details and views for all the common sites.

Basic angiography set

Almost every procedure requires the same basic set of tools for initial access. Additional equipment is added to this for more complex cases. To avoid repetition the essential items are outlined below, and specific items are discussed in the relevant chapters.

Essential items:

- **Arterial puncture needle**: 21 G for 0.018 inches wire (3Fr); 18 G for 0.035 inches wire (4Fr).
- **Guidewire**
  - For a 4Fr catheter, use a 150–180 cm-long 0.035 inch wire with a 3 mm J tip.
  - For a 3Fr catheter, use a 0.018 inch wire, which is usually supplied with the set.
- **Arterial sheath**: when catheter exchanges anticipated and for angioplasty.
- **Catheter**: pigtail catheters are the safest for high-flow flush injections. Straight catheters should be used in small vessels and whenever it is anticipated that the catheter will be pulled back into the iliac artery, e.g. pressure measurements.
  - 3Fr catheters have restricted flow rates; a 30 cm straight catheter has a maximum flow of only 6–8 mL/s.
  - 4Fr catheters have flow rates that are dependent on their length; a 60 cm catheter has a maximum flow of 18–20 mL/s. Use the shortest catheter that will reach the target.
  - 4Fr 60 cm for abdominal angiography from the femoral approach.
  - 4Fr 90 cm for arch aortography or abdominal angiography from the brachial approach.
  - 4Fr 120 cm for the radial approach.
- **High-pressure connector**: this is a sterile extension to attach the pump to the catheter. The catheter stays clean and the pump is out of the way!
- **Injector**: loaded with 100 mL of 300 mg/mL non-ionic contrast. Set maximum psi, flow rate and pressure rise time according to catheter recommendations.

Tip: Time spent on reconnaissance is never wasted. Ensure that you have all the equipment you anticipate needing before starting the case.

PRESSURE MEASUREMENTS

Vascular stenoses are haemodynamically significant when they narrow the vessel diameter by 50%; this corresponds to a 75% reduction in cross-sectional area. A significant stenosis is flow limiting and results in a pressure drop across it. Some vessels are readily assessed angiographically – e.g. the SFA – whereas others are tortuous and prone to eccentric plaques, and thus the degree of stenosis is harder to establish; this is particularly true in the iliac circulation (Fig. 11.1). Pressure gradients are used to demonstrate the significance of stenosis before and after treatment. Venous pressure measurements are less frequently used.

Equipment

- Basic angiography set.
- Arterial sheath: 1 Fr size bigger than the catheter.
- Catheters: straight catheters with end- and sideholes are used to measure pressures.
- Pressure measurement transducers: you must use non-compliant lines designed for pressure recording.
- Pressure monitor and recording.
- Vasodilator drugs: tolazoline, papaverine or glyceryl trinitrate (GTN).

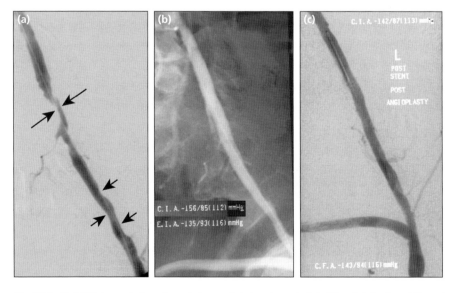

Fig. 11.1 ■ (a) High-grade iliac stenosis (arrows), 'minor irregularity' of the distal external iliac artery (EIA) is noted (short arrows). (b) Following angioplasty and stenting of the proximal lesion a 21 mmHg pressure gradient persists. Pullback measurements show this to be across the distal EIA. (c) Following distal EIA angioplasty, the pressure drop has been abolished.

Setting up

We cannot help you too much here: you have to know how to use the system in your catheter laboratory. Here are some general points:

- Flush the transducer system thoroughly to get rid of air bubbles, as these will cause damping and affect measurement.
- Tighten all connections; these not only cause leaks, but also affect measurements.
- Flush the system regularly to prevent pericatheter thrombosis.
- Zero the system to atmospheric pressure with the transducer at the level of the right atrium.
- Calibrate the system and set an appropriate scale to display the waveform trace.

Procedure

Access As always this depends on the target. Ipsilateral retrograde access is normally used to assess iliac arterial disease.

Catheterization The stenosis is crossed using standard angiography techniques (see Angioplasty, p. 139). The aim is to record the arterial pressure on either side of the stenosis. This can be achieved in three ways:

1. Simultaneous recording from the catheter and the sheath, with the catheter across the stenosis. Theoretically, the catheter should not be across the stenosis; in practice it usually is, but this does not affect the measurement unless the stenosis is very tight, in which case measurement is usually unnecessary.
2. Simultaneous recording from two catheters: one ipsilateral distal to the stenosis and one contralateral proximal to the stenosis. Theoretically better than option 1, but involves more arterial punctures for little practical advantage.
3. A single catheter is pulled back through the stenosis and changes in pressure are recorded. This technique is the least accurate, as beat-to-beat variations in blood pressure will affect it. In addition, access across the stenosis is lost when the catheter is withdrawn.

Runs Angiography is performed to demonstrate the stenosis. The straight catheter is positioned so that the proximal sidehole is above the stenosis and the sheath tip below the stenosis. Pressure gradients are recorded 'at rest' and following the administration of a vasodilator to reduce peripheral resistance and augment flow.

Interpretation

There is no consensus as to what constitutes a significant trans-stenotic arterial pressure gradient. Several alternatives have been proposed:

- ≥20 mmHg peak systolic gradient following vasodilation
- ≥15% peak systolic gradient following vasodilation
- ≥10 mmHg mean pressure gradient following vasodilation.

None of these measurements is ideal, and the science of pressure measurement is imprecise. Choose your preferred method and stick to it. You can use consensus if you prefer and have the time to make multiple measurements.

Venous pressures These are not measured as often as arterial pressure gradients. They are measured in the same way as arterial pressures, but without vasodilation.

The interpretation is different: a trans-stenotic pressure drop of 3 mmHg is considered significant in the venous system.

Portal systemic pressures

WEDGED PORTAL VEIN PRESSURE   The portal systemic gradient is often measured in the assessment of patients with liver disease to evaluate portal hypertension. Normal resting portal vein pressures are between 5 and 10 mmHg and only a few mmHg above the systemic venous pressure. The pressure gradient can be measured directly during a TIPS procedure, or can be estimated from the wedged hepatic vein pressure. Wedged pressure measurement is analogous to using the pulmonary artery wedge pressure to measure the left atrial pressure.

An endhole catheter is passed into a peripheral hepatic vein branch. If the catheter is wedged there is often a reassuring slurping sound when the wire is removed. This can be confirmed by contrast injection (Fig. 11.2), which will opacify the liver parenchyma if the catheter is wedged. If all the contrast passes back up the hepatic vein, put the wire back and try again. On rare occasions when a wedged position cannot be obtained, use either an angioplasty balloon or an occlusion balloon to occlude more centrally. Following this, the catheter is positioned more centrally in the hepatic vein and the 'free' pressure measured. The portal systemic gradient is the difference between the wedge pressure and the pressure in the IVC. There is portal hypertension when the portal pressure is above 12 mmHg. TIPS shunts should have a pressure gradient of less than 12 mmHg across them. Elevated free hepatic vein pressures indicate venous outflow obstruction.

Troubleshooting

Problems are most commonly caused by incorrectly set up equipment. Develop a systematic approach to reviewing the system to detect and rectify these faults.

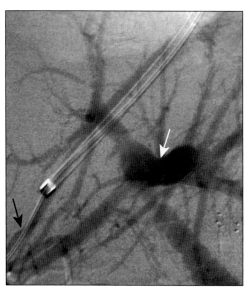

Fig. 11.2 ■ Carbon dioxide wedged hepatic venogram. A Cobra catheter (black arrow) has been wedged in a distal hepatic vein branch. CO_2 has refluxed through the hepatic sinusoids to opacify the portal vein (white arrow).

Bizarre or wildly fluctuating pressures   The equipment has probably been set up incorrectly. There may be an air bubble in the pressure line. Flush the line thoroughly and recalibrate the system.

Loss of pressure trace   Usually this is due to something simple, such as the three-way tap being off, or the catheter blocking or kinking. Check the set-up again to identify the problem.

The distal pressure is greater than the proximal pressure   This is not an uncommon finding (we told you that this was an imperfect science) and is due to changes in vessel diameter – reflected waves cause higher pressures in small vessels. Pulling back the upstream catheter can help; measure the pressures close to the stenosis (1–2 cm is ideal) at points where the arterial diameters are comparable.

Unexpectedly, there is no pressure gradient   That's life! The reason you measured the gradient was because you were unsure of the significance of the lesion.

The gradient is significant by one but not all of the criteria   The three techniques do not always agree; that's why you choose a method and stick to it.

LOWER LIMB ARTERIOGRAPHY

Indications

Peripheral angiography is most frequently requested to investigate chronic ischaemia (intermittent claudication, rest pain and ulceration) or acute ischaemia (Fig. 11.3). Less common reasons are trauma, vascular malformation and tumour.

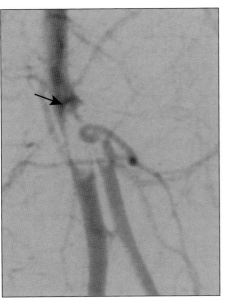

Fig. 11.3 ▮ Typical appearance of an embolus involving the bifurcation of the common femoral artery. The filling defect has a convex meniscus and is sited at a bifurcation. The underlying artery is normal and there are no collaterals.

Table 11.1 Typical parameters for a lower limb angiogram

View	Contrast volume (mL)	Injection rate (mL/s)	Frame rate (fps)	Field size (cm)	Inject delay (s)	X-ray delay (s)
AP aortoiliac	15	8	2	40	1.5	0
Oblique aortoiliac	15	8	2	28	1.5	0
AP proximal thigh	10	5	2	40	0	0
AP distal thigh	10–15	5	1	40	0	Increase as necessary
AP calf vessels	10–20	5	1	40	0	Increase as necessary
Lateral foot	10–20	5	1	28	0	Increase as necessary

AP, anteroposterior; fps, frames per second.

Equipment

- Basic angiography set.
- Catheter: pigtail or straight, 3Fr 30 cm length, 4Fr 60 cm, 90 cm or 120 cm (femoral, brachial and radial approaches, respectively). Always use the femoral route unless contraindicated.

Procedure

Access Use the symptomatic leg unless the femoral pulse is absent or very weak. This gives optimal images of the affected side. Straight catheters can be pulled back into the external iliac artery for single leg views. There is no risk to the asymptomatic limb.

Catheterization Position the catheter below the renal arteries unless there is a reason to image them, i.e. renal impairment or hypertension.

Runs Our standard angiogram covers from the infrarenal abdominal aorta to the ankle (Table 11.1). Tailor the examination to the individual patient. Lateral foot views are mandatory if distal reconstructive surgery is being considered.

To obtain high quality views of the aortoiliac segments, always paralyse the bowel using buscopan and use breath-holding or multimasking to eliminate misregistration.

Additional views

Oblique views are not really additional and are routinely used in the iliac arteries. In other circumstances use your skill and judgement to decide whether they are required. A problem commonly occurs because of prosthetic joints obscuring a vessel. It sometimes seems as if there is invariably a stenosis in the popliteal artery behind a total knee replacement, and only a true lateral view will show it (Fig.11.4).

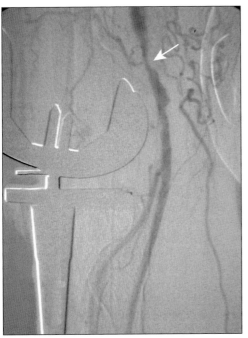

Fig 11.4. ■ High-grade stenosis (white arrow) seen on the lateral knee view. This was not seen on AP or shallower obliques.

Tip: The contralateral leg will often compromise a lateral knee view, especially if there are bilateral knee replacements. Flex the contralateral knee to give an unimpeded view of the side of interest.

Iliac obliques The iliac vessels are tortuous and oblique views are essential to allow full assessment − 25° side of interest down, i.e. LAO 25° for the right iliac system.

Profunda oblique The profunda femoris origin is often superimposed on the CFA. The profunda origin can usually be assessed 30–50° side of interest raised, i.e. RAO 30–50° for the right profunda.

Focal stenoses Any stenosis can be more accurately assessed if an additional oblique view is taken. Experiment with 30° obliques in either direction to try to profile the lesion.

Lateral foot views
(a) 'Charlie Chaplin' – place both heels together, turn toes out; 40 cm field.
(b) Single foot – externally rotate the foot and rotate C-arm to obtain lateral projection; 28 cm field.

Troubleshooting

Unable to advance the guidewire through the iliac artery
- Insert a 4Fr dilator to secure vascular access.
- Make sure blood can be aspirated from the dilator.

- Using fluoroscopy, gently inject contrast to confirm intraluminal position.
- Perform a hand-injected angiogram to identify the problem.
- Use a hydrophilic guidewire +/− shaped catheter (e.g. Cobra II) to negotiate stenoses and tortuous segments.

Poor views of the distal runoff

- Collimate to a single limb.
- In the ipsilateral limb, pull back a straight, multi-sidehole catheter into the external iliac artery to direct all of the contrast to the area of interest.
- In the contralateral limb, use a shaped catheter (e.g. Cobra II or RDC) to catheterize the contralateral external iliac artery (EIA).
- Use a vasodilator such as tolazoline or GTN.
- Consider performing an antegrade puncture so that contrast will be directed solely to the runoff vessels.
- Increase the volume/strength of the contrast. Consider using iso-osmolar contrast in patients with critical ischaemia. These patients are in pain and are often more sensitive to the heat associated with contrast injection. This effect is almost non-existent with iso-osmolar contrast; in consequence, the patient will keep still and you will save time and obtain diagnostic images!

GRAFT ANGIOGRAPHY

Graft angiography can be difficult. Success is much more likely if you spend time ascertaining the graft anatomy, material, and the results of the Duplex ultrasound before you start.

Aims of graft angiography

Grafts fail for many reasons. Remember Virchow's triad: stenoses, slow flow and hyper-coagulability states are often contributory factors. Angiography is a prelude to treatment and aims to demonstrate mechanical problems; these will nearly always have been detected on Duplex surveillance:

- Anastomotic stenoses caused by neointimal hyperplasia. Usually within the first year.
- Intragraft stenosis, particularly at valve cusps and in composite vein grafts.
- Progression of disease in the arterial inflow or outflow. Usually after the first year.
- Graft kinking during knee flexion. This should always be excluded following thrombolysis if no other abnormality is found (Fig. 11.5). The graft usually kinks a few centimetres above the knee joint; this is best appreciated in the lateral projection.

When synthetic grafts are being punctured the patient should be given prophylactic antibiotics, e.g. cefuroxime 750 mg IV.

Equipment

- Basic angiography set.
- 4Fr sheath.

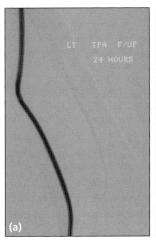 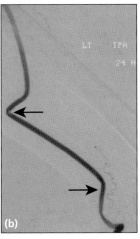

Fig. 11.5 ■ Following thrombolysis, lateral views with the knee straight (a) and flexed (b) reveal kinking (arrows) as the underlying problem.

Table 11.2 Access sites for graft angiography

Graft configuration	Angiography approach	Intervention approach	Tips
Axillofemoral	Radial or brachial*	Brachial for proximal lesions Graft or CFA for distal problems	
Aortofemoral	CFA or brachial*	CFA or brachial	
Iliofemoral crossover	Donor side CFA	Either CFA or graft	Angulation at origin, use Amplatz wire, Arrowflex sheath or guide-catheter
Femorofemoral crossover	Donor CFA	Either CFA or graft	Use ultrasound to avoid direct graft puncture at groin
Femoropopliteal/ distal	Antegrade CFA	Antegrade CFA for distal problem, retrograde for inflow	Cobra or RDC useful to access graft origin

* Consider MRA whenever there are no femoral pulses and it would be necessary to use the arm approach.

Procedure

Access Use Table 11.2 as a guideline.

Catheterization The majority of at-risk grafts will be infrainguinal, and antegrade puncture is usually required. Most grafts come off the CFA anteriorly. Steep ipsilateral anterior oblique views are useful to profile their origins and to guide selective catheterization (Fig. 11.6).

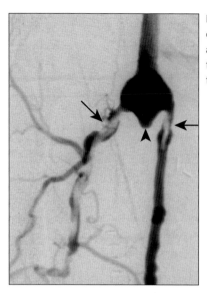

Fig. 11.6 ▨ Oblique view showing non-occlusive thrombus in the profunda femoris artery (black arrows) and origin of the femoropopliteal vein graft. The stump of the native SFA lies in between.

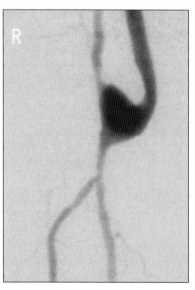

Fig. 11.7 ▨ Profile view of the distal cuff of a below-knee femoropopliteal vein graft. The popliteal artery is diffusely narrowed below the graft.

Runs A satisfactory angiogram must show the graft inflow and runoff, and include magnified views of the proximal and distal anastomoses in profile (Fig. 11.7). Magnified oblique views should be used to demonstrate stenoses. When imaging vein grafts, demonstration of contrast jetting as a result of valve cusps requires runs at 6 fps. These should be viewed with a wide contrast window (Fig. 11.8).

Tip: The Doppler is right! If the lesion cannot be identified at angiography, it should be marked under ultrasound guidance.

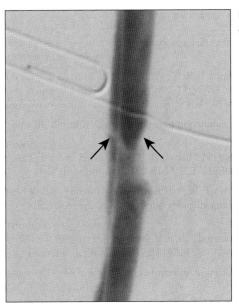

Fig. 11.8 ▦ Valve cusp (arrows) which was causing significant stenosis in a vein graft.

Troubleshooting

Difficulty inserting the sheath Remember the basics of vascular access. Insert plenty of wire, as it will often coil in the CFA. Heavy scarring at the puncture site is often a problem. Keep the guidewire taut and push and twist the catheter from close to the skin. Try a 4Fr dilator. A judiciously inserted Amplatz wire is often helpful.

Difficulty catheterizing the graft origin Remember to use a steep oblique projection; roadmap or fluoroscopy fade are invaluable for guidance. A shaped catheter, usually a Cobra or RDC, can be directed towards the graft origin.

Difficulty visualizing the graft origin Contrast in the CFA patch, the stump of the SFA or the PFA may obscure the graft origin. Position the catheter with its tip in the proximal graft; contrast can then be refluxed to show the graft origin. A frame rate of ≥2 fps is necessary. Laterally running grafts are best shown with the ipsilateral posterior oblique view.

UPPER LIMB ANGIOGRAPHY

Upper limb ischaemia represents only 4% of peripheral vascular disease and is not as frequently associated with generalized atherosclerosis as is lower limb ischaemia. Disease is usually focal, affecting the origins of the great vessels. In thoracic outlet syndrome (TOS), vascular compression by bone or ligament is associated with distal embolization, Raynaud's syndrome and subclavian aneurysm.

Arch aortography and selective catheterization of the great vessels carry a risk of stroke, so particular care must be taken during catheter and wire manipulation and catheter flushing.

Never flush a blocked catheter. Consider MRA for studies of the aortic arch and proximal great vessels.

Equipment

- Basic angiography set.
- Catheters: 90 cm 4Fr pigtail, Berenstein, Headhunter, Sidewinder.
- Guidewires: angled hydrophilic guidewire.
- GTN or other vasodilator.

Procedure

Access Diagnostic angiography is normally performed from the femoral approach. Therapeutic intervention is often easier from the brachial artery, or with combined femoral and brachial access.

Catheterization Use a pigtail catheter for arch aortography. A Berenstein catheter will engage the vast majority of arch vessels if used properly. Use a guidewire to advance the catheter tip beyond the target vessel. Withdraw the guidewire and rotate the catheter until the tip points cranially; the tip will flick into the vessel origin as it is withdrawn. More distal catheterization requires the catheter to be advanced over a guidewire.

Runs Begin with an arch aortogram to show the origins of the great vessels. Additional views may be needed to show the proximal subclavian arteries, particularly when they are tortuous. In suspected TOS, perform runs with the arms raised and also in the Roos position (elbow flexed 90°, shoulder abducted 90° and dorsiflexed). It is possible to see as far as the elbow from an arch injection. A selective catheter should be advanced peripherally to image the distal arm vessels. Use iso-osmolar contrast, or warn the patient that the contrast injection may be painful; this can be kept to a minimum by using half-strength contrast.

Tip: To obtain high-quality images of the digital arteries, place the hand on the image intensifier and immobilize it with a sandbag. Use a vasodilator to increase flow (Fig. 11.9).

Interpretation

Vascular compression during postural manoeuvres occurs in about 30% of normal subjects; subclavian artery irregularity or aneurysm is a more valuable sign of TOS (Fig. 11.10). Diffuse atheroma affecting the subclavian and axillary arteries is most commonly carried by radiotherapy. A proximal high-grade stenosis or occlusion may cause a subclavian steal. The reversed flow in the vertebral artery will only be seen on late images from the arch aortogram.

The radial and ulnar arteries may arise from the axillary or brachial arteries – failure to recognize this will lead to misinterpretation.

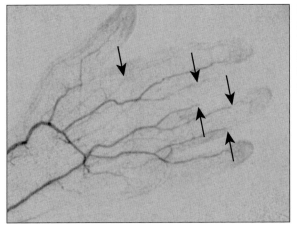

Fig. 11.9 ■ 'Blue digit syndrome': hand arteriogram following intra-arterial GTN. There are several digital artery occlusions (arrows) secondary to microemboli from a subclavian stenosis. The middle finger is particularly ischaemic.

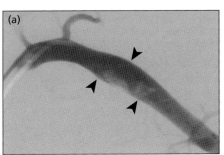
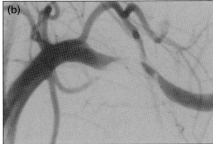

Fig. 11.10 ■ Thoracic outlet stenosis presenting with distal embolization. (a) There is a subclavian aneurysm containing thrombus (arrowheads). (b) Arm abduction results in marked compression of the subclavian artery.

Troubleshooting

Unable to catheterize an arch vessel

- Remember the basic rules: identify the target vessel on an overview.
- If the arch is unfolded, the Berenstein catheter may be difficult to control; try using a Headhunter 1 catheter, which has a wider primary curve.
- If the target vessel is angulated backwards, then a reverse-curve catheter such as a Sidewinder may be helpful.

Poor visualization of the distal vessels

- Use a vasodilator to increase flow, and also to discriminate spasm from irreversible fibrosis.
- Use iso-osmolar contrast and try increased contrast strength.

AORTIC ARCH AORTOGRAPHY

Arch aortography is performed in trauma patients with possible aortic rupture, and also as a preliminary stage of arm and carotid angiography to display the origins of the great vessels (Fig. 11.11). Aortic dissection is now almost always investigated by CT and MRI.

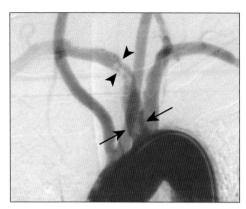

Fig. 11.11 ▦ 30° LAO projection showing an aberrant right subclavian artery origin (arrows). The patient presented with 'blue digit syndrome' secondary to emboli from the subclavian artery stenosis (arrowheads).

Table 11.3 Suggested runs for arch aortography

View	Contrast volume (mL)	Injection rate (mL/s)	Frame rate (fps)	Field size (cm)
LAO 30°, LAO 60° AP	40	18–25	2–4	28–40

Equipment

- Basic angiography set.
- Catheter: 90 cm 4Fr or 5Fr pigtail.

Procedure

Catheterization Position the pigtail catheter in the ascending aorta just above the aortic valve.

Runs 30° LAO to show aortic arch and origin of the great vessels (centre on the aortic arch). 60° LAO may be helpful in trauma cases (Table 11.3).

Interpretation

Look for irregularity in the lumen in the region of the ligamentum arteriosum, as this is the usual site of injury (Fig. 11.12). If there is evidence of dissection, demonstrate the origin of the dissection flap and the site of re-entry into the aortic lumen, and document visceral artery involvement.

Troubleshooting

The ductus bump can mimic aortic rupture. It appears as a smooth bulge at the site of the ligamentum arteriosum.

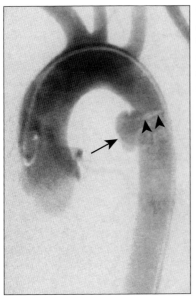

Fig. 11.12 ■ Aortic trauma: the chest X-ray showed upper rib fractures and mediastinal widening. Arch angiography shows a false aneurysm (black arrow) distal to the left subclavian artery and associated intimal irregularity (arrowheads).

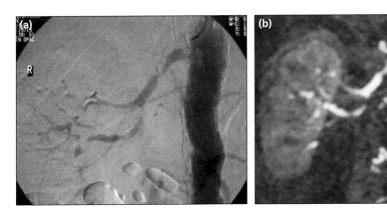

Fig. 11.13 ■ Multifocal renal artery stenosis. (a) DSA. (b) MRA. Note that the MRA does not demonstrate the calcification in the aorta and renal arteries.

RENAL ANGIOGRAPHY

Renal angiography is being replaced by magnetic resonance angiography (MRA). Angiography remains the 'gold standard' and is still required in case of doubt, or to demonstrate distal disease such as fibromuscular dysplasia (Fig 11.13). Renal angiography is most frequently requested to investigate renal artery stenosis (RAS). The occurrence is low in the general population, but up to 40% of patients with generalized vascular disease will have RAS, particularly those with renal impairment or hypertension.

The remainder of referrals are for trauma, tumour, pretransplant assessment, or rarely arteritis. This group of patients will often require selective catheterization.

Table 11.4 Typical parameters for renal angiography

Run	Field size (cm)	Catheter position	Contrast volume (mL)	Injection rate (mL/s)	Frame rate (FPS)
AP aortogram	40	L1	15–20	15	2
20° Oblique	28		15–20	15	2
Selective	28–20		10	5	2

 Tip: Remember, 15% of people will have accessory renal arteries; these may arise almost anywhere in the abdominal aorta or iliac arteries.

Equipment

- Basic angiography set.
- Flush aortogram: 4Fr pigtail catheter.
- Selective angiography: Cobra II, RDC, Sidewinder II.

Procedure

Access The right CFA is usual for diagnostic angiography; the contralateral CFA often provides better access for selective angiography and intervention, as the catheters tend to deflect towards the contralateral side of the aorta.

Catheterization Start with a flush arteriogram! This is good, safe practice; an aortic injection will answer most questions. Position the catheter at L1.

Runs See Table 11.4.

Selective catheterization should be avoided when there is RAS, as it increases the risk of thrombosis and embolization. Use selective renal angiography to resolve detailed intrarenal anatomy, or in rare instances when the renal artery origin cannot be seen in profile.

Flush aortogram Aim to show the origins of the renal arteries in profile (Fig. 11.14). The renal arteries arise at L1/2. On a clock face, the right renal artery typically arises from the aorta at 10 o'clock and the left renal artery at 3 o'clock. In theory, an LAO 15° projection should suffice. Unfortunately, this does not hold true in the diseased or aneurysmal aorta. In practice, other projections are frequently necessary. In these cases, rotational angiography is helpful if it is available.

Selective angiography A Cobra II or RDC catheter will usually select the renal artery and should be the first choice of catheter. Occasionally, a Sidewinder will be necessary to deal with an acutely angled artery. Hand-injection of 10 mL of contrast is usually satisfactory.

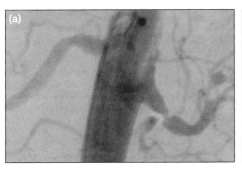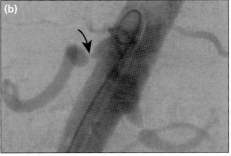

Fig. 11.14 ■ (a) The right renal artery appears normal on first run (RAO) but the origin is not seen. (b) The LAO view reveals a high-grade stenosis of the right renal artery. It is essential to obtain views of both renal artery ostia in profile. The same applies to MRA images.

Troubleshooting

Only one kidney seen
- Ensure the catheter is high enough.
- Fluoroscope to check for an ectopic kidney.
- Check late-phase angiogram for renal perfusion via collaterals.

Contrast in the superior mesenteric artery (SMA) obscures the right renal artery   If the catheter is too high, contrast fills the SMA. For subsequent runs, pull back the catheter and try alternative oblique tube positions.

Unable to profile the renal artery ostia   If all else fails, catheterize selectively.

RENAL TRANSPLANT ANGIOGRAPHY

In established transplants, chronic deterioration in function or hypertension may indicate RAS. In a recent transplant, angiography usually follows an abnormal MRA, Duplex or isotope scan. Acute graft failure occurs secondary to rejection, thrombosis of the artery or vein or, less commonly, a poorly fashioned anastomosis.

Equipment
- Basic angiography set.
- Catheters: 4Fr straight, RDC for selective angiography.
- Wires: 3 mm J, Terumo.

Procedure

Access   Ipsilateral CFA for diagnosis; the contralateral CFA is often better for intervention.

Table 11.5 Suggested runs for renal transplant angiography

Position	View	Contrast volume (mL)	Inject rate (mL/s)	Field size (cm)	Centring
Above renal artery	AP, multiple obliques	10–15	5	28–20	Over renal artery and kidney

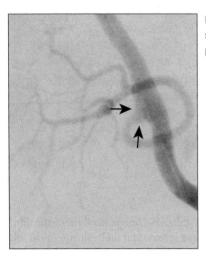

Fig. 11.15 ■ Cadaveric renal transplant showing typical appearance of the Carel patch (arrows).

Catheterization Contrast in the internal iliac artery or the contralateral iliac artery often obscures the transplant renal artery. To minimize this, use a hand-injection run to establish the position of the catheter just proximal to the transplant artery.

Runs A hand injection is mandatory for selective catheterization (Table 11.5).

Interpretation

In adults, cadaveric transplants are often taken with an aortic patch (Carel patch, Fig. 11.15) and anastomosed to the side of the EIA. Transplants from live related donors may be anastomosed to the internal iliac artery. In children, because of the small calibre of the iliac vessels, the graft is often anastomosed to the lower aorta. RAS occurs at the anastomosis, and focal smooth stenoses distal to this are often clamp injuries (Fig. 11.16). In transplant rejection there is pruning of the intrarenal vessels. If there is early venous filling look hard for a post-biopsy arteriovenous fistula.

Troubleshooting

The transplant artery is tortuous or overlapped by other vessels

- Craniocaudal tilt and rotational angiography may be necessary.
- If satisfactory views cannot be obtained, try selective catheterization. Contrast can be refluxed to show the anastomosis.
- Try a higher frame rate.

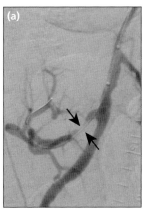 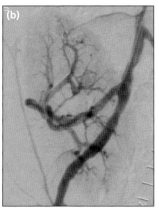

Fig. 11.16 ▨ (a) Transplant renal artery stenosis (arrows) distal to the anastomosis owing to a clamp injury during surgery. (b) Excellent result of angioplasty.

Can't get over the bifurcation
- Use a reverse-curve catheter, e.g. Sidewinder.
- A shaped sheath such as the Balkan can be invaluable for intervention.

HEPATIC ANGIOGRAPHY

Diagnostic angiography has largely been superseded in the assessment of hepatic malignancy by CT, MRI and ultrasound. Angiography is requested only when cross-sectional imaging suggests vascular involvement that would affect surgery, or when embolization is an option. Patients with haemobilia often have a focal bleeding source, usually secondary to percutaneous transhepatic cholangiography (PTC) or biopsy.

Equipment
- Basic angiography set.
- Catheters: Cobra II, Sidewinder II (hydrophilic Cobra catheter, microcatheter).
- Guidewires: 3 mm J, angled Terumo.

Procedure
Access Usually the right CFA.

Catheterization The coeliac axis arises anteriorly from the aorta at T12/L1. A Cobra catheter will be successful in most cases. Perform a diagnostic angiogram to ensure the arterial anatomy is conventional. Anatomical variants of the hepatic arterial supply are common (Fig. 11.17). Transplant vascular anatomy may be surprising: the transplant hepatic artery may be anastomosed to the recipient hepatic artery or via a conduit to the aorta or iliac artery. Check the operative notes before starting! Selective catheterization of the common hepatic artery and its branches may be required, particularly when assessing tumours or embolizing.

Runs Runs should be centred to include all of the liver, including the right hemidiaphragm and chest wall. Less contrast is required for distal selective angiograms. Magnified oblique views of the liver hilum are often required (Table 11.6).

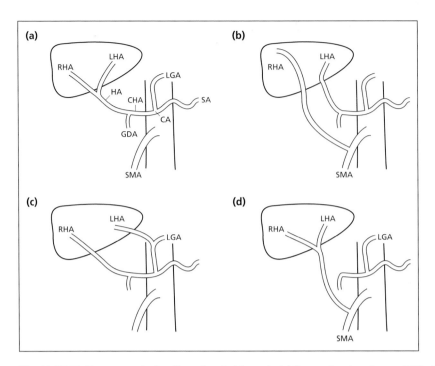

Fig. 11.17 ■ Common variants of hepatic arterial supply. (a) Conventional anatomy – 55%. (b) Replaced right hepatic artery (RHA) arises from the superior mesenteric artery (SMA) – 16%. (c) Replaced left hepatic artery (LHA) arises from the left gastric artery (LGA) – ~20%. (d) Replaced common hepatic artery (CHA) arising from the SMA – ~2%. CA, coeliac artery; GDA, gastroduodenal artery; HA, hepatic artery; SA, splenic artery.

Table 11.6	Typical parameters for hepatic angiography					
Catheter position	Contrast volume (mL)	Injection rate (mL/s)	Frame rate (FPS)	Field size (cm)	Projection	Run length (s)
Coeliac axis	32	8	2 → 1	40	AP	To portal vein = 20
Selective hepatic artery	5–15	Hand	2	20–28	AP and RAO 20°	=5
Splenic artery	20	5	2 → 1	40	AP	To portal vein = 20

 Tip: Catheters often pass preferentially into the splenic artery, which comes more anteriorly off the coeliac axis. A Terumo wire can usually be negotiated into the hepatic artery, and the catheter will follow it.

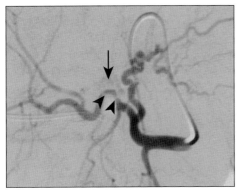

Fig. 11.18 ■ Encasement of the right hepatic artery by cholangiocarcinoma (arrowheads); there is minimal tumour blush (arrows).

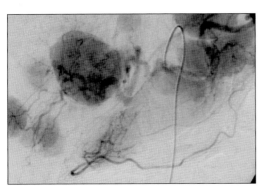

Fig. 11.19 ■ Carcinoid syndrome. Late arterial phase image from a coeliac axis injection showing multiple hypervascular liver metastases.

Interpretation

Most secondary liver tumours are hypovascular and angiographic signs are subtle. Mass effect displaces vessels; constant vessel irregularity or occlusion suggests arterial invasion (Fig. 11.18). Vascular tumours (e.g. hepatoma and carcinoid) show neovascularity and an abnormal parenchymal stain (Fig. 11.19). Arterial injury following PTC usually manifests as small pseudoaneurysms, which can almost always be selectively embolized.

Tip: The hepatic artery is prone to spasm when catheterized. Take care not to misdiagnose this as encasement.

Troubleshooting

Unable to pass a guidewire into the hepatic artery

- Check that the catheter tip is not in the splenic artery by gently injecting contrast and avoiding reflux.
- If the Cobra catheter is pushed out by the wire, try a reverse-curve catheter.

Unable to selectively catheterize the hepatic artery

- Put plenty of guidewire into a peripheral hepatic branch or the gastroduodenal artery.
- Keep the wire under tension while gently turning the catheter from side to side; only apply gentle forward pressure, and let the catheter find its own way in.
- Try a softer catheter, e.g. a hydrophilic Cobra.
- Try from the radial or brachial artery: the caudal angulation of the mesenteric vessels lends itself to this approach.
- If all else fails, dust off a 7Fr Sidewinder III – the superior torque control often helps.

MESENTERIC ANGIOGRAPHY

The production of satisfactory mesenteric angiograms is challenging, particularly in patients with acute gastrointestinal bleeding. The patient is often elderly, agitated, potentially haemodynamically unstable, and the study is performed out of hours by relatively inexperienced staff. Using a systematic approach to acquire and interpret the images will greatly increase the chances of success.

Equipment

Personal preference is important here!
- 5Fr sheath.
- Catheters: 4Fr pigtail catheter for flush aortography; Cobra II, RDC, Sidewinder, Sos Omni for selective catheterization.
- Hydrophilic guidewire.
- A hydrophilic catheter may be useful for distal catheterization.

Procedure

Access Right CFA is easiest.

Catheterization Start with the vessel of interest and perform an overview of each target arterial territory before proceeding to more selective angiography. It is generally held that in colonic bleeding the examination should start with the inferior mesenteric artery (IMA) to avoid bladder contrast obscuring the detail of the sigmoid arteries. However, do not spend all day trying to catheterize a tiny IMA; if difficult, move to the SMA first. Selective catheterization of the mesenteric vessels can be frustrating for even the most experienced angiographer. Start with the right tools.

A skilled angiographer will usually manage the whole study with a Sidewinder II; however, there are alternatives for the less coordinated. The IMA arises acutely from the anterolateral aspect of the distal aorta (Fig. 11.20). Perform a steep RAO angiogram of the distal aorta to show its origin. Catheterization is easiest with a short reverse-curve catheter such as the Sos Omni or Sidewinder I.

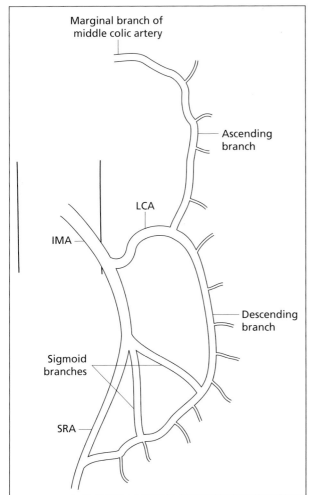

Fig. 11.20 ■ The inferior mesenteric artery (IMA). LCA, left colic artery; SRA, superior rectal artery.

Marginal branch of middle colic artery

Ascending branch

LCA

IMA

Descending branch

Sigmoid branches

SRA

The SMA can usually be catheterized with a Cobra II. It can be advanced distally over a hydrophilic wire for superselective views of the ileocolic and right colic arteries, which are the most common sites of bleeding (Fig. 11.21).

A Cobra II will often engage the coeliac axis (Fig. 11.22). If this fails, try a Sidewinder II.

The gastroduodenal artery is most easily catheterized with a forward-facing catheter such as the Cobra II or RDC.

For a virtuoso finish, the left gastric artery (LGA) can be catheterized using a Sidewinder II. The catheter is initially advanced into the splenic artery and then slowly pulled back until the tip flicks up and engages the LGA. In reality, this vessel is seldom catheterized unless there is a very strong clinical suspicion of gastric bleeding.

Runs Paralyse the intestine. If you cannot abolish peristalsis with buscopan or glucagon, there is little hope of success!

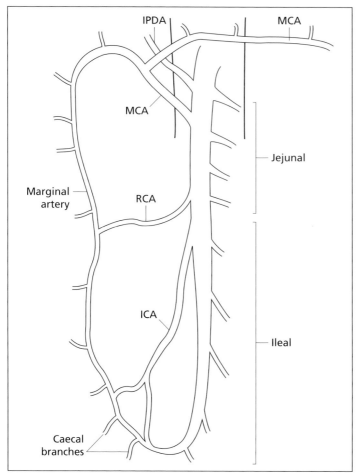

Fig. 11.21 ■ The principal branches of the superior mesenteric artery: ICA, ileocolic artery; IPDA, inferior pancreaticoduodenal artery; MCA, middle colic artery; RCA, right colic artery. The origin of the ICA marks the transition between jejunal and ileal branches.

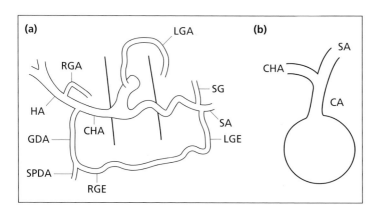

Fig. 11.22 ■ The coeliac artery (CA). (a) Principal arterial branches. (b) Cross-section showing why catheters and wires preferentially enter the splenic artery (SA). CHA, common hepatic artery; GDA, gastro-duodenal artery; HA, hepatic artery; LGA, left gastric artery; LGE, left gastroepiploic artery; RGA, right gastric artery; RGE, right gastroepiploic artery; SG, short gastric artery; SPDA, superior pancreaticoduodenal artery.

Table 11.7 Suggested runs for mesenteric angiography

Run	Field size (cm)	Centring	Contrast volume (mL)	Injection rate (mL/s)	Frame rate (fps)
SMA AP	40	Mid-abdomen	30	6	2 → 1
IMA AP	28	Rectosigmoid	10	Hand	2 → 1
IMA RAO 25°	28	Rectosigmoid	10	Hand	2 → 1
IMA LAO 30°	28	Ascending colon and splenic flexure	10	Hand	2 → 1
Coeliac axis	40	Epigastrium	30	6	2 → 1
Gastro-duodenal artery	28	Epigastrium	15	Hand	2
LGA	28	Epigastrium	8–10	Hand	2

Use breath-holding if the patient's condition permits. If not, wake the radiographer and try multimasking (Table 11.7).

Gastrointestinal bleeding – what to look for

A few conditions are responsible for the majority of cases of acute and chronic gastro-intestinal blood loss. Bleeding is usually intermittent and contrast extravasation is not frequently seen unless the patient is actively bleeding, i.e. haemodynamically unstable. In these cases, it is sometimes possible to identify the causative lesion on the angiogram.

The usual suspects

Angiodysplasia Almost universally suspected in the elderly but less frequently convincingly demonstrated. Angiodysplasia most often occurs in the caecum and ascending colon, though it can occur elsewhere, and is seen as a focal area of increased vascularity with dilated tiny arterioles with a prominent early draining vein (Fig. 11.23).

Diverticular disease Bleeding is often venous and therefore difficult to demonstrate. Inflamed diverticulae will give a patchy hyperaemic blush.

Meckel's diverticulum Bleeding rarely occurs in the absence of ectopic gastric mucosa, hence the diagnosis is usually made on technetium isotope scanning. The feeding vitelline artery characteristically extends beyond the mesenteric border, has no side branches, and ends in a corkscrew appearance (Fig. 11.24).

Tumour A rare cause of acute gastrointestinal bleeding. Angiographic signs of bowel tumours are often subtle. Examine the venous phase carefully – veins are larger and thinner walled than arteries, and are therefore involved earlier. Look for vascular displacement, encasement (constant narrowing – be careful not to misdiagnose spasm) and truncation (Fig. 11.25).

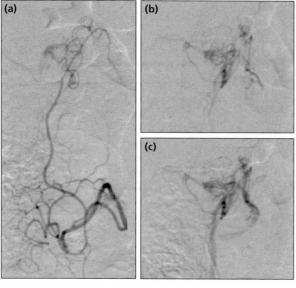

Fig. 11.23 ▪ Angiodysplasia in the ascending colon. (a) Early arterial phase shows a subtle blush. (b) Midarterial phase: note dilated arterioles and venous staining. (c) Late arterial phase – prominent draining veins.

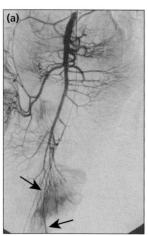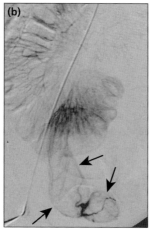

Fig. 11.24 ▪ Meckel's diverticulum. (a) The superior mesenteric artery run shows a vessel (arrows) extending beyond the mesentery; not all of the vessel is seen. (b) The subsequent run shows the typical blush (arrows) of a large Meckel's diverticulum; the vessel is the vitelline artery.

Interpretation

Examine the run frame by frame, looking carefully at the whole field. Take the time to remask each image. Review each phase of the angiogram looking for the following abnormalities:

1. **Arterial phase**
   - Active bleeding: extravasation appears as an irregularly shaped contrast stain (Fig. 11.26) that persists beyond the arterial phase of the angiogram. Is the bleeding from a named vessel? This will localize the site of bleeding and aid the surgeon.
   - Structural vascular abnormalities: look for arterial encasement, displacement or occlusion (Fig. 11.25).
   - Early venous return: the appearance of a vein in the arterial phase is abnormal and may indicate angiodysplasia (Fig. 11.23). The ileocolic vein often opacifies before other mesenteric veins in normal subjects.

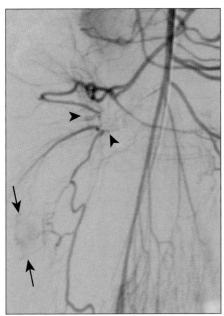

Fig. 11.25 Carcinoid tumour. There is a blush in the right iliac fossa (arrows). Invasion of the mesentery is demonstrated by occlusion of the ileocolic artery and distortion of the adjacent vessels (arrowheads).

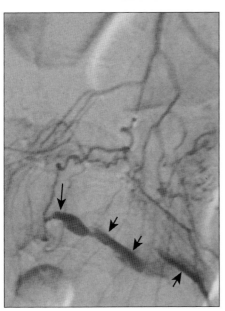

Fig. 11.26 Active bleeding from the inferior mesenteric artery; contrast is extravasating (arrows) into the sigmoid colon.

2. Capillary phase

- An area of increased capillary stain may indicate angiodysplasia or inflammatory or neoplastic involvement; look for supporting evidence. Beware: in the normal intestine the capillary phase may appear patchy, particularly in the large bowel.
- Remember, areas of overlapping bowel can simulate increased vascularity – be particularly careful in the sigmoid colon. If there is a genuine lesion, the abnormality will be seen on every view.

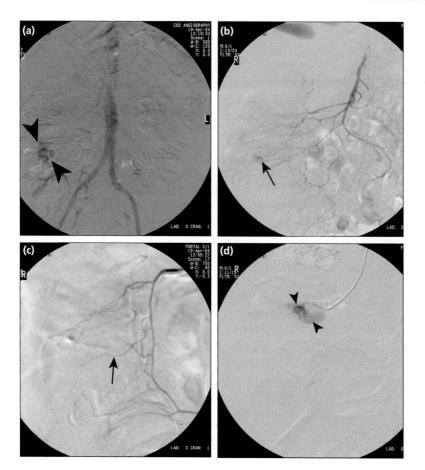

Fig. 11.27 ■ Intermittent GI bleeding. (a) Initial aortic run CO_2 angiogram showing extravasation in the caecum (arrowheads). (b) Selective SMA contrast angiogram the extravasation is just visible (arrow). (c) Highly selective run from the right colic artery. The bleeding has stopped (arrow = target artery). (d) Extravasation (arrowheads) is seen again immediately prior to embolization.

3. **Venous phase**
    *   Look carefully for evidence of venous invasion, occlusion or hypertrophied collateral veins, as these may be the first angiographic evidence of a tumour.
    *   Normal veins have a similar branching pattern to the arterial tree; tumour venous circulation is often chaotic and tortuous.

Acute gastrointestinal bleeding

A conundrum: GI bleeding is often intermittent (Fig. 11.27): the diagnostic yield is highest when the patient is bleeding. Balance the need for resuscitation against delay reducing the chance of locating the bleeding point. Make sure that there is someone from the clinical

Table 11.8 Likely sources of gastrointestinal bleeding

Blood loss	Likely source	Target vessel
Red blood PR	Left colon	IMA
	Right colon	SMA
Altered blood PR	Small intestine	SMA/Coeliac axis
Haematemesis/ malaena*	Oesophagus, stomach or duodenum	Coeliac axis SMA (pancreaticoduodenal arcade)

*The patient should have oesophagogastroduodenoscopy first.
PR, per rectum.

team available to manage the patient's haemodynamic status, as you will be concentrating too hard on the angiogram to do this.

Before starting:
- Ensure that the patient is adequately resuscitated, has large-calibre IV access, and that there is appropriate blood product and electrolyte replacement available.
- Target the angiogram to the suspected source of bleeding (Table 11.8).
- Check the plan of action for the patient. What will happen if the angiogram is positive or negative? Will embolization or laparotomy be appropriate? Has the patient given appropriate consent?

What to look for:
- Active bleeding
- Spasm
- Early venous filling
- Abnormal vessels.

If a bleeding site is identified:
- Inform the surgeon (ideally the surgeon will be watching from the control room).
- Embolize the bleeding vessel if it can be catheterized highly selectively – you will certainly need to be competent with microcatheters and coils. Non-selective embolization is likely to result in bowel infarction in the colon, and may not be effective in the small intestine because of collateral flow. Remember, the surgical alternative is likely to be quite extensive bowel resection, e.g. hemicolectomy.
- Small bowel lesions are harder to identify surgically; consider marking the area with coils or leaving a microcatheter in situ to permit injection of methylene blue in theatre.

 Tip: CO_2 may demonstrate the site of extravasation from a flush aortogram and will sometimes display bleeding that is not readily shown with conventional contrast (Fig. 11.27).

Troubleshooting

The commonest causes for failing to spot an identifiable lesion are due to poor imaging:

- Failure to get good subtracted images owing to peristalsis and respiratory artefact.
- Missing out part of the intestine.
- Failing to image through to the venous phase.
- Lack of understanding of the relevant pathologies.
- The patient has stopped bleeding: consider repeating the angiogram when bleeding is clinically apparent.

Chronic gastrointestinal bleeding

The patient's history may give important clues to the source of the bleeding. There are two forms of long-term blood loss:

- Repeated episodes of brisk bleeding are often associated with a structural lesion such as angiodysplasia. Herald symptoms, typically abdominal pain, are usually associated with heavy bleeding, e.g. from a pseudoaneurysm. These cases should be treated as repeated episodes of acute bleeding, and angiography performed during active bleeding.
- Chronic insidious blood loss. In these patients, a cause is less likely to be found. The patient will already have had multiple negative investigations, so do not expect to solve the problem in 5 minutes. Angiography should be performed as an elective procedure by the most experienced gastrointestinal angiographer available.

Tip: Do not perform angiography for insidious blood loss until you have the results from all previous investigations, including barium studies and endoscopy of the whole gastrointestinal tract!

In either case, catheterization of all three main visceral arteries and multiple selective views will be necessary. Even with excellent technique, no lesion will be found in 30–50% of patients!

Mesenteric ischaemia

Once again MRA is becoming the first-choice investigation. At least two of the visceral arteries will be diseased, and the SMA and coeliac axis are both almost always involved. Doppler ultrasound is a helpful screening test, as most lesions are ostial. Visceral angiography is still required to confirm the diagnosis and look for more distal disease.

Equipment

- Basic angiography set.
- 4Fr pigtail catheter.

Procedure

Access Right CFA.

Catheterization Begin with a pigtail catheter above the coeliac axis (T11/12).

Runs Start with a lateral flush aortogram. The visceral arteries arise anteriorly from the aorta. Contrast layers posteriorly in the aorta, so it is sometimes necessary to use a larger, faster contrast bolus (20–30 mL at 15–20 mL/s). Centre on L2/3 just anterior to the spine and use filters to eliminate flare caused by bowel gas. An additional AP flush aortogram is often all that is required to demonstrate the integrity of the distal SMA.

Tip: Mesenteric ischaemia should be suspected when a large marginal artery of Drummond is seen during peripheral angiography (Fig. 11.28).

Troubleshooting

A vessel is seen on the AP arteriogram but cannot be identified on the lateral aortogram This is usually due to proximal occlusion with reconstitution via collaterals. The coeliac axis and superior mesenteric artery often communicate via a hypertrophied pancreaticoduodenal arcade (Fig. 11.29): this may be confusing at first sight.

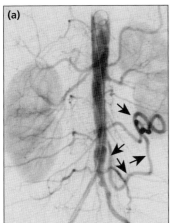
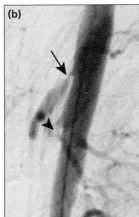

Fig. 11.28 ▪ Angiograms from a patient with 'intestinal angina'. The AP view (a) shows hypertrophy of the inferior mesenteric artery (IMA) (arrows). Branches of the superior mesenteric artery (SMA) are filling via the IMA. Lateral flush aortogram (b) showing high-grade stenosis of the coeliac axis (arrow) and occlusion of the SMA (arrowhead).

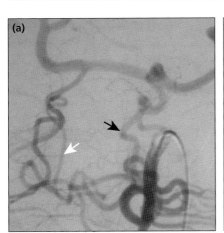
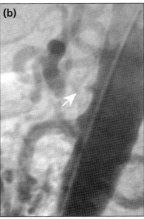

Fig. 11.29 ▪ (a) SMA injection showing filling of the coeliac axis via hypertrophied pancreaticoduodenal (white arrow) and pancreatic collaterals (black arrow). (b) Lateral flush aortogram showing occlusion of the coeliac axis (white arrow).

A smooth impression is seen on the superior aspect of the coeliac axis   This is the result of extrinsic compression by the median arcuate ligament of the diaphragm. The diagnosis is confirmed by showing a normal appearance on a lateral flush aortogram with the patient in the right lateral decubitus position. This finding is seen in 20% of asymptomatic patients. A few patients have severe compression of both coeliac axis and SMA, and are candidates for surgery.

 Tip: Selective catheterization is only required when distal disease is suspected on the flush angiogram.

ARTERIOPORTOGRAPHY

The portal vein can be assessed with ultrasound CT and MRI. Arterioportography is seldom required when these modalities are available, but it is the best method for assessing the anatomy of the portal and mesenteric venous systems, particularly in candidates for surgical portosystemic shunting (Fig. 11.30a). It still has a small role to play in the assessment of hepatobiliary tumours for resection (Fig. 11.30b).

Equipment

- Basic angiography set.
- Catheters: Cobra, Sidewinder (end- and sidehole).

Procedure

Access Right CFA.

Catheterization SMA and coeliac axis/splenic artery. Advance the catheter sufficiently far into the artery to avoid recoil and reflux of contrast out of the vessel.

Runs Runs are obtained to show the region of interest, which is usually the main portal vein and its branches. AP and RAO 20° views centred to the right hypochondrium are usually sufficient. It is frequently necessary to use multimasking, as runs are usually 20 seconds or longer. It is traditional to acquire the arterial phase of the run at 2 fps, so change to 1 fps for the portal venous phase.

 Tip: Every angiographer has been frustrated by the run terminating just as the portal vein starts to fill! Check that you are set up for a run of at least 40 seconds' duration.

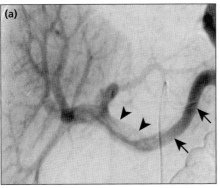
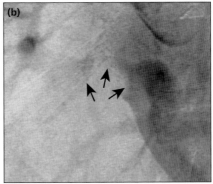

Fig. 11.30 ▦ (a) Normal arterioportogram from a selective splenic artery injection. Opacified blood returns via the splenic vein (arrows). Note the effect of unopacified blood returning from the superior mesenteric vein (arrowheads). (b) Tumour invasion of the right portal vein (arrows).

Troubleshooting

Poor opacification of the portal venous system   Try:
- Vasodilation – tolazoline 25 mg directly into the target vessel.
- Increasing the injection volume and rate.
- Increase contrast density by using 370 mg/mL contrast.

Your machine has too few megabytes for a 40 s run   Try imaging at 1 frame every other second, or introduce a delay between injection and imaging, even though this may compromise the mask images available.

PULMONARY ANGIOGRAPHY

Pulmonary angiography is used relatively infrequently in the UK. The principal indication is the diagnosis of pulmonary thromboembolism (Fig. 11.31), but the vast majority of patients are investigated with V/Q scanning or spiral CT. Pulmonary angiography tends to be used when the V/Q scan is indeterminate, or when an immediate diagnosis is essential secondary to cardiopulmonary collapse.

Equipment
- 5Fr sheath.
- 3 mm J guidewire.
- 5Fr 90–100 cm-long pigtail catheter.
- Terumo wire.
- ECG monitoring and pressure kit required.

Procedure

Do not puncture a grossly swollen leg – embolization of the underlying ileofemoral thrombus may cause embarrassment to both the patient and you. Stop and consider alternative access points, such as the other groin, the jugular vein or the basilic vein.

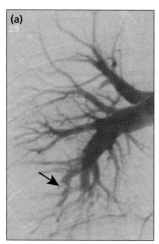
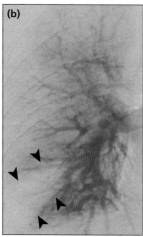

Fig. 11.31 ▪ Early and late arterial phase images from a pulmonary angiogram showing thrombus truncating a right lower lobe artery (arrow) and a wedge-shaped defect in the parenchymal enhancement (arrowheads).

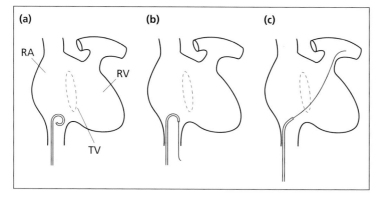

Fig. 11.32 ▪ Technique for pulmonary artery catheterization. (a) Pigtail and hydrophilic wire at the upper inferior vena cava. (b) Advance the guidewire, which opens the pigtail loop. (c) The wire usually goes through the tricuspid valve into the pulmonary artery. RA, right atrium; RV, right ventricle; TV, tricuspid valve.

1. Access can be from either the femoral vein or the basilic or jugular veins. Most practitioners use femoral venous access.
2. Obtain an IV cavogram. Use a hand injection of 20 mL non-ionic contrast via the side-arm of the sheath. Use buscopan or glucagon to paralyse the gut. If there are filling defects within the IVC, use an alternative access point from above.
3. Advance the 5Fr pigtail catheter over the J wire until the loop of the pigtail lies at the level of the suprarenal IVC.
4. Insert the Terumo wire into the pigtail catheter and advance (Fig. 11.32). The wire will progressively unfurl the pigtail until the wire points to about 1 o'clock, almost invariably straight at the pulmonary trunk. Advance the wire carefully across the tricuspid valve – get your assistant to watch the ECG – and the wire almost always goes into the left main pulmonary artery. Advance the catheter until it is in the left main pulmonary artery.

5. Measure the pulmonary artery pressures (see pressure measurements, p. 96):
   - systolic pulmonary artery pressure <50 mmHg, then angiography is safe.
   - systolic pulmonary artery pressure >50 mmHg, then pull the catheter back into the right ventricle.
   - measure the right ventricular pressures – if the right ventricular end-diastolic pressure (RVEDP) is greater than 20 mmHg, non-selective pulmonary angiography is dangerous.

   If this is your first pulmonary angiogram, now is a good time to shout very loudly for help. If you remain determined, selective pulmonary angiography with hand injections of contrast into areas identified by the V/Q scan may be very useful.

6. Give a test injection with 10 mL of contrast, and make sure the end of the pigtail catheter is not in a small pulmonary artery branch. Connect the catheter to a pump injector. Set the pump for 40 mL at 20 mL/s.

7. Assuming you are using DSA, ask for 6fps – the faster frame rate will help overcome misregistration secondary to cardiac motion. Start with an AP view.

8. Look carefully through the first run. If you have definitely identified an embolus, then you have finished the examination and may proceed to item 12.

9. Proceed to perform further runs in RAO 30° and LAO 30°.

10. Pulling the pigtail catheter back into the pulmonary trunk then gently advancing it, the Terumo guidewire enters the right pulmonary artery. The guidewire often loops into the right pulmonary artery; by gently manipulating the wire, a right lower lobe pulmonary artery can be entered with the wire. Make sure you advance the catheter well into the right main pulmonary artery at least as far as the hilum, as the catheter always tends to come back slightly when the wire is withdrawn.

11. Repeat the AP, LAO and RAO projections for the right lung.

12. Look through the standard projections. If there are any questionable areas, consider a repeat run, possibly magnified or in a different projection.

13. Before withdrawing the catheter, straighten out the pigtail with the Terumo wire. This prevents an unnecessary thoracotomy to retrieve a catheter firmly entangled in the chordae tendinae of the tricuspid valve.

Troubleshooting

Failure to catheterize the pulmonary artery   Bad luck! Did you really use the rules outlined earlier in the procedure section? Enlarged right ventricles can cause difficulty with the wire repeatedly entering the apex of the right ventricle. Carefully use a Headhunter or Berenstein catheter with a Terumo wire to manipulate into the pulmonary artery.

Pulsatile injection with poor peripheral pulmonary artery filling despite 40 mL at 20 mL/s   Check the PSI rate on the pump – fast injections require higher PSI. The catheter packaging will tell you the maximum rate for that catheter. Rarely 50 mL at 25 mL/s is required.

Breathless patient and poor DSA images   Ask the radiographer to get more mask images at the beginning of the run. It may be better to do a run at 2 fps with the patient breathing, or consider selective angiography of relevant areas from the V/Q scan.

Complications

Pulmonary angiography is a relatively safe procedure. Overall mortality rate is 0.2%.

- Cardiopulmonary collapse is the main cause of death. It usually occurs in patients with severe pulmonary hypertension and RVEDP >20 mmHg or right ventricular strain diagnosed echocardiographically.
- Right ventricle perforation 1% – usually no sequelae.
- Symptomatic persistent arrhythmia.

CAROTID ANGIOGRAPHY

Carotid and cerebral angiography are diagnostic tests that until recently were frequently used in the investigation of cerebrovascular disease. Advances in CT, MRI and ultrasound have now greatly reduced the indications for angiography. In most centres, carotid angiography is now reserved to assess those patients with carotid artery disease in whom ultrasound and MRI are discordant, or where MRA is contraindicated. Cerebral angiography is mainly performed as part of the investigation and treatment of aneurysmal disease and vascular malformations.

Equipment

- Basic angiography set.
- 5Fr sheath.
- Catheters: non-selective, 90° cm 4Fr pigtail; selective, personal preference is important; options include Berenstein, Headhunter, Sidewinder and Mani.
- Guidewires: 3 mm J and angled Terumo.

Procedure

Access Normally via the right CFA.

Catheterization In the presence of carotid disease there is an approximately 2% stroke risk associated with selective carotid angiography. The risk of cerebrovascular accident (CVA) is probably less for aortic arch injection, but image quality is reduced. It is best practice to avoid catheterizing the carotid and vertebral arteries unless absolutely necessary for the test. To minimize the risk of CVA, scrupulous angiographic technique and attention to catheter flushing are mandatory.

Arch aortogram Position a pigtail catheter in the ascending aorta just above the aortic root.

Carotid and vertebral artery catheterization The difficulty of this procedure depends on the curvature of the aortic arch and the presence of any disease within it. In general, it is easiest to start with an LAO 30° projection to 'open up the arch'. An arch aortogram may help to localize the vessel ostia. Choose the most suitable catheter for the configuration of the arch; remember the basic rules of catheter selection. The Berenstein catheter is forward facing and can be used for most arch vessels unless they are angled acutely retrogradely.

Table 11.9 Typical parameters for carotid angiography

Position	Runs	Contrast volume (mL)	Injection rate (mL/s)	Frame rate (fps)	Centring	Field size (cm)
Aortic arch	LAO 30°	30–40	15–20	2	Aortic root upwards	40–28
Carotid bifurcation	AP and lateral	10	Hand	2	Over carotid bifurcation (ant to C4)	28
Internal carotid extracranial	AP and lateral	10	Hand	2	Over ipsilateral carotid	28–40
Internal carotid intracranial	AP and lateral	10	Hand	2–1 for venous phase	Lateral skull and Townes view	28–40
Vertebral	AP and lateral	10	Hand	2–1 for venous phase	Intracranial – lateral skull and Townes view	28–40

In unfolded arches, or when the vessel is awkwardly angulated, use the Headhunter, Sidewinder or Mani catheters.

When selective catheterization is necessary to investigate carotid stenosis, position the catheter in the common carotid artery (CCA). For a vertebrobasilar problem, start with the catheter in the proximal subclavian artery to show vertebral origin. Then perform selective vertebral catheterization. Cerebral angiography requires selective internal carotid artery (ICA) catheterization.

Runs The runs performed depend on the clinical indication. Perform the minimum number of runs to achieve a diagnostic examination (Table 11.9). Additional runs may be required to demonstrate specific intracerebral vessels. These are beyond the scope of this book and may be found in textbooks of neuroradiology.

Interpretation

Stenoses should be measured accurately using calipers and analysed according to the NASCET or ECST study criteria, which form the basis for treatment (Fig. 11.33). Dissection of the carotid artery causes string-like narrowing (Fig. 11.34).

Flush catheters in the descending aorta whenever possible; that way, any emboli will not affect the cerebral circulation. Make sure that there are no air bubbles in the flush solution. Never flush a blocked catheter in the aortic arch!

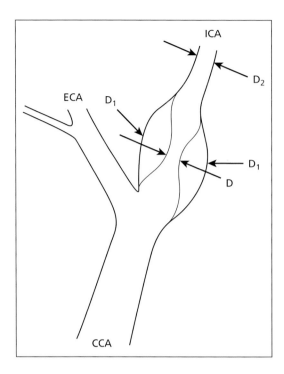

Fig. 11.33 ▦ NASCET and ECST criteria. Note that percentage stenosis varies with the method of measurement.

NASCET = $[1 - (D/D2)] \times 100\%$
ECST = $[1 - (D/D1)] \times 100\%$

(Note: D1 is estimated, as it is not seen on the angiogram.) CCA, common carotid artery; ECA, external carotid artery; ICA, internal carotid artery.

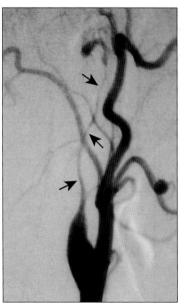

Fig. 11.34 ▦ Lateral view from a selective carotid angiogram. The internal carotid artery has a 'string-like' appearance (arrows) typical of dissection. (Image courtesy of Dr P Turner.)

Troubleshooting

Catheter 'jumps' around the aortic arch   This is usually a consequence of the catheter being held under tension in the aortic arch (Fig. 11.35). Turn the catheter to face appropriately and pull it back slowly, trying not to 'bridge' the catheter. Occasionally, it may be

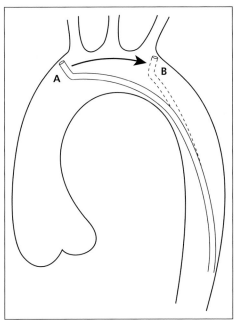

Fig. 11.35 ■ In position A, the catheter is under tension against the inner curve of the aortic arch. As it is withdrawn it suddenly springs, making controlled catheterization impossible.

necessary to use a larger-calibre catheter, particularly if initial attempts were with a 4Fr. A reverse-curve catheter such as the Sidewinder can be useful in this situation.

Unable to catheterize an arch vessel   Perform a run in the LAO 30° projection and use this to confirm the anatomy and exclude an origin stenosis. Choose an appropriately shaped catheter.

Unable to advance catheter into arch vessel   Once again, this is usually a consequence of the catheter being held under tension in the aortic arch. Try advancing more wire into the artery to increase stability, perform a run to establish the anatomy, and avoid passing the wire up the internal carotid artery. Make use of the subclavian and axillary arteries to get 'a good purchase'. It is rarely necessary to resort to using a larger catheter or a guide-catheter. If you are in trouble, pull the catheter back into the descending aorta and get help!

The external carotid artery superimposes on the internal carotid artery   This is fairly common on the AP projection. Try a 15° ipsilateral anterior oblique projection. Another common problem is for dental fillings to project over the ICA. This can also be solved by a suitable oblique projection.

CALIBRATED ANGIOGRAPHY

Calibrated angiography is usually performed as a prelude to stent-grafting. Accurate measurements of vessel diameters and lengths are required to choose the correct size graft. Modern CT angiography and MRA are replacing the need for calibrated angiography, but the same measurements are required (Fig. 11.36).

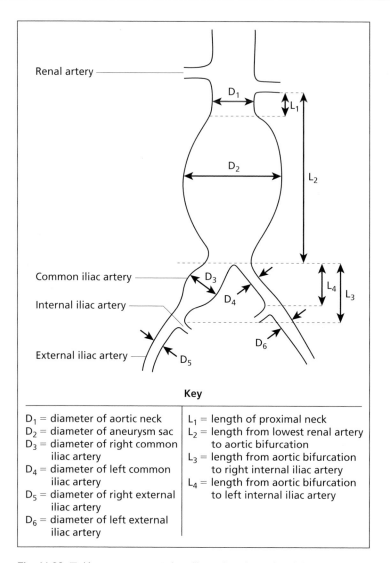

Fig. 11.36 ▪ Key measurements in calibrated angiography of abdominal aortic aneurysm.

Equipment

- Basic angiography set.
- Sheath: optional, but required if planning embolization of lumbar arteries or the IMA.
- Catheters: 5Fr calibrated pigtail catheter with 1cm markings over 15cm.
- Consider placing a radio-opaque ruler under the patient to the left of the spine.

Procedure

Access Choose the CFA from which the stent-graft procedure is planned.

Table 11.10 Suggested runs for calibrated angiography					
Position	**Runs**	**Contrast volume (mL)**	**Injection rate (mL/s)**	**Centring**	**Field size (cm)**
Aorta	AP and lateral	30	20	Coeliac axis – bifurcation	40–28
Iliac	AP, obliques and lateral	15	8	Aortic bifurcation – CFA	28

Runs Position the catheter so that the upper marker is at the level of the lowest renal artery. The calibration markings will probably just reach into the iliac artery. Perform AP and lateral runs in this position. Perform additional views as necessary to show incidental pathology, e.g. RAS (Table 11.10).

Pull the catheter back to the distal aorta. Image the iliac arteries. AP, both 25° obliques (and lateral projection if the vessels are tortuous). Finally image the femoral vessels to the knees.

Interpretation

Confirm patency of the coeliac axis and SMA. Look for accessory renal arteries and try to estimate how much of the kidney they supply, as these vessels may be covered by the stent-graft. Patent lumbar arteries and the IMA may require embolization. Look for any iliac artery stenoses and calcification which may impede passage of the stent-graft. Lengths and diameters should be measured as shown in Figure 11.36. Measurements can be made from the printed film using calipers or on the angiography system console. The stent-graft diameter should be approximately 10–20% greater than the luminal diameter.

TRAUMA ANGIOGRAPHY

Trauma includes a wide range of physical insults, from penetrating wounds to massive blunt injury. Angiography may be required in three circumstances:
* When there is clear evidence of a vascular injury – haemorrhage or ischaemia.
* When the mechanism of the trauma makes a vascular injury likely.
* When endovascular therapy is indicated – embolization or stent-grafting.

The most important consideration is the patient's condition. The patient must be adequately triaged by an experienced clinician. Do not waste time performing angiography when the patient needs emergency surgery. Major life-threatening injuries must be dealt with before attending to less severe problems. You cannot perform angiography and resuscitate the patient at the same time. Make sure that there is adequate clinical support to manage potentially unstable patients.

Once the decision to perform angiography has been made, establish the objectives of the study and discuss them with the referring clinician. Plan the study so that the important information is obtained as quickly as possible. Look at the major targets first and do not be distracted by minor abnormalities. You can always return to these later if they are relevant. You may be asked to 'Just look at … while you're here.' This is inappropriate unless it is of immediate clinical relevance.

We are principally concerned with the diagnosis and management of arterial injury, but do not forget that veins are thinner walled and more easily damaged than arteries. The angiographic signs of arterial injury are discussed below. The abnormality depends on the mechanism of injury, the severity of the injury, the general condition of the vessel and the condition of the patient. In essence, vessels are damaged either by penetrating injury or by stretching and tearing. The injury may affect the full thickness of the vessel wall or just one of the component layers.

Signs of vascular injury

Penetrating injury This is usually manifest by contrast extravasation or false aneurysm. Occasionally, there will be a significant adventitial and medial tear in the absence of intimal injury, and the result is an almost normal angiogram. Sometimes, bleeding will have stopped. Look out for spasm and the presence of vascular deviation caused by haematomas.

Blunt injury The mechanisms of injury are vascular compression and stretching. These actions can tear the intima, media or adventitia, and may lead to the formation of intramural haematomas. Minor injury causes spasm; more severe injuries are manifest as dissections of increasing severity, leading ultimately to occlusion (Fig. 11.37) or rupture. It is essential to demonstrate the distal runoff to allow planning of any surgical reconstruction. As smaller muscular arteries commonly go into spasm when injured, consider giving an antispasmodic drug to reveal the true condition of the underlying vessel.

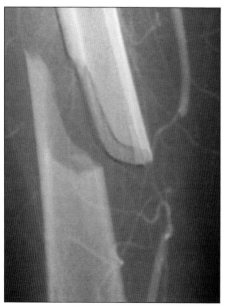

Fig. 11.37 ▥ Acute occlusion of the superficial femoral artery secondary to femoral fracture. At surgery there was extensive dissection causing the obstruction; the patient made an uneventful recovery after a short jump graft was inserted.

Blunt aortic injury   Aortic trauma is a life-threatening injury and the majority of patients with significant ascending aortic injury die at the scene of the accident. The aorta is injured either by direct compression and rupture (usually fatal), or because of shearing forces during injuries to the upper chest. Angiography or CT is requested for patients with signs of mediastinal haematoma on the chest X-ray. Spiral or multislice CT with 3D reconstruction and MRI give more information about other injuries and will rarely miss an aortic abnormality, and have largely replaced diagnostic angiography. In reality the choice depends on the local expertise and availability: remember that angiography is a simple procedure which will rapidly confirm or exclude a significant aortic injury (see Aortic arch angiography, p. 107). Whichever modality is chosen must allow stent-graft repair to be planned, as this is becoming the first-choice treatment option.

Hepatic and splenic injury   Blunt hepatic and splenic trauma is usually diagnosed on CT, and if intervention is required it will usually be surgical. Angiography is usually requested to investigate persistent postoperative bleeding. Start with a flush aortogram to ensure that there is no other obvious bleeding source and then perform selective hepatic and splenic arteriograms and portal vein studies. If an arterial bleeding source is identified, embolization is often the treatment of choice.

Renal injury   Renal trauma is usually diagnosed on CT, so angiography is not usually performed in the acute setting. Occasionally, angiography is necessary when there is persistent haematuria after blunt injury. Selective arterial embolization may allow treatment of a focal arterial injury without loss of the affected kidney.

Pelvic injury   Major pelvic fractures are invariably associated with massive blood loss, often from venous injury. Management is surgical; the fracture is stabilized and the pelvis may be operatively explored. Angiography is indicated if there is persistent bleeding which fails to settle after the fracture has been stabilized by external pelvic fixation. Bleeding can occur at any of the pelvic arteries, but the lateral sacral artery seems particularly prone to injury. These lesions can most often be readily treated by embolization.

Peripheral vascular injury   Blunt traumatic injury can occur as the result of direct trauma or dislocation, e.g. the popliteal artery. Angiography may demonstrate dissection, disruption or occlusion. Penetrating wounds, either manmade or fracture fragments, may cause acute bleeding, with extravasation or pseudoaneurysm formation. Selective embolization may be appropriate if the injured vessel is not vital.

SUGGESTIONS FOR FURTHER READING

Standards of Practice Committee, Society of Cardiovascular and Interventional Radiology. Standard for diagnostic arteriography in adults. J Vasc Intervent Radiol 1993;4:385–395.

Pressure gradients
McWilliams RG, Robertson I, Smye SW et al. Sources of error in intra-arterial pressure measurements across a stenosis. Eur J Endovasc Surg 1998;15:535–540.
Practical points about pressure measurements.

Tetteroo E, van Engelen AD, Spithoven JH et al. Stent placement after iliac angioplasty: comparison of hemodynamic and angiographic criteria. Radiology 1996;201:155–159.
A discussion of the criteria used in the Dutch iliac stent trial. Full of references for the enthusiast.

Renal
Wijesinghe LD, Scott DJA, Kessel D. Analysis of renal artery geometry may assist in the design of new stents for endovascular aortic aneurysm repair. Br J Surg 1997;84:797–799.
The position of renal arteries as demonstrated in a cadaver study.

Mesenteric
Bakal CW, Sprayregen S, Wolf EI. Radiology in intestinal ischaemia: angiographic diagnosis and management. Surg Clin North Am 1992;72:125–139.
Rollins ES, Picus D, Hicks ME et al. Angiography is useful in detecting the source of chronic gastro-intestinal bleeding of obscure origin. AJR 1991;156:385–388.
Confirms that the best angiography will reveal a source of bleeding in about 50% of cases. Some required repeat angiography.

Rosen RJ, Sanchez G. Angiographic diagnosis and management of gastrointestinal hemorrhage. Radiol Clin North Am 1994;32:951–967.
Whitaker SC, Gregson RHS. The role of angiography in the investigation of acute or chronic gastro-intestinal haemorrhage. Clin Radiol 1993;47:382–388.
A good pictorial review.

Hepatic
Soulen MC. Angiographic evaluation of focal liver masses. Semin Roentgenol 1995;30:362–374.
A beautiful pictorial review.

Pulmonary
Grollman JH. Pulmonary arteriography. Cardiovasc Intervent Radiol 1992;15:166–170.
Knows so much about the subject they named a catheter after him! Describes the use of angled pigtail catheters.

Hudson ER, Smith TP, McDermott VG, et al. Pulmonary angiography performed with iopamidol: complications in 1434 patients. Radiology 1996;198:61–65.

Carotid angiography
Fox AJ. How to measure carotid stenosis. Radiology 1993;186:316–318.

Calibrated angiography
Thurnhur SA, Dorffner R, Thurnher MM et al. Evaluation of abdominal aortic aneurysm for stent graft placement: Comparison of gadolinium enhanced MR angiography versus helical CT angiography and digital subtraction angiography. Radiology 1997;205:341–352.
Describes the techniques for imaging of AAA and demonstrates the measurements required.

Trauma
Pais OS. Diagnostic and therapeutic angiography in the trauma patient. Semin Roentgenol 1992;27:211–232.
White CS, Mirvis SE. Imaging of traumatic aortic injury (pictorial review). Clin Radiol 1995;50:281–287.
How to recognize aortic trauma on plain film, cross-sectional imaging and angiography.

Chapter Twelve

Angioplasty and stenting

Angioplasty and stenting are cornerstone techniques in interventional radiology and have widespread applications, both vascular and non-vascular. The key skills and equipment choices remain largely the same regardless of the site.

Basic principles

Atherosclerotic plaque is incompressible. Concentric plaque splits during balloon angioplasty and the intima and media stretch and tear (Fig. 12.1). When there is eccentric plaque, the tears occur at the interface between the plaque and the adjacent normal artery (Fig. 12.2). This often causes deep clefts and occasionally results in distal embolization of the plaque. Balloon dilation stimulates nerve fibres in the adventitia, causing discomfort. Severe pain usually indicates that the vessel is being excessively dilated and at risk of rupture. Luminal gain occurs because progressive dilation irreversibly stretches the adventitia. Over a period of weeks, the damaged intima undergoes a period of 'remodelling'. This involves neointimal hyperplasia, which restores the smooth intimal surface.

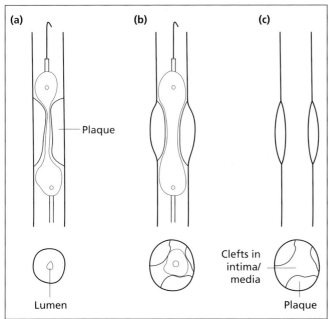

Fig. 12.1 ■ Angioplasty of concentric plaque. (a) Balloon 'waisting' in stenosis before plaque rupture. (b) Balloon dilation – the plaque is ruptured but the plaque volume unchanged. (c) Balloon deflation – the luminal area is increased because of stretching of the media/adventitia and intimal clefts.

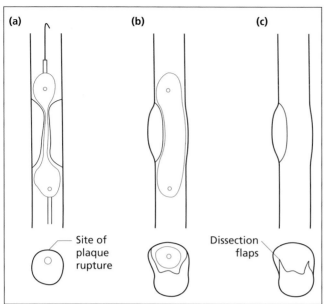

Fig. 12.2 ■ Angioplasty of eccentric plaques. (a) Balloon 'waisting' in stenosis before plaque rupture. (b) Plaque has ruptured at its thinnest point – eccentric media/adventitia stretching. (c) Postangioplasty dissection flaps in eccentric lumen. Plaque volume is unchanged.

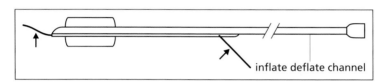

Fig. 12.3 ■ Schematic view of a monorail angioplasty balloon. The guidewire (arrows) enters the catheter at the tip and exits after about 15 cm. The remainder of the catheter shaft is the inflate/deflate channel (chevron).

Equipment

Over the years changes in materials have led to a decrease in both the size of the catheter shaft and the physical bulk of the angioplasty balloon. This allows angioplasty to be performed through smaller sheaths. Low-profile balloons up to 6 mm in diameter will pass through a 4Fr sheath. The balloons will cross virtually any lesion and will sometimes pass through stenoses and occlusions that cannot be traversed by a 4Fr catheter.

Monorail ('rapid exchange') systems are typified by cardiology angioplasty balloons and stents. In a monorail system the guidewire channel does not run the length of the catheter: instead, it exits after about 15 cm (Fig. 12.3). This allows the use of shorter guidewires and can improve control. Remember, you will need a guide-catheter or sheath to perform angiography, as the catheter does not have a lumen. In practice they are most useful for specialist applications such as carotid angioplasty and stenting. Monorail systems simplify the introduction and withdrawal of the catheter, as the wire is controlled very close to the sheath. To remove a monorail system the guidewire is fixed; the catheter can then be pulled back until it stops at the point at which the wire channel exits. After this the last portion is handled in the same way as normal.

Angioplasty catheters are available in a range of diameters, from 2 mm to over 25 mm, and in lengths from 60 to 120 cm. Variations in balloon materials, coatings and catheter

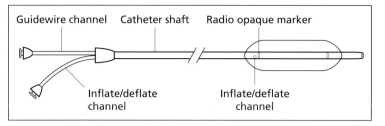

Fig. 12.4 Typical angioplasty balloon construction. Note the balloon length refers to the distance between the markers, over which the balloon is of its rated diameter. The catheter shaft comprises the guidewire lumen and the inflation channel. Smaller shaft sizes can be achieved with thinner materials and smaller inflate/deflate channels.

construction give a range of catheters, from everyday workhorses (Fig. 12.4) for SFA angioplasty to thoroughbreds which are capable of negotiating the most tortuous circulation. Some balloons even have razor blades in their walls. In day-to-day practice, balloon choice is dictated by a few simple concepts.

Balloon diameter The diameter of the arterial segment immediately adjacent to the lesion should be measured on the pretreatment angiogram. Always be careful to avoid measuring an area of poststenotic dilation. In practice, most operators use an approximate guide:

- Aorta   10–15 mm
- Common iliac   8 mm
- External iliac   7 mm
- CFA, proximal SFA   6 mm
- Distal SFA   5 mm
- Popliteal   4 mm
- Crural   2–3 mm.

Scale the balloon size up or down to suit the patient, e.g. a small elderly woman is likely to have smaller vessels than a large, muscular man.

Balloon lengths To minimize intimal damage to the adjacent vessel wall, choose the shortest balloon length that allows treatment of the diseased segment. An exception to this principle is when a short balloon cannot be held in a stable position during inflation. This phenomenon is akin to what happens when you pinch a lemon pip between your fingers and it shoots out. In these circumstances a longer balloon will add stability.

Tip: To minimize balloon migration ask your assistant to inflate the balloon while you hold the catheter and wire to maintain the balloon in the correct position. This is an active process performed under fluoroscopic control.

Shaft lengths The shaft length of an angioplasty balloon is always longer than the 'working' length. The presence of the side-arm for balloon inflation means the balloon cannot be inserted up to the hub. The bulk of work in the iliac or femoral circulation can be reached with a 75 cm balloon shaft. For other sites and approaches, consider the lengths of both the

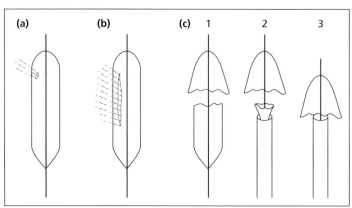

Fig. 12.5 ■ Burst angioplasty balloons. (a) 'Pinhole' tear: common and of no significance. (b) 'Longitudinal' tear: rare and seldom a problem. (c) 'Circumferential' tear: very rare but serious, as balloon will impact in sheath when it is withdrawn.

balloon catheter and the guidewire you will need. Remember to ensure that the guidewire is long enough to allow catheter exchange.

Sheaths Always use angioplasty balloons through a sheath; the balloon profile is lovely when it goes in, but even the best balloon has 'wings' when deflated that will cause an irregular arteriotomy on removal. The manufacturer records the appropriate sheath size on the balloon packet, so it is always worth checking. The sheath size will always be larger than the shaft diameter, so as to accommodate the balloon flaps. It may be possible to squeeze a virgin balloon through a smaller sheath, but it will be a devil to remove through the same sheath later.

Under pressure A consequence of the wide variety of balloon materials available is that balloons vary in their compliance. A balloon rated as 6 mm will be 6 mm at the recommended inflation pressure (another piece of information on that discarded packet); if the pressure is increased, a compliant balloon will progressively expand. The majority of modern balloons have a limited compliance range, but occasionally, particularly with the latex balloons provided with stent-grafts, compliance can be a problem.

Angioplasty balloons have a maximum-rated inflation pressure. If this is not exceeded, the manufacturer has 95% confidence that 99.9% of their balloons will not burst. Balloons may rupture in stents and very tight calcified stenoses. As the balloon is designed to tear longitudinally, this rarely has any significant sequelae (Fig. 12.5). Less than 1% of balloons will tear circumferentially (Fig. 12.6). This does pose a problem during withdrawal through the sheath, akin to backing through a doorway with an open umbrella!

Inflation The only way to be certain a balloon is being used at the correct pressure is to use an inflation handle with a pressure gauge (Fig. 12.7). The syringe barrel in this device has a thread and the syringe plunger is screwed into the barrel with a progressive and controlled increase in balloon pressure.

Use approximately one-third strength contrast to inflate the balloon. Manual inflation using a standard syringe was favoured by the founding fathers of intervention, but even the strong will find it impossible to exert a sustained pressure. In addition, it hurts the delicate skilled hand and may result in a hernia. Certainly for small vessel balloons and for lesions likely to require prolonged or high-pressure inflation, an inflation handle and gauge are recommended.

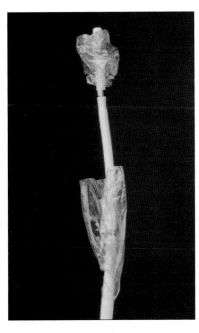

Fig. 12.6 ■ Example of a circumferential balloon tear; the distal balloon has crumpled up as it was pulled into an 8Fr reinforced sheath.

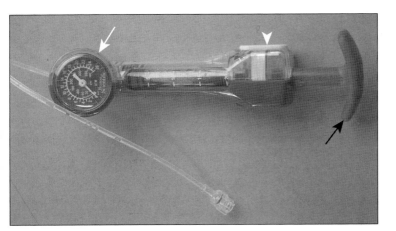

Fig. 12.7 ■ Inflation handle. The balloon is inflated by screwing the handle (black arrow) clockwise until the gauge (white arrow) shows the appropriate pressure. Pressing the button (arrowhead) releases the screw thread. The handle can then be pulled back to deflate the balloon. Further aspiration with an empty 20 mL syringe may be needed to empty the balloon completely.

The dilating force is related to the diameter of the balloon; therefore, for the same pressure a larger balloon will apply a greater force on the vessel wall. In practice, 3 mm balloons are often inflated to 12 atm, whereas 15 mm balloons only require a pressure of 4–6 atm.

Fluoroscope during balloon inflation – check the balloon remains in position and that it has completely 'de-waisted'.

The duration of inflation varies from operator to operator and between lesions:
- For a stenosis, inflate for 1 min.
- For an occlusion, allow 2–3 min.
- For a dissection flap, 3–5 min at low pressure.

Deflation   Contrast is viscous and can be slow to aspirate from the balloon – the inflation handle will not always deflate the balloon completely. Before removal, aspirate the balloon as completely as possible using an empty 20 mL syringe. Clockwise rotation of the balloon during withdrawal will help wrap the wings on to the catheter shaft and reduce the profile. If the balloon is reluctant to come out of the sheath, STOP. Do not impact the balloon, as it will cause the sheath to concertina. Try to aspirate the balloon again, if necessary with a 50 mL syringe, and confirm on fluoroscopy that the balloon is deflated. Very rarely a balloon will not deflate. Do not panic, but simply puncture the balloon with a Chiba needle.

Procedure

There are four stages to angioplasty and stenting:
- Vascular access
- Crossing the lesion
- Dilating the lesion
- Completion angiography.

Vascular access   As always, plan the procedure before starting. Use the preintervention angiogram to determine the best point of access; a good rule is to use the shortest, straightest route possible. The fewer curves the angioplasty balloon has to negotiate, the better.

Crossing the lesion   Angioplasty can be used to treat either stenoses or occlusions.

A stenosis must narrow the lumen by 50% before it becomes haemodynamically significant; a 50% diameter reduction results in a 75% reduction in the luminal cross-sectional area. Even the tightest stenosis can be negotiated with patience, a little skill and the right tools. Simple stenoses are readily negotiated with a guidewire alone: either a curved hydrophilic wire or a Bentson (Fig. 12.8).

More complex stenoses can be a challenge, and the key is to steer through the narrow segment using a shaped catheter and a curved hydrophilic wire. A pin-vice is invaluable to turn the wire in the correct direction. Take your time and never use force. If the wire starts to buckle, there is a good chance it will cause a dissection. If the wire starts to spiral down the artery, it is dissecting (Fig. 12.9)! Hydrophilic wires are great for crossing the lesion and equally easy to pull out; exchanging for a conventional wire after negotiating the lesion is infinitely safer. To exchange the wire, pass a catheter through the lesion, inject contrast to confirm intraluminal position, and then put in a suitable wire such as a 3 mm J wire.

 Tip: Use a pin-vice to help steer the hydrophilic wire. If you have not got one, then dry the wire to allow you to grip it. Be careful! A dry wire will stick to your gloves and is easily pulled out!

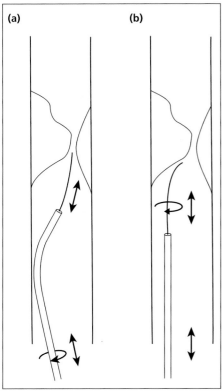

(a) (b)

Fig. 12.8 ■ Crossing a stenosis. Obtain a decent angiogram to use as a 'route map'. Use fluoroscopy fade or roadmap if available. (a) Straight wire and curved catheter. Turn the catheter to direct the wire through the stenosis. (b) Angled hydrophilic wire and straight catheter. Turn the wire, giving it space to rotate outside the catheter.

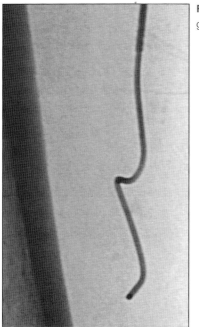

Fig. 12.9 ■ Typical spiral appearance of a guidewire that is dissecting.

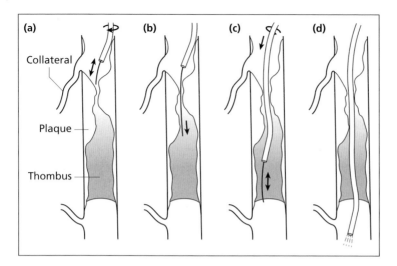

Fig. 12.10 ■ Crossing an occlusion. Occlusions occur where there is thrombus at the site of a stenosis. The thrombus propagates to the next collateral. (a) Gently probe the 'apex' of the occlusion with a straight wire using a curved catheter to steer. (b) Typically the wire will enter the thrombosed lumen with a slight give in resistance. (c) Advance the catheter into the occlusion to support and steer the wire through. (d) Perform an angiogram to confirm intraluminal position.

Crossing **occlusions** is more complex and requires a little more patience. It is vital to obtain a high-quality angiogram at the start. Look at the shape of the vessel at the point of occlusion. The artery often tapers to a point – this is your target. Start with a straight wire and use a Cobra catheter to direct it to the apex of the occlusion (Fig. 12.10). The wire will often pass straight through the occlusion with minimal resistance. If there is no obvious point to enter the occlusion, gently probe it with a straight wire using a shaped catheter to direct it. Once the wire enters the occlusion, proceed as above.

When the guidewire has crossed the lesion, treat it with care and respect; keep a wire across the lesion until the end of the procedure. This will allow rescue if the wheels come off. Always take the opportunity to perform an angiogram to prove you are in the target vessel. It is possible to be fooled by a wire position in a small collateral vessel behind the target vessel, with disastrous results. The choice of support wire depends on the anatomy, but as a rule, the more curves to negotiate, the stiffer the wire required, e.g. for a standard SFA a 3 mm J wire is fine, but for a tortuous iliac segment an Amplatz wire may be necessary. J wires are the safest support wires as the end of the wire inevitably moves during catheter exchanges.

Make sure that the tip of the wire is always visible to avoid damaging the distal vessels!

After crossing the lesion, give a bolus of heparin, usually 3000–5000 units.

Dilating the lesion   There are a variety of different techniques used to mark the area for angioplasty:

- If you are lucky, there is an obvious bony landmark at the site of the lesion, although this is rarely the case in the SFA.
- Inject contrast during fluoroscopy and position sponge forceps to mark the stenosis; either apply a metallic marker to the thigh or use a chinagraph pencil to mark the

position on the screen. Confirm this is in the correct position with another angiogram. Do not move the table after marking.

- On modern X-ray machines, use the roadmap or fluoroscopy fade facility to position the balloon. Roadmaps need a cooperative patient and operator, and it is essential that no movement occurs.

Use an appropriate balloon size for the target vessel. The balloon length may be shorter than the target length, and overlapping dilations will be necessary. It does not really matter whether this is started proximally or distally.

Completion angiography   Post angioplasty remove the balloon catheter, but remember you haven't finished yet. Always leave the wire through the lesion in case a bail-out procedure is necessary (remember how long it took you to cross the lesion in the first place!). A completion angiogram should be performed to assess the treated segment and the distal runoff. Look for:

- **Residual stenosis**: less than 30% residual stenosis is the aim.
- **Dissection flaps**: most angioplasty sites will have a minor dissection, which appears as a small linear defect; this will heal in time. Occasionally, the intimal–medial interface has been very disrupted and a flap extends into the lumen that reduces flow distally.
- **Venous filling**: venous opacification sometimes occurs, extending from the angioplasty site into the adjacent vein. This is rarely of any consequence and can safely be left alone.
- **Runoff**: final angiograms must include the circulation distal to the angioplasty site. Compare with the preintervention angiogram, looking particularly for distal embolization.

Never inject with an endhole-only catheter adjacent to an angioplasty site. There is a significant risk of lifting an intimal flap and causing vessel occlusion.

Subintimal angioplasty is a technique best avoided in the early stages of an interventional career. It would more appropriately be called extraluminal angioplasty, or even 'who knows where you are angioplasty'. It is likely that many occlusions are traversed extraluminally without the operator knowing. In an occlusion it is difficult to know what plane you are in within the artery wall. There are two distinct strategies to extraluminal angioplasty.

Most commonly an attempt is made to traverse the occlusion in the standard way, but the guidewire does not make progress. If this happens, reach for your friend the Terumo wire and advance it until it forms a loop beyond the catheter tip (Fig. 12.11). If the loop can now be advanced with relatively little resistance, this is fine. Only go as far as the point where the artery reforms. Now comes the clever bit, re-entering the true lumen of the vessel! Frequently the wire drops spontaneously straight back in; if not, this can take a considerable time using a shaped catheter and wire.

The alternative is to deliberately enter the vessel wall above the occlusion. You will usually need a straight wire and a shaped catheter such as the Berenstein to do this. Sometimes it is necessary to use the 'wrong end' of the wire: to manage this use great care, as the alternative is transmural angioplasty! Extraluminal position can be confirmed by injecting a small amount of contrast into the wall. Once this has been achieved a hydrophilic wire is advanced in a loop as above.

The outcome of extraluminal angioplasty is akin to the false lumen in an aortic dissection. The channel communicates with the true lumen via tears at the entry and re-entry sites.

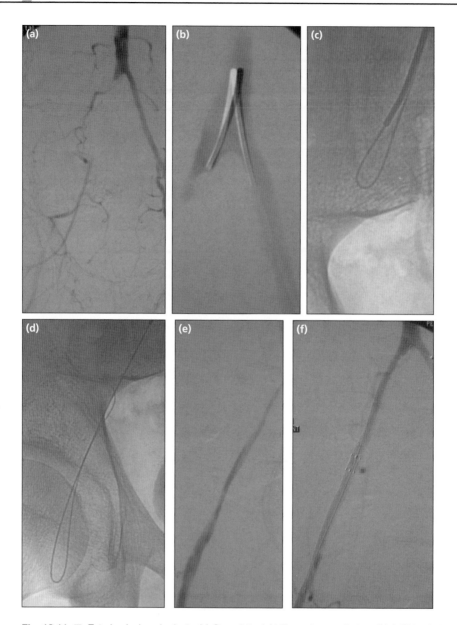

Fig. 12.11 ▪ Extraluminal angioplasty. (a) Complete right iliac artery occlusion. (b) A Sidewinder catheter is used to engage the origin of the CIA. (c) A loop has been formed in a hydrophilic wire and is advanced through the occlusion. (d) The loop has re-entered the arterial lumen in the CFA. (e) Injection around a 0.018 inch guidewire shows the extraluminal tract. (f) Completion angiogram following stenting.

There are a few caveats to 'extraluminal angioplasty':

- 'Extraluminal angioplasty' is seldom successful in heavily calcified vessels.
- Closely observe the diameter of the guidewire loop. If it starts to exceed the expected vessel diameter you are at best 'subadventitial' and will not succeed. STOP: you can always try again another day!

- Don't propagate the false lumen far beyond the point at which the vessel reconstitutes, as you will only occlude it.
- Consider using a stiff/supportive guidewire such as the stiff Terumo to help the catheter overcome friction when it is advanced.
- Consider using a low-profile angioplasty balloon catheter. They are excellent for dilating the lesion and can also be used to cross the lesion when a conventional catheter has failed.

Supporters of the extraluminal approach claim better long-term patency rates, particularly for long segment disease, because of the smooth subintimal lining. The downside of the technique is that it can be very difficult to re-enter; there is a higher incidence of vessel perforation and collaterals are occluded – important if the subintimal tract fails.

Angioplasty consent The main issues to be considered during consent are:
- **The 3Bs of arterial access**: bruising , bleeding and blockage at the puncture site.
- **Generic angioplasty related**: vessel occlusion, rupture or dissection usually fixed by stent or stent-graft, distal embolization 1–4% (often of no clinical importance). About 1% of patients will require surgery.
- **Site specific**: obviously emboli to the brain or the kidney are going to be much more important.

Troubleshooting

Unable to cross the lesion despite exhaustive efforts   Stop! In most situations it is possible to come back on another day, and sometimes the lesion seems effortless on the second attempt. Consider whether it might be possible to cross it coming from the other side, e.g. with a popliteal puncture.

A guidewire perforation occurs   This is likely to settle spontaneously. Simply pull back and repeat the angiogram after waiting for a couple of minutes to ensure there is not persistent extravasation (Fig. 12.12).

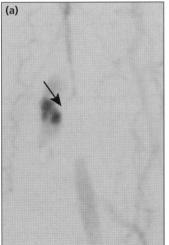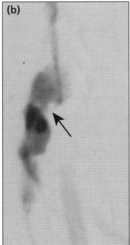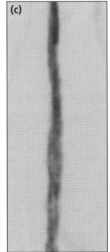

Fig. 12.12 ▢ (a and b) Guidewire perforation of the superior femoral artery. (c) The extravasation resolved following satisfactory angioplasty.

The wire crosses the lesion but the catheter will not follow This is particularly likely in heavily calcified lesions. Hold the guidewire as taut as possible and try to push and rotate the catheter through the stenosis. If this fails, use the lowest-profile catheter available; a tapered Van Andel catheter is ideal. Rarely it may be necessary to cross the lesion with a 0.018 inch guidewire; a low-profile angioplasty balloon can be used to predilate the lesion to 3 mm.

A dissection flap is seen post angioplasty Most sites show angiographic evidence of dissection after angioplasty. A dissection is only significant if it impedes distal flow; in the iliac segment, this can be assessed with pressure measurements. If a flow-limiting dissection is present:

- First try a low-pressure balloon inflation for 3–5 minutes across the dissection flap. This often 'tacks' the flap back into position.
- Persistent dissections can be readily treated by stenting across the flap.

There is a greater than 30% residual stenosis Residual stenosis can occur because the lesion has been underdilated or secondary to elastic recoil.

- Measure the adjacent target artery and repeat the inflation with a balloon 1 mm larger than this vessel.
- If possible, measure the pressure gradient across the lesion. If no gradient is present, stop.
- Many stenoses will remodel after angioplasty, and if there is a 30–50% residual stenosis in a non-critical vessel it may be appropriate to leave it.
- If elastic recoil occurs (the angioplasty balloon expands completely, but the lesion recoils on deflation), then arterial stenting is indicated. Do not stent lesions that it has not been possible to 'de-waist' during angioplasty, as you will simply line a stenosis with a stent!
- The balloon waist cannot be abolished. This occurs in really tough lesions, most commonly in dialysis access and in grafts. DO NOT be tempted to just increase the inflation pressure, as this is likely to burst the balloon. The resulting explosion will probably rupture the vessel. Instead, either use a high-pressure balloon to overcome the stenosis, or use a cutting balloon.

Cutting angioplasty balloons These are ballons developed for treating restenosis in coronary arteries. They have mini razor blades incorporated into the wall which make small cuts, the fibrous tissue allowing dilatation. Cutting ballons should be undersized unless you wish to see brisk extravasation.

Distal embolization occurs

- Obtain good-quality angiograms to assess the runoff and the presence of any collaterals.
- Assess the clinical status of the limb. If the limb is well perfused and the embolus is into a non-critical branch vessel, then further intervention is inappropriate.
- Obtain ipsilateral access and perform clot aspiration (see Thrombosuction, p. 188).

Extravasation occurs postangioplasty Extravasation indicates disruption of all layers of the arterial wall and prompt action is essential. Brisk haemorrhage can occur, particularly in the iliac segment, and aggressive resuscitation may be required.

- Reintroduce the balloon and perform a low-pressure inflation proximal to the rupture to tamponade the bleeding. Sometimes this is sufficient to allow a small hole to seal.
- Contact a friendly vascular surgeon and warn them you may need their skills.
- Put in a large drip and set up a saline infusion. Monitor the patient's pulse, BP and oxygen saturation. Take blood for a coagulation screen and cross-match.

- Wait for 5 minutes, then repeat the angiogram. If extravasation persists, reinflate the balloon to maintain haemostastic control.
- If expertise and equipment permit, a stent-graft can be inserted (Fig. 12.13). This will not only rescue the situation but also prolong your increasingly tenuous friendship with the vascular surgeon. If nothing works, the patient will need immediate surgical intervention!

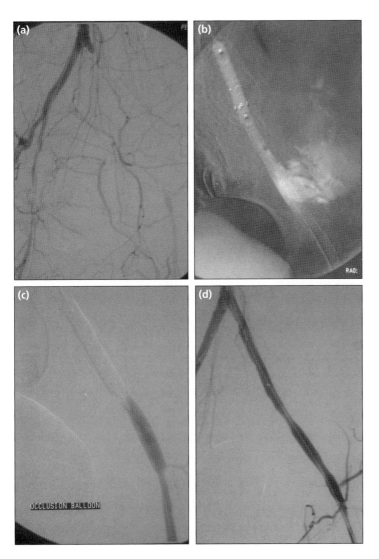

Fig. 12.13 ■ Managing iliac artery rupture. (a) Long iliac artery occlusion which was traversed from the contralateral femoral artery. (b) Following stenting there was severe pain during EIA angioplasty. The balloon was immediately inflated in the CIA (arrows). Angiography demonstrated EIA rupture with extravasation (arrowheads). (c) Balloon inflated to tamponade the rupture site. Brisk extravasation persisted despite prolonged inflation. (d) A stent-graft has been deployed via the ipsilateral femoral artery. The occlusion balloon was pulled back to the CIA during deployment.

ANGIOPLASTY AND STENTING OF SPECIFIC SITES

This section outlines the clinical and technical steps for successful angioplasty/stenting of the most common indications.

The key determinants of successful angioplasty are:
- Arterial inflow and outflow.
- Lesion morphology: stenosis or occlusion, length, calcification, plaque distribution.
- Net lumen gain: a balance between vessel diameter and elastic recoil.

As a general rule, you can expect a good outcome for a focal stenosis in a large vessel with good inflow and runoff, and a poor result in a long occlusion of a small, blind-ending vessel.

Many of the complications are common to all angioplasty procedures:
- Puncture site haematoma: 2–3% commoner with larger sheaths, obesity and hypertension.
- Distal embolization: overall ~2%.
- Angioplasty site thrombosis: overall ~1%.

Unless particularly relevant, these will not be discussed for each site.

Aortas

Focal infrarenal aortic stenoses are ideal for angioplasty and have a technical success rate exceeding 95%, with excellent 5-year patency rates. Stents can be reserved for cases in which there is elastic recoil, recurrent stenoses, and when the aorta is heavily calcified. Lesions that involve the aortic bifurcation should be treated with bilateral simultaneous common iliac balloons extending into the aortic bifurcation (Fig. 12.14).

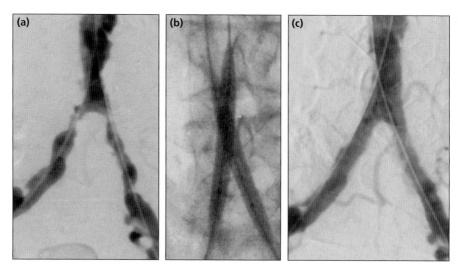

Fig. 12.14 ■ (a) Stenosis involving the distal aorta and common iliac arteries. (b) Kissing angioplasty balloons. (c) Completion angiography.

Pressure measurements are essential in the initial assessment of these lesions. Frequently, apparently severe stenoses on angiography do not produce a significant pressure drop.

Procedure

Access Bilateral femoral access is often used for lesions involving the distal aorta and its bifurcation; these lesions are not suitable for treatment with a single aortic balloon.

The taper on a 15–18 mm aortic balloon may extend 1–2 cm beyond the balloon marker and will wreak havoc if it is in an iliac artery! If a lesion is in the distal infrarenal aorta, either ensure the aortic balloon has a short taper or use bilateral balloons extending from the common iliac arteries into the distal aorta.

Catheterization These lesions always look easy to cross, but in practice it can be quite tricky to negotiate a 1–2 mm channel in a 12 mm artery. Safety first: once you have traversed the stenosis with a hydrophilic guidewire this should be exchanged for a stiffer wire, e.g. an Amplatz superstiff, prior to balloon insertion.

Runs Always perform AP and lateral runs to allow angiographic assessment before intervention. Identify the IMA if it remains patent. In most patients, occlusion of the IMA during angioplasty will have no consequence; however, rarely, the IMA is hypertrophied secondary to disease in the SMA, and occlusion must be avoided. If necessary, angioplasty can be performed with a protection balloon in the IMA from the brachial route.

Complications

The principal risk is distal embolization secondary to treatment of a large atherosclerotic plaque. Iliac trauma from the balloon is an avoidable risk with good angiographic technique.

Iliac arteries

Angioplasty is an effective treatment for symptomatic iliac atherosclerotic disease. Initial technical success rates of 90–95% are achievable in suitable patients; 80–90% 5-year patency rates are achieved for stenoses <5 cm in length. Patency rates are lower for occlusions, heavily calcified lesions and stenotic disease that exceeds 10 cm in length, and in these circumstances primary stenting should be considered.

Iliac diameters are usually between 7 and 8 mm; however, take particular care in the female external iliac, which can be small and is prone to dissection, spasm and rupture. Remember to measure the size of the target vessel before dilation. If the external iliac artery is narrowed throughout its length, it may well be because of vasospasm (Fig. 12.15). Inject 100 mg of nitroglycerin via the sheath and repeat the angiogram after a few minutes.

A single balloon is ineffective for lesions involving the distal aorta and impinging on the origin of the common iliac artery (Fig. 12.14). In this situation simultaneous inflation of a balloon in each common iliac artery origin – 'kissing balloons' – is needed. Kissing balloons are also used to prevent embolization of plaque into the contralateral iliac system. This is most likely to occur when using a balloon expandable stent to treat a common iliac artery occlusion.

The internal iliac artery may be occluded if angioplasty or stenting is performed across its origin. In a male patient with a unilateral internal iliac this may cause impotence, and you will not have done his buttock claudication any favours! Protect the internal iliac artery by inserting a guidewire into it from the contralateral route. If the internal iliac artery origin is diseased, then angioplasty it as well (Fig. 12.16) – a male patient may be very grateful. If the internal iliac is at risk of occlusion, make sure you discuss the potential implications of this during consent.

Pressure measurements (p. 96) are invaluable for assessing the significance of iliac lesions. Pullback pressure measurements are particularly useful in multifocal disease.

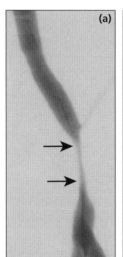
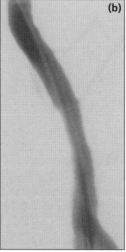

Fig. 12.15 ▨ (a) Apparent stenosis of the external iliac artery (arrows). Note the smooth outline characteristic of spasm. (b) Appearance following intra-arterial administration of 200 mg of GTN.

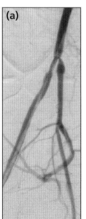
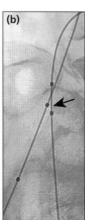
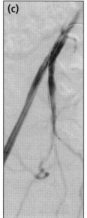

Fig. 12.16 ▨ (a) Stenosis involving the external iliac artery (EIA) and the origin of the solitary internal iliac artery (IIA). (b) Angioplasty balloons in situ; the balloon (arrow) has been placed from the contralateral approach. (c) Completion angiography.

Procedure

Access Use the ipsilateral common femoral artery whenever possible. If the common femoral is difficult to palpate, use an ultrasound-guided puncture to gain access.

Catheterization Sometimes it is impossible to negotiate a lesion from the retrograde approach. Use a Sidewinder or Sos catheter to manipulate over the bifurcation, and try to cross the lesion from above. If successful, the wire can either be snared or manipulated through the sheath (Fig. 18.4) or permit the ipsilateral passage of balloons.

Runs Initial angiograms from the aorta tend to overestimate the length of occlusions. Perform a run with simultaneous injections from both the aorta and the ipsilateral sheath. Always perform obliques, and use the run that shows the lesion in profile during attempted catheterization.

Complications

Complications are more frequent in occlusions than in stenoses, and are considerably more frequent in the external than the common iliac artery. In particular, distal embolization occurs more frequently in occlusions and is often impossible to treat by clot aspiration because of the pre-existing 7Fr retrograde puncture used to perform the angioplasty. Primary stent insertion minimizes the risk by trapping atheroma and thrombus against the vessel wall.

Iliac rupture can occur after angioplasty, particularly of the external iliac artery. Blood loss can be very rapid and prompt balloon tamponade is essential. It is now that you realize the importance of having a stent-graft available for 'endovascular rescue'. If this fails, seek immediate surgical assistance.

Common femoral artery

CFA stenoses are often the result of large calcified eccentric plaques. As the CFA is superficial, lesions are often treated by endarterectomy rather than angioplasty. If the stenosis is postsurgical then try angioplasty instead. For angioplasty, access often has to be from the contralateral groin, and protection may be necessary if the lesion involves the profunda origin. Try to avoid stents in the CFA as they will be prone to repeated flexion and will preclude arterial access and complicate any future surgery.

Superficial femoral artery

Angioplasty of the SFA for claudication is bread and butter for most radiologists, despite the results being no better than supervised exercise programmes. Overall patency rates for SFA disease are around 50% at 3 years. As always, short non-calcified stenoses offer the best long-term results: 5-year patency 70%. The results of angioplasty in stenoses or occlusions longer than 10 cm are much poorer, but angioplasty may be appropriate if the patient is not a surgical candidate and has rest pain or tissue ischaemia. Stents are usually reserved for bail-out procedures and are best avoided in the popliteal artery (flexion again). Stent-grafts in the SFA remain largely unproven compared to surgical alternatives.

Doppler ultrasound is very useful to identify whether stenoses are haemodynamically significant prior to angioplasty, particularly in multifocal disease, or to follow up interventions.

Procedure

Access The ipsilateral groin provides the shortest, straightest route. Perform an antegrade puncture using the guidelines on page 73. Rarely, a lesion cannot be crossed from the antegrade route and a popliteal puncture may provide a more favourable route.

Catheterization Stenoses are usually negotiated with a hydrophilic guidewire. Occlusions may be more readily traversed with a straight wire and shaped catheter. Always perform a run after successfully crossing the lesion to confirm re-entry into the target vessel. Dilating a collateral will cause havoc, and few things are more embarrassing than creating a 5 mm hole through the side of the SFA.

Runs In difficult lesions, manipulate a catheter and guidewire to the target lesion and then perform a magnified view to optimize the chances of steering through the lesion. Choose the largest magnification that allows visualization of the lesion and the target runoff vessel, as this keeps the wire in view at all times.

Complications

The most frequent complications are puncture site haematoma (2%), distal embolization (2–3%) and angioplasty site thrombosis (1%).

Vessel perforation occasionally occurs during femoropopliteal angioplasty, but seldom has clinical consequences. Anticoagulation should be reversed if necessary; balloon tamponade, stent-grafting or, rarely, coil embolization should be used if bleeding fails to settle.

Tibial vessels

Tibial angioplasty is a useful technique for ulcer healing and rest pain in patients who are not surgical candidates. The durability and the risks make it inappropriate for the treatment of claudication. Small-calibre low-profile balloons (2–4 mm) and 0.014–0.018 inch guidewires are required. These vessels are extremely prone to vasospasm, and the use of antispasmodic agents is essential. As always, the elusive single focal non-calcified stenosis does best, but more diffuse disease can be treated successfully and may stay open long enough to permit ulcer healing. Extraluminal angioplasty can be particularly effective in crural vessel occlusion (Fig. 12.17).

Renal artery

Renal artery angioplasty and stenting is a complex procedure; access can be difficult, and when there is a problem the consequences are rapid and serious – there may be renal loss even with immediately available surgical support. Renal angioplasty should only be attempted by angiographers who are already competent at all aspects of peripheral angioplasty.

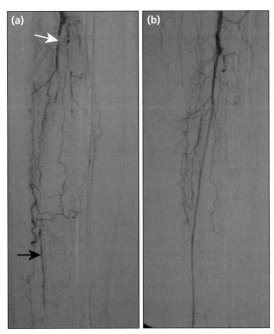

Fig. 12.17 Extraluminal angioplasty of the posterior tibial artery. (a) Diseased tibioperoneal trunk (white arrow) and posterior tibial artery (black arrow). (b) Following extraluminal recanalization of the posterior tibial artery in line runoff is restored.

Renal angioplasty

The main issues for consent are:
- The 3Bs of arterial access. Risk of CVA if using the arm approach
- General risks of angioplasty
- Specific to kidney – renal loss resulting in need for dialysis overall about 2% if treating entire renal mass
- Unpredictable clinical outcome in terms of renal function and blood pressure control.

Renal angiosplasty is undertaken for the treatment of either ischaemic renal failure or hypertension. The clinical outcomes are poorly understood and are currently the subject of a large multicentre randomized trial (the ASTRAL trial).

The clearest indications for renal angioplasty/stenting are:
- **Flash pulmonary oedema** The aetiology of this condition is incompletely understood, but treating the underlying renal artery stenosis is usually very effective.
- **Hypertension refractory to treatment** A few patients will have hypertension which is poorly controlled despite maximal drug therapy, malignant hypertension, or do not tolerate the antihypertensive medication. In these patients it is worth trying renal artery angioplasty and stenting, with the caveat that there will be no improvement in about one-third of patients.

- **Rapidly decreasing renal function with preserved renal size** These patients are going to require renal replacement therapy in the near future and have nothing to lose. They are the least likely to benefit from revascularization therapy.

The majority of renal stenoses are secondary to atherosclerotic lesions that tend to involve the proximal renal artery or its ostium (Fig. 12.18a). Fibromuscular dysplasia can affect any part of the renal artery and has a characteristic beaded appearance at angiography (Fig. 12.18b). Angioplasty success rates are highest with fibromuscular dysplasia, moderate with non-ostial atherosclerotic stenoses (Fig. 12.19), and poorest with ostial lesions. Ostial lesions are due to aortic wall atheroma and are prone to elastic recoil. Most angiographers will opt for a primary stent placement when dealing with an ostial lesion.

Ischaemic nephropathy can only occur when the stenosis affects the whole functional renal mass. In the presence of two kidneys, renal impairment in the presence of unilateral RAS indicates another renal pathology. Frequently, one of the renal arteries is already occluded, with a significant stenosis in the contralateral artery. The risk of progression to renal occlusion is at least 11% within 2 years, and therefore patients are treated to prevent progression

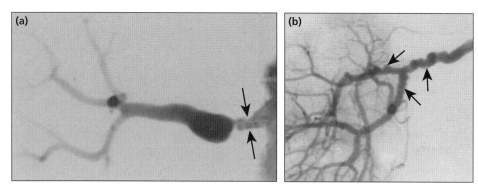

Fig. 12.18 ▪ (a) Atheromatous ostial renal artery stenosis (arrows) with post-stenotic dilation. (b) Typical beaded appearance of fibromuscular dysplasia (arrows) involving the distal renal artery and its branches.

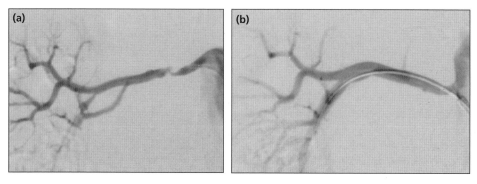

Fig. 12.19 ▪ Atheromatous stenosis in the midrenal artery (a) before and (b) after angioplasty. Hypertension was cured but returned 2 years later, and was again successfully treated.

to renal failure. Preintervention assessment must include creatinine clearance and ultrasound assessment of renal length. When the creatinine is greater than 300 mmol, the damage is seldom reversible. Similarly, a kidney smaller than 8.5 cm is unlikely to develop useful function in response to angioplasty.

Primary technical success rates for renal artery angioplasty exceed 90% in most series; clinical success is considerably poorer. It is difficult to predict which patients with hypertension will benefit from angioplasty; 'suck it and see' is often the only answer. Typically, young patients with fibromuscular hyperplasia respond well, and patients with unilateral disease do better than those with bilateral disease. Hypertensive patients are only 'cured' in 15–20% of cases, although blood pressure control is often improved. The results for ischaemic nephropathy indicate that in appropriately selected patients (i.e. reasonable renal function at the time of percutaneous transluminal angioplasty) approximately 30% improve renal function, with a further 20% stabilizing renal function.

Equipment

- Basic angiography set.
- Cobra, RDC and Sidewinder catheters for the CFA approach. Berenstein or Multipurpose catheters from the arm.
- 4/5Fr sheath – renal artery stenting can be performed through a 4Fr sheath using low-profile balloons and stents.
- Low-profile 5–7 mm × 2 cm angioplasty balloons (make sure that they are long enough if you are using the brachial or radial approach).
- Supportive guidewire – the author's favourite is the 0.018 inch Platinum Plus wire with a 3 cm floppy tip. This allows positioning angiography to be performed around the guidewire. Alternatives: TAD II guidewires (and extension).
- Renal stent: 15 mm × 5 or 6 mm for most patients; used by most operators as the primary treatment for ostial disease, and essential for a bail-out procedure.
- Antispasmodic agents: nifedipine, GTN.

Procedure

Review the aortogram/MRA and plan the access. Patients with a steeply angled renal artery or with severe aortoiliac disease may require treatment from a brachial or radial approach. If the aorta has gross atherosclerotic plaque, then plan to do the procedure through a guide-catheter to minimize the risk of cholesterol embolization.

Access Tailor this according to the renal artery geometry. Use the arm approach for caudally angulated vessels, and in the presence of abdominal aortic aneurysm or severe aortoiliac disease.

Tip: It is often best to approach the renal artery from the contralateral CFA.

Catheterization The stenosis is crossed with a hydrophilic wire; this is subsequently exchanged for a supportive wire such as the Platinum Plus. When learning the procedure it is helpful to be able to image while the balloon/stent is being positioned. This can be achieved in three ways:

- Injection around a guidewire using a Tuohy Borst adapter. This works best when using CO_2, or when using a balloon with a 0.035 inch lumen (see Fig. 12.19).
- Bilateral access. This has several advantages, including the ability to position the balloon and perform postangioplasty images from a contralateral pigtail catheter.
- A guide-catheter can be used to permit per-procedural imaging.

Dilation Always measure the required balloon size, taking care not to include an area of poststenotic dilation; if the entire renal artery is dilated, measure the contralateral renal artery (Fig. 12.20). In practice, most males require a 6 mm balloon and small female patients need a 5 mm dilation. Warn the patient that it is normal to experience mild loin pain during angioplasty. Ask them to let you know when discomfort is felt, and be careful if dilating more than this.

Complications

- **Transient renal insufficiency** Prevention is better than cure: prehydrate the patient, give N-acetyl cysteine; use carbon dioxide or iso-osmolar non ionic contrast (iodixanol) and minimize contrast volume; perform diagnostic and therapeutic examinations separately.
- **Flow-limiting dissection** Readily treated with stent insertion.

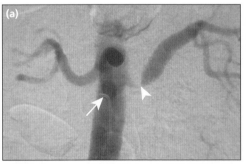

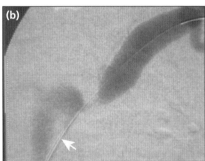

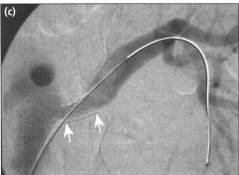

Fig. 12.20 ▦ Renal artery stenting for severe hypertension. (a) CO_2 angiogram using a Cobra catheter in the aorta (arrow), high-grade ostial stenosis with poststenotic dilatation affecting the entire renal artery. (b) The stenosis has been crossed, and angiography performed by injection through the Cobra catheter (arrow) around 0.018 inch guidewire. (c) Completion angiogram obtained as in (b). Note that the stent (arrows) has been dilated to 6 mm to match the diameter of the contralateral renal artery.

- **Vasospasm** Use oral nifedipine 10 mg as a pretreatment and intra-arterial GTN 100 mg aliquots.
- **Intrarenal embolization** Thrombus may be treated with in situ thrombolysis.
- Renal artery rupture. Secondary to either overdilation or subintimal balloon passage. Reinflate the balloon within the renal artery to tamponade the hole. Sometimes this is sufficient to allow a small defect to close. When this fails, reach for your friend the stent-graft and deploy it over the defect. If this doesn't work, leave the balloon inflated. It is good to have a strategy for this rare eventuality worked out before starting the procedure. Either accept the most likely outcome and embolize the kidney, or call your ex-friend the vascular surgeon. The warm ischaemia time for a kidney is fairly short (approximately 40 minutes) and therefore renal loss is likely.

Supra-aortic angioplasty and stenting

Roughly speaking, supra-aortic angioplasty and stenting can be divided into treatment of upper limb ischaemia and treatment of cerebral ischaemia (carotid and vertebral arteries). Both carry a risk of stroke. This is advanced intervention and should not be attempted without proper training and supervision.

Supra-aortic angioplasty

The main consent issues are:
- The 3Bs of arterial access.
- General risks of angioplasty.
- Specific to supra-aortic – risk of causing CVA is approximately 5% for carotid angioplasty and stenting, but probably less for arm ischaemia. As with carotid endarterectomy the patient may prefer medical treatment alone.

Upper limb angioplasty

Subclavian stenoses and occlusions can be successfully treated in 90% of patients, and over 80% of patients have sustained clinical improvement at 3 years. Occlusions are best approached from the brachial route and are frequently stented to minimize the risk of cerebral embolization. Patients with subclavian steal usually have retrograde flow in the vertebral artery, which offers some degree of protection against cerebral embolization. Patients with antegrade vertebral flow can still undergo subclavian angioplasty, though some angiographers would opt to protect the vertebral circulation with an additional balloon.

Carotid angioplasty

Carotid angioplasty and stenting are increasingly being used as an alternative to surgery for symptomatic carotid artery stenosis. Patients should be assessed in conjunction with a neurologist and carefully worked up. The risk of stroke is around 5%; this must be discussed in advance. Patients should be started on clopidogrel (75 mg/day) a week before the procedure.

The key to success is obtaining a stable position in the common carotid artery. Before starting, obtain an MRA to assess the aortic arch and carotid arteries. If the aorta is unfolded and the carotid arteries are tortuous seek expert guidance, as not all carotids can be treated by endovascular means. The technique of carotid artery stenting is rapidly evolving. Low-profile monorail (rapid exchange) angioplasty balloons and stents are used. Cerebral protection devices are becoming popular, but although attractive they remain unproven. These devices have different properties and discussion of their use is beyond the scope of this book. The basic principles of carotid angioplasty and stenting are set out below.

Ten key steps to carotid intervention

- Obtain common femoral artery access; heparinize the patient fully.
- Catheterize the symptomatic common carotid artery and perform a lateral carotid angiogram.
- Catheterize the distal external carotid artery and introduce a 1 cm tip Amplatz wire.
- Introduce an 80 cm reinforced sheath into the common carotid artery and perfuse this from a bag of pressurized heparinized saline run slowly.
- Place a coin of known diameter over the ipsilateral mandible close to but not obscuring the ICA. This is used to measure the diameter of the carotid artery. Perform another lateral carotid angiogram and measure the diameters of the ICA and CCA, and the length of the diseased segment.
- Give atropine 1.2 mg into the sheath. This will cause the ipsilateral pupil to dilate. Warn the patient and ward staff that this is not a cause for concern.
- Cross the stenosis with a steerable 0.014 or 0.018 inch guidewire. This may be part of the cerebral protection device if one is being used. Use a 3 mm balloon to predilate lesions with a diameter less than 3 mm.
- Pass the stent across the lesion and deploy it, and dilate to an appropriate diameter – usually 4–6 mm.
- Perform a check angiogram to demonstrate the treatment site. Carefully remove the cerebral protection device if one was used.
- Use a closure device at the common femoral artery puncture site. This is a prime indication to use a closure device; large sheath, heparinized patient, clopidogrel.

Vertebral artery intervention

The majority of symptomatic carotid artery disease is due to embolic phenomena, hence the need for primary stenting and cerebral protection. Vertebrobasilar insufficiency is usually a flow-related phenomenon and angioplasty alone may be sufficient. Short balloon-expandable stents are used for recoil and restenosis.

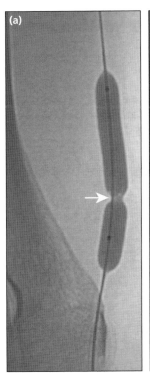
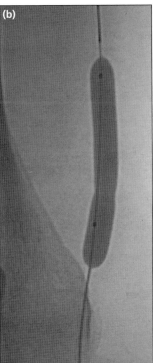

Fig. 12.21 ■ High-pressure inflation to treat basilic vein stenosis. (a) Persistent waist (arrow) in conventional angioplasty balloon at 8 atm. (b) Following use of a high-pressure balloon inflated to 20 atm the stenosis is abolished. Remember, do not exceed the rated pressure for the balloon or it will rupture.

Venous angioplasty

Venous angioplasty has been used extensively in the treatment of central venous stenoses and dialysis outflow lesions. Recurrence is much more frequent in the venous system. Dialysis stenoses are particularly resistant and may require high-inflation pressures with a suitably strong balloon, or the use of a cutting balloon (Fig. 12.21; see also Fig. 17.4).

SUGGESTIONS FOR FURTHER READING

Peripheral angioplasty

Bosch JL, Hunink MG. Meta-analysis of the results of percutaneous transluminal angioplasty and stent placement for aortoiliac occlusive disease. Radiology 1997;204:87–96.
A review of all the published reports of iliac angioplasty and stenting confirms what we all believed: that iliac angioplasty is worthwhile.

Bradbury AW, Ruckley CV. Angioplasty for lower limb ischaemia: Time for randomised controlled trials. Lancet 1996;347:277–278.
A thought-provoking surgical perspective.

Casteneda-Zuniga WR, Formanek A, Tadavarthy M et al. The mechanism of balloon angioplasty. Radiology 1980;135:565–571.
How angioplasty actually works, demonstrated in an experimental model. Shows the importance of plaque rupture and wall stretching.

Chetter IC, Spark JI, Kent PJ et al. Percutaneous transluminal angioplasty for intermittent claudication: evidence on which to base the medicine. Eur J Vasc Endovasc Surg 1998;16:477–484.
Outcomes of angioplasty from the patient's perspective based on quality of life parameters. Provokes thought on patient selection.

Dotter CT, Judkins MP. Transluminal treatment of arteriosclerotic obstruction: Description of a new technique and a preliminary report of its application. Circulation 1964;30:654–670.
The start of an era, pioneer work, a must for historians.

Houghton AD, Todd C, Pardy B et al. Percutaneous angioplasty for infrainguinal graft related stenoses. Eur J Vasc Endovasc Surg 1997;14:380–385.
Angioplasty seems to be the treatment of choice for short vein graft stenoses.

Johnston KW. Femoral and popliteal arteries: Reanalysis of results of balloon angioplasty. Radiology 1992;183:767–771.
Johnston KW. Iliac arteries: Reanalysis of results of balloon angioplasty. Radiology 1993;186:207–212.
Still the best studies of outcome in angioplasty. Honesty, clear follow-up and defined outcome measures.

Pentecost MJ, Criqui MH, Dorros G et al. Guidelines for peripheral transluminal angioplasty in the abdominal aorta and lower extremity vessels. Circulation 1994;89:511–531.
Tonnesen KH, Bulow J, Holstein P et al. Comparison of efficacy in crossing femoro-popliteal artery occlusions with movable core and hydrophilic guidewires. Cardiovasc Intervent Radiol 1994;17:319–322.
Do not use hydrophilic wires as your first choice.

Weitz JI, Byrne J, Clagett P et al. Diagnosis and treatment of chronic arterial insufficiency of the lower extremities: A critical review. Circulation 1996;94:3026–3049.

Upper limb angioplasty

McNamara TO, Greaser LE, Fischer JR et al. Initial and long-term results of treatment of brachiocephalic arterial stenoses and occlusions with balloon angioplasty, thrombolysis and stents. J Invas Cardiol 1997;9:372–382.
A useful overview of the technique and outcomes.

Renal angioplasty

Pohl MA. Natural history of renal artery stenosis: When to intervene. J Vasc Intervent Radiol 1999;10 (Suppl 2):144–150.
Most of what you need to know regarding patient selection for renal angioplasty and stenting, extensively referenced.

Complications of angioplasty and stenting

Belli A-M, Cumberland DC, Knox AM et al. The complication rate of percutaneous peripheral balloon angioplasty. Clin Radiol 1990;41:380–383.
Matsi PJ, Manninen HI. Complications of lower limb percutaneous transluminal angioplasty: A prospective analysis of 410 procedures on 295 consecutive patients. Cardiovasc Intervent Radiol 1998;21:361–366.
These articles help to set standards for acceptable practice.

Chapter Thirteen

Stents and stent-grafts

Stents

Stents are metal scaffolds used to support a vessel wall. They are introduced in a compressed state and then expanded to line the vessel. Stent-grafts are stents covered with graft material and function as vascular conduits. Stents are used to treat stenotic and occlusive disease, and stent-grafts to treat aneurysms and arterial rupture.

Indications for stenting

A procedure may be undertaken with the intention of deploying a stent – so-called primary stenting. Iliac artery occlusions are often primarily stented to reduce the incidence of distal embolization (Fig. 13.1). Most angiographers will primarily stent ostial RAS without trying angioplasty because of the inevitability of elastic recoil.

A stent may be deployed to salvage an unsuccessful procedure. This is secondary stenting and is the commonest reason to use a stent. The most frequent indication is failed iliac angioplasty with residual pressure gradient, stenosis or flow-limiting dissection (Table 13.1).

Stent types

Most catheter laboratories will keep a selection of stents of different types and sizes on the shelf. This allows the operator a choice for different circumstances. In most cases the exact

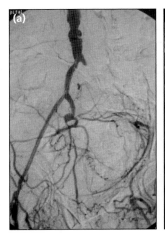
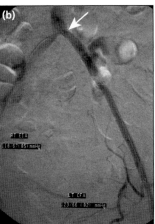

Fig. 13.1 ■ (a) Typical long iliac occlusion. (b) Two overlapping stents have been deployed from the contralateral approach. Note the proximal stent position at the iliac bifurcation and the distal at the inguinal ligament. Unilateral stents can be used to treat these patients provided they are accurately deployed and do not cover the contralateral iliac artery origin.

Table 13.1 Indications for arterial stenting		
Indication	**Primary**	**Secondary**
Failed angioplasty	X	✓
Risk of embolization	✓	X
Iliac occlusion	✓	X
Ostial RAS	✓	X
Restenosis	✓	X
Carotid artery	✓	X

stent chosen is less important than selecting the correct size and deploying it accurately. Choice of which stent to keep on the shelf is influenced by several factors:

- **Evidence of superior effectiveness** The immediate and long term technical and clinical effectiveness should be the most important factors. Unfortunately, in a rapidly evolving market no manufacturer ever has any long-term data to support their product. Until they do, you have to assume that the device is indeed a stent.
- **Ease of use** There is not much point in a device that is complicated or unreliable in its deployment.
- **Profile** The expansion ratio of stents is improving all the time, which means that larger devices can be delivered through smaller sheaths. In practice most stents up to about 12 mm will pass through a 6Fr sheath; some will even pass through a 5Fr sheath, and a few smaller stents pass through a 4Fr sheath.
- **Trackability and flexibility** The ability of a stent to reach its target site and to conform to the vessel anatomy. Some stents pass readily over the aortic bifurcation and can be deployed in the contralateral iliac system; others don't manage this even with a stiff wire (Fig. 13.1).
- **Cost** In many circumstances any stent will do; in this case the choice is pragmatic and the cheapest may well be the best. Obviously you will not be swayed by the offer of a sportscar or equivalent.

There are many stents on the market but all fall into two basic types: balloon-mounted or self-expanding. Most balloon-expandable stents and the Wallstent are made of stainless steel; virtually all new self-expanding stents are made of nickel titanium alloys (Nitinol). Nitinol has a 'thermal memory' and expands to a preset diameter at body temperature. As Nitinol is not very radio-opaque, many stents have platinum or tantalum markers on their crowns. Early Nitinol stents tended to shorten by about 5% on expansion. This has largely been overcome with newer designs, and modern stents can be deployed very precisely.

In a crowded market everyone has their own favourite stents, but there is not a great deal to choose between manufacturers. The list we mention is not comprehensive, nor does inclusion indicate an endorsement or exclusion imply a criticism; rather, the examples are chosen to illustrate the types of device available.

Balloon-mounted stents   Balloon-mounted stents, e.g. Bridge (AVE), Saxx (Bard), Genesis (Cordis), LifeStent (Edwards), Herculink (Guidant), and stent grafts e.g. JOSTENT (JOMED) are usually made of stainless steel; balloon dilation is necessary to expand them to their working diameter. Once deployed, most have high radial strength. There is usually some shortening during deployment, but this is very predictable unless the stent is expanded beyond its recommended working range, in which case marked shortening will occur. Balloon-mounted stents tend to be less flexible than their self-expanding counterparts. More rigid devices are less suited for use in tortuous vessels or at points of flexion. Stents are typically oversized by 1 mm to ensure secure fixation when deployed. Balloon-expandable stents can be 'flared' within their rated range of diameter by using balloons of different sizes to deploy them; if this is important, start with the smaller diameter!

Balloon-mounted stents may be purchased separately and manually crimped on to an appropriately sized balloon at the time of the procedure. This is becoming unpopular, and most people are opting for stents premounted on an angioplasty balloon. This requires a greater stock of devices to cater for different diameters and lengths.

A properly mounted stent grips securely on the balloon: this is essential to prevent migration. If the stent slides on the balloon, STOP; do not attempt to deploy it, as both you and the stent will 'come unstuck'.

Some stents require an introducer to pass through the sheath's haemostatic valve. Failure to do so will result in the stent dislodging from the balloon. This may also occur during the stent's passage to the deployment site, and is one of the reasons for using guide-catheters.

Tip: Many angioplasty balloons have a hydrophilic coating to help them pass through tight strictures. This virtually guarantees that the stent will not stay in place. Try inflating and deflating the balloon before crimping the stent in place. Increased friction is obtained at the price of a slight loss of profile.

Troubleshooting

There are some well-known potential pitfalls with balloon-mounted stents which can sometimes be prevented or salvaged if recognized early. When things do go wrong, try to keep the situation in perspective. Remember not to cause more harm than necessary. It is often best to summon a more senior colleague or obtain surgical help.

The stent moves proximal or distal to the balloon markers prior to deployment
(Fig. 13.2)   Prevention is better than cure, and this tends to occur either during passage through heavily calcified stenoses or around sharp corners; predilation and the use of guide-catheters are useful. Do not attempt deployment if either end of the stent has moved outside the balloon markers. If there has been significant stent movement, asymmetrical balloon inflation will push the stent off the balloon.

If the whole stent remains on the balloon:
- Partially inflate the balloon with contrast, as this helps the stent to grip the balloon.
- Attempt to reposition the stent over the stenosis.

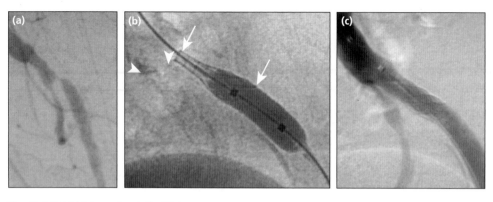

Fig. 13.2 ■ (a) High-grade calcified EIA stenosis prior to femoropopliteal grafting. (b) During deployment the balloon has 'been pushed out' of the stent (arrows); note the stent has not moved and remains perfectly placed in relation to the origin of the IIA (chevrons). In this case the balloon was deflated and repositioned to deploy the remainder of the stent. (c) Completion angiogram.

- If the stent begins to migrate, deflate the balloon and gently try to recapture the stent. If this fails, then it is probably best to deploy this stent either where it is or, even better, at a safe site such as the common iliac artery.
- If repositioning is successful, slowly inflate the balloon. Deploy the stent as normal if it remains in position.

If the stent has come off the balloon:
- Find the stent! It is usually on the catheter shaft or in the groin sheath. Some stents are poorly opaque and it may be necessary to take spot radiographs to locate them.
- Withdraw the stent into the sheath, then remove sheath and catheter and insert a new sheath (use one that you have prepared earlier). Do not forget to crimp the stent on this time when you reuse it!
- If you are unlucky, the stent has come completely off the balloon but is still on the wire. This is much harder! Pass a 4Fr straight catheter through the stent and exchange for a 0.018 = wire. Try to capture the stent with a small vessel balloon.
- Alternatively, pass a gooseneck snare alongside the guidewire and snare the stent by lassoing the wire.

Self-expanding stents and stent-grafts   In their compressed state, these devices are constrained by a sheath or membrane which prevents them from expanding. The stent automatically expands when the sheath is withdrawn (Fig. 13.3).

Deploying self-expanding stents

All of the current systems deploy in one of the following ways; none is complicated once the basic principles have been grasped. In essence, the stent is held in a compressed state in a sheath or on the delivery catheter. The sheath is progressively withdrawn, allowing the stent to expand and deploy.

- **Pusher and sheath,** e.g. Gianturco stent (Cook). Basically a simple spring, nowadays this is rarely used as a stent but forms the basis of the Cook aortic stent-graft. The pusher and sheath system was the original technique, and variations on the theme are the basis for most systems. Several aortic stent-grafts and IVC filters also function in

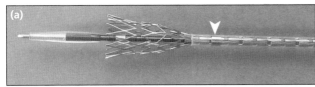

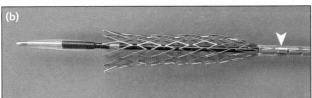

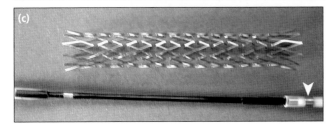

Fig. 13.3 ■ A self-expanding stent opening as the outer sheath is retracted. Note that the distal marker (arrows) moves back with the sheath, but the stent remains in the original position.

this way. A long sheath is placed at the target deployment site. The 'device' comes separate from the delivery sheath. It is typically held in a cartridge and introduced into the delivery sheath using a 'pusher' – a blunt-ended dilator. The pusher is used to advance the stent to the end of the sheath. The action now changes completely: the pusher is held completely still to maintain the position of the stent and the sheath is retracted progressively, releasing the stent as it is exposed (Fig. 13.4).

- **Pusher and sheath incorporated into a single delivery catheter**, e.g. Wallstent-Uni and Wallgraft (Boston Scientific), Fluency stent-graft (Bard), Zilver (Cook), SuperFlex (Pyramed). To deploy the stent the central component of the catheter is fixed in position and the outer sheath manually pulled back (Fig. 13.5).
- The Wallstent offers a particular challenge. Although there are advantages in the flexibility of this stent, its construction leads to significant shortening during deployment. Because of this it is best restricted to situations where precise positioning is not critical. The deployed length of the Wallstent depends on final diameter: a chart on the back of the packaging will help you to predict how long the stent will be, e.g. a 10 × 68 mm long Wallstent is roughly 95 mm long when constrained; it will shorten to 83 mm long at its minimum recommended diameter of 7 mm, 77 mm long at 8 mm, and 69 mm at 9 mm. The markers at the end of the Wallstent delivery catheter bear little relation to the final position of the stent (Fig. 13.6). The critical marker lies closer to the proximal end, and indicates the limit to which the stent may be deployed if it is to be resheathed, and roughly where the proximal end of the unconstrained stent will shorten to.

Tip: It is common practice to start with the distal end of the Wallstent well beyond the target site. When the stent has opened it can be pulled back until the 'critical' marker is in position. This is fine in TIPS or in SVCO, but is best avoided in an occluded iliac artery unless you are intending to embolize the runoff.

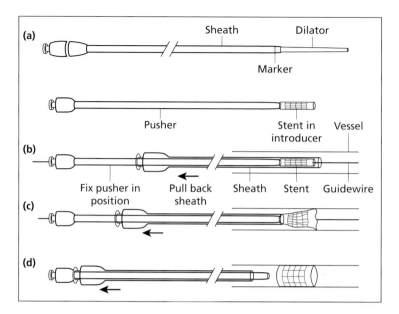

Fig. 13.4 ■ Principles of the pusher and sheath introducer system. (a) The outer sheath is inserted just beyond the target site using a tapering dilator. The dilator is removed and the pusher used to introduce the stent into the sheath. (b) The pusher is advanced until the stent is at the target site. The pusher is then fixed in position and the sheath pulled back. (c) Continue pulling back the sheath to progressively deploy the stent. (d) When the sheath is fully retracted, the stent is deployed.

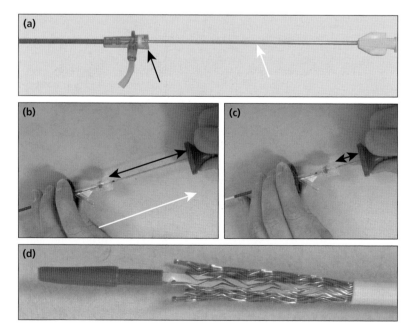

Fig. 13.5 ■ Deploying a stent using an integrated pusher and sheath delivery system. (a) Delivery sheath (black arrow) pusher (white arrow) (b and c). The pusher is fixed and the sheath pulled back (white arrow) until the stent is deployed. (d) Stent opening as it is unsheathed.

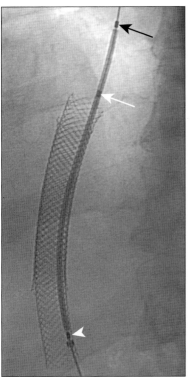

Fig. 13.6 ▪ Wallstent markers shown during a TIPS revision. The distal marker (white arrowhead), the proximal marker (black arrow) and the 'critical marker' (white arrow) which indicates roughly the point to which the stent will shorten, and the limit of deployment for resheathing.

- **'Trigger' and 'screw' systems**, e.g. Luminexx 3 stent (Bard), SMART (Cordis), LifeStent NT (Edwards), Absolute (Guidant). All these systems are a modification of the pusher and sheath and incorporate either a trigger mechanism or a screw mechanism to gradually unsheath the stent. Trigger systems can be operated one-handed, and less coordination is required to deploy them.
- **Ripcord system**, e.g. Hemobahn, Viator and Excluder (Gore). This is currently employed on some types of stent graft manufactured by Gore for use in aortic aneurysm and the peripheral circulation. The stent is held constrained by a fabric cover rather than a sheath. Pulling the ripcord undoes the seam and releases the stent-graft.

Alarm: Beware! The positioning markers are different in different systems! On some systems the markers are on the stent; on some they are on the delivery catheter, and on others a combination of both. Check that you are familiar with the device you have chosen, especially if the markers do not correspond to the final position of the stent. Failure to appreciate this will lead to malpositioning.

Choosing that stent

Basically, you will use what your boss likes, but there are some factors which influence whether you reach for a balloon-expandable or self-expanding stent. The following should be considered in individual cases (Fig. 13.7).

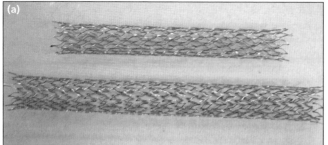

Fig. 13.7 ■ Differences in stent properties. The shorter stent (Sinus-Repo, OptiMed) has higher radial force and can be resheathed, but is more prone to kinking (arrow). The longer stent is more flexible (Sinus-SuperFlex, OptiMed).

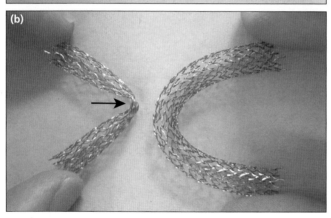

Strength of the stent Balloon-expandable stents tend to exert the greatest radial force. This can be advantageous in calcified lesions.

Precise positioning The Wallstent is probably best avoided in these circumstances, as it can shorten unpredictably even in experienced hands. In the past critical positioning was an indication to choose a balloon-mounted stent. This is no longer the case: most self-expanding stents can be deployed as accurately as their balloon-mounted counterparts (see Fig. 13.1). The reasons for this are enhanced visibility of the stent and near-elimination of shortening with modern designs.

Conformability In general, self-expanding stents are better at conforming to the vessel wall, particularly where there are changes in calibre or there is tortuosity: the Wallstent scores particularly highly here. However, newer balloon-expandable stents tend to be less rigid. Balloon-expandable stents can be dilated to different diameters (obviously this requires more than one balloon), but as the smallest balloon is used first the potential for migration is greater.

Risk of compression post deployment Avoid balloon-expandable stents and think hard whether you really want a stent at all. There have been several reports of balloon-expandable stents being deformed by external compression, e.g. in the carotid, subclavian and popliteal arteries. In these circumstances a self-expanding stent is better, but even these may be damaged by repeated compression.

Future imaging If MRA is part of your plan for follow-up then stick with Nitinol: the latest designs will cause minimal artefact. Forget about using a stainless steel stent, as the susceptibility artefact will obscure all the vascular detail (Fig. 5.5).

Tip: Nitinol stents must be accurately sized. Unlike balloon-mounted stents, they cannot be overexpanded as they will recoil back to their nominal diameter! A Nitinol stent needs to be 1–2 mm larger in diameter than the target vessel.

Guide to safe stenting

Stenting is usually a straightforward procedure.
- Obtain the best possible angiogram, centred over the deployment site.
- Use fluoroscopy fade or bony landmarks to identify the deployment site. A useful technique is to ask an assistant to mark important landmarks on the monitor with a chinagraph pencil. The stent can then be deployed relative to these. Remember to stand in the same position to avoid parallax.
- Never move the table or image intensifier once in position. Parallax will affect the landmarks.
- Consider protecting vital vessels with guidewires or balloons.
- Measure the lesion length and the diameters of the normal vessel proximal and distal to it. Choose the correct size stent. Most modern angiography equipment has the facility to make measurements. If this is not available, then use either a calibrated catheter or balloon or an external ruler.
- Position the stent.
- Perform a check angiogram to confirm the position of the stent and markers before deployment (Fig. 13.8).
- Use continuous fluoroscopy while deploying the stent. Take your time!

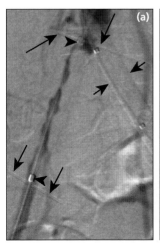
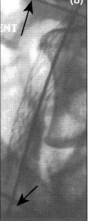

Fig.13.8 High-grade stricture of the right common iliac artery. (a) Needles (long arrows) have been placed on the drapes to mark the stenosis and the stent markers (arrowheads) have been aligned with these. Note the contralateral angioplasty balloon (short arrows) to prevent embolization over the bifurcation. (b) Accurate stent placement between the markers.

- Screen during withdrawal of the delivery system.
- Use angioplasty to 'tailor' the stent to the vessel wall. All stents, including self-expanding stents, need a balloon for complete deployment.
- Perform completion angiography and pressure measurements, and check runoff vessels for distal embolization.

Stent-grafts

One of the most important indications for using stent-grafts is the treatment of vessel rupture during angioplasty. All catheter laboratories should keep one or two stent-grafts in reserve specifically to treat this eventuality. Your patient and their lawyer will expect you to know how to use it!

Covered stents reline the vessel and hence treat ruptures, exclude aneurysms, and may prevent restenosis (Fig. 13.9). They are an attractive concept, but are still evolving.

Various stent coverings are available, the most common being Dacron (polyester) and ePTFE (polytetrafluorethylene). Polycarbonate, woven Nitinol and autologous vein have also been used. In order to reduce the profile of the delivery catheters the graft material is thin walled compared to conventional surgical grafts, and in the long term their durability is uncertain. The proximal and distal portions of the device are often uncovered to improve anchorage.

Stent-grafts come in two basic configurations: straight tube and bifurcated. Straight grafts are most commonly used in iliac artery aneurysm or to repair post-traumatic false aneurysm or

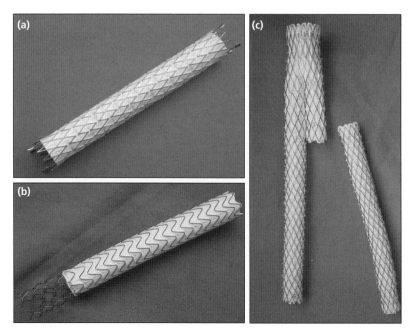

Fig. 13.9 ▦ Three different types of stent graft. (a) Peripheral – Fluency (Bard). (b) TIPS – Viator (Gore). (c) Aortic – AneuRx (Medtronic).

arterial rupture. Bifurcated stent-grafts are used to repair abdominal aortic aneurysms that extend into the common iliac vessels. More complex 'fenestrated' and branching grafts are available and allow branch vessels to be treated; their use is beyond the scope of this book.

Stent-grafting – basic rules

Stent-grafting is not dissimilar to stenting, but the margins for error are smaller. For a stent-graft to be effective, it must fit precisely within the target vessel. An undersized graft will allow blood to flow between it and the vessel wall. Oversized devices will have creases in the graft material, which may adversely affect flow and promote thrombosis. Calibrated angiography and CT are usually used to measure the target vessel dimensions. In general, the stent-graft diameter should be 10–20% greater than the diameter of the implantation site. Length is also important: too long a covered stent may occlude important branch vessels.

Spontaneous and iatrogenic arterial rupture   Use similar principles to choosing a stent for occlusive disease. Choose a device that is long enough to cover the defect in the artery wall and is an appropriate diameter (i.e. oversized by at least 1 mm). Remember that it may be necessary to increase the size of your arterial sheath: most stent-grafts require at least an 8Fr sheath. Choose the stent graft which is simplest to use and most likely to do the job effectively.

Three devices to 'Get out of Jail Free' (Fig. 13.10)
- **Jomed**, a simple PTFE stent graft which is crimped on to an angioplasty balloon and deployed as a conventional balloon mounted stent. An advantage is that a Jomed graft can treat a range of diameters – e.g. 4–9 mm – when put on an appropriately sized balloon. Remember to choose a sheath at least 2Fr greater than the angioplasty balloon

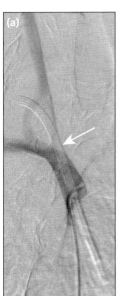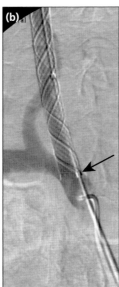

Fig. 13.10 ■ The great escape. (a) An 11Fr dialysis catheter has been placed in the right common carotid artery. The low puncture would necessitate a thoracotomy to repair surgically. (b) Following placement of a Wallgraft (Boston Scientific), the dialysis catheter was removed without bleeding after the graft was placed. Note the end of the graft overhangs the origin of the subclavian artery. Covering the hole was much more important than the potential for arm ischaemia.

to allow the device through. Unfortunately, this device is relatively inflexible and will not be suited to tortuous vessels.

- **Wallgraft**, a variation of the Wallstent. If you can use the Wallstent you can use this.
- **Fluency** (Bard) Deploys just like the Wallgraft, but is a Nitinol stent.

Occlusive disease   Stent-grafts are currently being evaluated for use in occlusive disease in situations where angioplasty and stenting are ineffective. The principal goal is the treatment of long segment stenosis or occlusion of the superficial femoral and popliteal arteries. There is no current evidence to suggest that stent-grafts are more effective than uncovered stents in the iliac arteries.

Aneurysms   Interest in the endovascular treatment of aortic and other aneurysms is increasing. The technique is evolving, and there have been rapid developments in the design of the grafts and improvements in the delivery systems.

THORACIC AORTIC ANEURYSM   The greatest advantage of endovascular repair is likely to be in patients with thoracic aortic aneurysm (TAA), acute aortic dissection with ischaemic sequelae, and in traumatic aortic rupture. Avoiding a thoracotomy reduces morbidity and mortality compared to surgical repair.

ABDOMINAL AORTIC ANEURYSM   With the currently available devices roughly one-third of patients with abdominal aortic aneurysm (AAA) will be relatively straightforward to treat and one-third will be untreatable, mainly owing to lack of suitable implantation sites, awkward angulation, or difficulty with access. The remainder may be treatable but would be expected to be complex.

There is no financial advantage in using stent-grafting to treat AAA. The patient benefits in terms of reduced physiological stress during the procedure (no aortic cross-clamping, less peripheral ischaemia, reduced blood loss) and also a shorter convalescence (no abdominal wound).

Evidence of long-term effectiveness of aneurysm exclusion is lacking, and patients should be recruited in ongoing trials if sufficient data are to become available.

Aneurysm exclusion with a straight stent-graft

Less than 10% of AAA will be suited to a tube graft. The main use for tube grafts will be the treatment of iliac aneurysm (Fig. 13.11) and false aneurysm repair (Fig. 13.12).

Branch vessels have important implications for stent-grafting and must be assessed on the preprocedural angiograms:

- The vessel may be indispensable, in which case it must not be covered. The stent length and anchorage points must take this into account.
- The vessel may adversely affect aneurysm exclusion, e.g. when treating an iliac artery aneurysm retrograde flow through a patent internal iliac artery would leave the aneurysm perfused. In these circumstances, the artery must be embolized prior to deployment of the stent-graft.

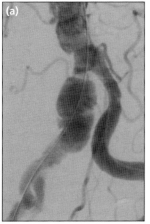
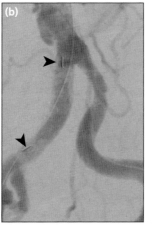

Fig. 13.11 ▨ (a) 4 cm common iliac artery aneurysm. (b) Following deployment of a tubular stent-graft (arrowheads), the aneurysm is excluded.

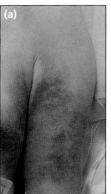
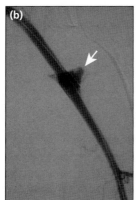
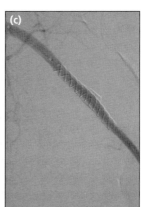

Fig. 13.12 ▨ (a) Extensive bruising following dislocation of the shoulder. (b) Brachial artery false aneurysm (arrow). (c) Completion angiogram following deployment of a Wallgraft from the brachial artery. Surgical cutdown was used due to the 9Fr sheath. Endovascular repair meant that surgery in the region of the haematoma could be avoided. (Picture courtesy of Dr Tony Nicholson.)

Assessment of AAA for endovascular stent-grafting

Endovascular aneurysm repair requires far more detailed assessment than is necessary for surgery. Ultrasound is used to identify aneurysms that are large enough to require treatment.

Computed tomography is an accurate technique used to measure the diameters of the aneurysm necks. More sophisticated 3D reconstructions are extremely helpful to assess the aneurysm morphology, and can accurately measure aneurysm length and dimensions.

MRI is not currently widely used to assess AAA, but is likely to become the modality of choice. Remember that Gd-MRA only shows the flowing lumen, and other sequences are required to assess the true extent of the aneurysm.

Calibrated angiography is used to measure aneurysm dimensions (see Chapter 11, p. 133). Mural thrombus will mask the true extent of the aneurysm. Angiography is likely to be superseded by non-invasive techniques.

Three areas are particularly important:

- **Access** Currently available devices are introduced via 21–28Fr sheaths. Diseased and tortuous iliac arteries will prevent passage of the delivery system.
    - **Contraindications**: Iliac artery diameter less than 8 mm, more than one = 90° angulation, heavily calcified iliac artery.
- **Anchorage sites** Suitable diameter and length for the proximal and distal stents.
    - **Contraindications**: Proximal neck length less than 15 mm, proximal neck angulation = 60°, tapering neck.
- **Adequate visceral blood supply** The stent-graft must not cover vital arteries to the intestine or kidneys.
    - **Contraindications**: Low renal artery origin. Diseased SMA; the IMA will be covered during stent-grafting. The IMA and large lumbar arteries are often embolized before the procedure. If the SMA is diseased, bowel infarction will be inevitable.

Deployment of a modular bifurcated stent-graft

This is a complex practical procedure that requires a well-integrated team of vascular surgeons and radiologists and cannot be learnt from a book. Training usually commences on a simulated aneurysm before performing in vivo deployment. The general concept of graft deployment will be considered, but details of individual devices will not be included.

Stent-graft deployment: a step-by-step guide

1. Surgical cutdown to access CFA to allow introducer placement.
2. A 4Fr pigtail catheter is placed at the level of the renal arteries from the contralateral groin.
3. Initial angiography to give an overview of the aneurysm.
4. Insertion of the delivery system to just above the renal arteries.
5. Magnified angiogram to demonstrate the position of the renal arteries. The table is locked in position and the exact level of the lowest renal artery is marked.
6. Using continuous fluoroscopy, start deployment of the stent-graft just proximal to the renal arteries. The device will shorten as the stent expands.
7. Repeat angiography to confirm satisfactory position.
8. Fully deploy the aortic component of the graft and ipsilateral iliac arterial limb.
9. Remove the introducer system and close the arteriotomy, leaving a 7Fr sheath in position.
10. The contralateral iliac limb stump must now be catheterized. Direct catheterization from the iliac artery can be difficult in a large aneurysm. An alternative is to approach from over the neobifurcation, in which case the wire can be snared in the aneurysm sac or navigated out through the iliac sheath.
11. Deploy the contralateral iliac limb.
12. Perform completion angiography in AP and oblique projections to exclude perigraft leakage.

SUGGESTIONS FOR FURTHER READING

Stents

Beek FJ, Kaatee R, Beutler JJ et al. Complications during renal artery stent placement for atherosclerotic ostial stenosis. Cariovasc Intervent Radiol 1997;20:184–190.
Scary stuff: honest reporting of the real results of renal angioplasty. You should be trained before trying this at home!

Blum U, Krumme B, Flugel P et al. Treatment of ostial renal artery stenosis with vascular endoprostheses after unsuccessful balloon angioplasty. N Engl J Med 1997;336:459–465.
Describes the technique for renal artery stenting as a bail-out procedure and reports encouraging results.

Bosch JL, Hunnink MGM. Meta-analysis of the results of percutaneous transluminal angioplasty and
stent placement for aortoiliac occlusive disease. Radiology 1997;204:87–96.
Overviews of outcomes of stents and stent-grafting.

Tetteroo E, van der Graaf Y, Bosch JL et al. Randomised comparison of primary stent placement
versus primary angioplasty followed by selective stent placement in patients with iliac artery
occlusive disease. Lancet 1998;351:1153–1159.

Westcott MA, Bonn J. Comparison of conventional angioplasty with the Palmaz stent in the treatment
of abdominal aortic stenoses from the STAR registry. J Vasc Intervent Radiol 1998;9:225–231.
Short focal lesions do as well with angioplasty alone.

Stent-grafts

Gunther RW, Vorwerk D (eds). Stent grafting. Semin Intervent Radiol 1998;15.
A whole issue dedicated to stent grafting.

Chapter Fourteen

Thrombolysis and thrombectomy

Thrombolysis

Arterial thrombosis, in both native or graft vessels, is usually secondary to an underlying stenotic lesion. The aim of thrombolysis is to break down blood clot, restore perfusion and reveal the vascular anatomy. The thrombolytic agent is delivered directly into the thrombus; systemic thrombolysis is much less effective and is only used in the treatment of myocardial infarction and pulmonary embolism (PE).

When the vessel has been cleared, an underlying lesion should be carefully looked for and treated. Even partial clearing of the vessels may simplify any subsequent surgical procedure. The agents used for thrombolysis are discussed in Chapter 4 (p. 29). Only rt-PA is discussed in this chapter, but the principles apply equally to the other agents.

Indications

It was hoped that thrombolytic therapy with fibrin-specific agents would be akin to a magic bullet and prevent patients requiring surgery. This has not proved to be the case, however, and consequently thrombolysis is not as popular as it was a few years ago. The principal indications for thrombolysis are:

- Acute or acute-on-chronic critical limb ischaemia (Table 14.1). Thrombolysis is not usually clinically indicated more than 6 weeks after the thrombotic event.
- Graft thrombosis.
- Thrombosed popliteal aneurysm – the aim here is to clear the runoff vessels to allow bypass grafting.
- Periprocedural thrombolysis – thrombosis may occur during interventional procedures and surgery. Acute thrombus is particularly likely to clear; thrombolysis may salvage the procedure.

Contraindications

Thrombolysis is not without risk, particularly bleeding and CVA; the risk–benefit ratio is so unfavourable in some patients that thrombolysis is contraindicated.

Absolute contraindications:

- Irreversible ischaemia.
- Major trauma, surgery or cardiopulmonary resuscitation within the past 2 weeks.
- CVA within the last 2 months; primary or secondary cerebral tumour.
- Bleeding diathesis.

Table 14.1 Clinical categories of acute limb ischaemia

Category	Description	Capillary return	Muscle paralysis	Sensory loss	Arterial Doppler signal	Venous Doppler signal
I Viable	Not immediately threatened	Intact	None	None	+	+
IIa Threatened	Salvageable, if promptly treated	Intact/slow	None	Partial	–	+
IIb Threatened	Salvageable, if immediately treated	Slow/absent	Partial	Partial	–	+
III Irreversible	Amputation regardless of treatment	Absent	Complete	Complete	–	–

Modified from the Consensus Report on Thrombolysis. J Intern Med 1996;240:343–355.

- Graft thrombosis within 4 weeks of surgery. Early graft failure is almost always due to a technical problem with the surgery, e.g. poor-quality vein, graft kinking.
- Pregnancy.
- Any obvious potential bleeding source, e.g. proven active ulceration, bladder tumour.

Relative contraindications:
- Age >80 years – these patients have the highest risk of stroke and haemorrhagic complications.
- The white limb – best treated by surgery.
- Anticoagulation.
- Knitted Dacron grafts – these rely on deposition of thrombus to be impermeable; hence they become porous during thrombolysis and marked extravasation may occur.
- Vein graft – the vein relies on perfusion for its viability, and after about 3 days the vein is irreversibly damaged. However, the runoff may be cleared, allowing subsequent regrafting.
- Recent thrombolysis with no underlying cause demonstrable. Rethrombosis is very likely.
- Thrombolysis with streptokinase within the previous 5 years. This is only relevant if using streptokinase, as antibodies persist for many years and limit the effectiveness of the treatment while increasing the risk of adverse reaction.
- Cardiac emboli – thrombolysis may lead to further embolization.

Equipment

As there are different techniques for performing thrombolysis, the equipment varies with the strategy being used:
- Basic angiography set.
- Infusion catheters: a 4Fr straight catheter with sideholes is suitable in most cases.
- A pump suitable for arterial infusion.

Table 14.2 Guidelines for best arterial access	
Site of occlusion	**Optimal arterial access**
Iliac artery	Ipsilateral CFA if patent, otherwise contralateral CFA
CFA	Contralateral CFA or, exceptionally, brachial
SFA, PFA or femoropopliteal graft	Ipsilateral CFA
Femorofemoral crossover	Direct graft puncture or inflow CFA
Axillofemoral graft	Consider surgery

- Infusion wires and microcatheters may be required.
- Pulse spray techniques require special catheters and pumps.

Procedure

Access The key to thrombolysis is knowing the vascular anatomy; this is obvious in native vessels, but can be obscure in the presence of bypass grafts. Always clarify what grafts are in situ, look for operation notes, and talk to the patient and a senior surgeon. Before puncturing an artery consider performing MRA or an IVDSA, as this will usually demonstrate the inflow anatomy and may even reveal the runoff vessels

The approach for thrombolysis can now be chosen. Make only a single arterial puncture (multiple punctures increase the risk of haemorrhage); the shortest most direct approach is usually the best, as it affords the greatest scope for adjunctive intervention (Table 14.2).

When performing antegrade femoral artery puncture, use ultrasound and fluoroscopy to ensure a safe puncture below the inguinal ligament. Always use ultrasound guidance to target the puncture, especially when puncturing a groin with multiple grafts, or when performing direct graft puncture. Use the contralateral approach in obese patients and when the femoral artery is occluded. If possible, avoid the brachial approach, as there is a risk of pericatheter thrombus causing cerebral embolization.

Infrainguinal grafts almost invariably arise from the anterior aspect of the CFA. Arterial puncture must be sufficiently proximal to allow manipulation of a shaped catheter (Cobra or RDC) to direct a straight guidewire toward the graft origin.

 Tip: To catheterize the graft origin, it is often helpful to obtain an angiogram in a steep oblique projection. Use roadmapping or fluoroscopy fade if these options are available.

Direct prosthetic graft puncture is sometimes helpful, e.g. in femorofemoral crossover grafts. When the graft is palpable, fix it between forefinger and thumb and then perform a single wall puncture in the conventional manner. There is a very distinctive give and fall in resistance as the needle enters the graft lumen. Depending on the direction of catheterization, direct graft puncture will preclude accessing either the origin or the outflow. Retrograde lysis often occurs, but sometimes it is necessary to use a crossed catheter technique.

Techniques and regimens

There are several different agents and methods for performing thrombolysis. All the techniques share a common principle: the delivery catheter is embedded in the thrombus. There is no evidence that any particular technique confers outcome benefit compared to the alternatives.

 TIP: If a guidewire cannot be passed through the thrombus it is probably organized, and is less likely to clear with thrombolysis.

The simplest technique is to infuse the lytic agent through a straight catheter. Variations on this theme have been developed to speed up the lytic process, but there is no evidence that this improves the clinical outcome and there are suggestions that complications such as bleeding and distal embolization may be more common. The dosages given below are for rt-PA. Heparin (250 IU/h) is usually administered concomitantly to minimize the risk of pericatheter thrombosis.

- **Low-dose infusion** rt-PA is infused directly into the thrombus at a rate of 0.5 mg/h (10 mg rt-PA in 500 mL of normal saline (0.02 mg/mL) run at 25 mL/h). The catheter tip is embedded into the proximal thrombus and the infusion started. Check angiography is performed every 4–6 hours, and the catheter is repositioned distally as necessary. This form of thrombolysis often takes 24–72 hours.
- **Bolus lacing followed by low-dose infusion** The catheter is advanced to the distal portion of the clot and then 5 mg of rt-PA is injected at high concentration (rt-PA 1 mg/mL) as the catheter is pulled back through the proximal clot. A check angiogram is performed every 15–30 minutes. The bolus lacing is performed up to a total of three times (15 mg of rt-PA). If thrombus persists after this, a low-dose infusion is initiated as above.
- **Bolus lacing followed by high-dose infusion** The technique is performed as above, but a high-dose infusion (rt-PA 10 mg in 100 mL, i.e. 0.1 mg/mL) is set up and run at 40 mL/h (4 mg/h) for up to 4 hours. Check angiography is performed every 60–90 minutes. After this, a low-dose infusion is used if indicated.
- **Pulse spray techniques** Pulse spray techniques use special catheters with multiple sideholes or slits. The catheter endhole is occluded with a guidewire and the drug is injected in repeated 0.5 mL (0.05 mg rt-PA) high-pressure pulses every 30 seconds through the sidearm of a Tuohy–Borst adaptor. This creates fissures in the clot, increasing the surface area exposed to the drug, and therefore speeds up lysis. Manual injections are made using a 1 mL syringe; a tame registrar is essential for this, but if none is available use a specialized pump.
- **Coaxial lysis** When there is extensive thrombus it is sometimes desirable to deliver the lytic agent at more than one site. Coaxial systems allow this. The simplest method is to infuse the drug through the arterial sheath into the proximal clot and through the catheter into the distal thrombus (Fig. 14.1). Microcatheters or infusion wires can be used to deliver the drug to the tibial circulation. Infusion wires are 0.035 inch wires with a hollow core (just like a 3Fr catheter); they are used for coaxial lysis.

Procedural care

The patient must be looked after in a high-dependency area where their condition can be closely monitored. This can be on the vascular ward if staffing levels and experience permit.

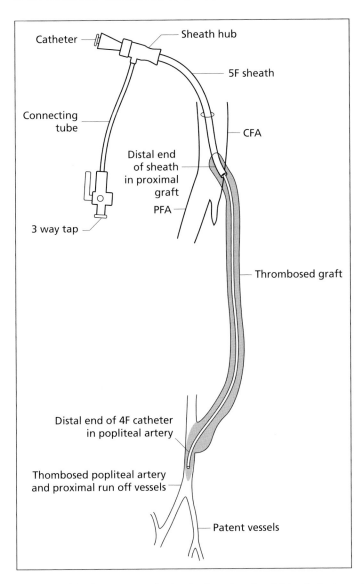

Fig. 14.1 ▮ In the presence of extensive thrombus the distal catheter is used to clear the runoff vessels while the sheath delivers the lytic agent to the graft. It is essential to secure the catheter and sheath. Failure to do so invariably leads to inadvertent removal, and the subsequent haemorrhage is extremely difficult to control. CFA, common femoral artery; PFA, profunda femoris artery.

The patient is nursed in bed as flat as possible. They may have a light diet unless surgery is imminent. The following must be checked:

- Arterial puncture sites every 15 minutes.
- Limb viability – perfusion, pulses, Doppler signal, movement and sensation.
- Urine output – the patient must be kept adequately hydrated. If necessary, IV fluids should be given and the patient catheterized.

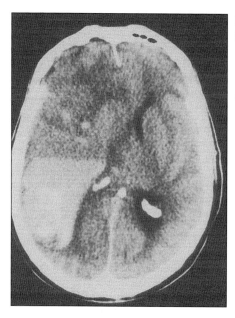

Fig. 14.2 ■ Fatal acute haemorrhagic cerebral infarct during thrombolysis.

- Pulse, BP and temperature 4-hourly.
- Daily FBC, coagulation screen and fibrinogen, urea and electrolytes, glucose.
- Analgesia should be regularly reviewed. Intramuscular injections must not be given.

Tip: It is essential to liaise closely with the surgical team. Keep the treatment plan under review, and be alert to the need for surgical or radiological intervention.

Endpoints

- If the patient's condition allows, thrombolysis is continued until the clot has cleared and flow has been restored. Try not to continue for more than 48 hours.
- Sometimes, there is no clearing of thrombus in between check angiograms. This is termed 'lytic stagnation' and is an indication to stop the procedure.
- Deterioration in the clinical status of the limb may necessitate urgent surgical revascularization.
- Bleeding occurs most commonly at the puncture site, but can occur elsewhere; intra-cerebral (Fig. 14.2) and retroperitoneal bleeding may be fatal. If bleeding occurs, stop the infusion immediately. Confusion and agitation can indicate bleeding; if there is a change in the patient's mental state, the infusion should be stopped pending a thorough assessment.

Adjunctive techniques

Successful thrombolysis usually reveals an underlying stenosis of occlusion. It is mandatory to correct these lesions by endovascular or surgical means. Failure to do so condemns the

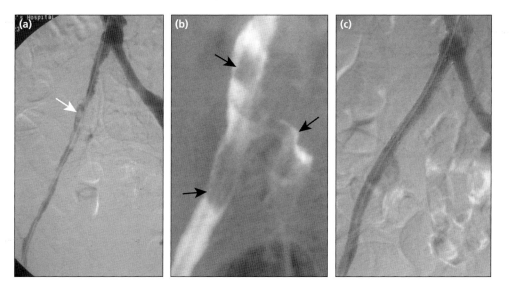

Fig. 14.3 ■ (a) Acute critical limb ischaemia with near occlusion of the right iliac artery (white arrow). (b) Non-subtracted view clearly demonstrates saddle embolus at the right iliac bifurcation. (c) The patient was warfarinized and had recently had a CVA, hence primary stenting was performed and a closure device used.

patient to rethrombosis. Thrombolysis alone may not be sufficient to restore flow. The following techniques may be helpful:

- **Angioplasty and stenting** Used to treat stenoses and occlusions following thrombolysis. In high-risk patients it is worth considering stenting directly over thrombus (Fig. 14.3).
- **Thromboaspiration** See below.
- **Surgical intervention** Embolectomy may be needed if there is distal embolization during thrombolysis. Fasciotomy is indicated if a compartment syndrome develops. This is most likely when there has been prolonged ischaemia and is recognized by painful swollen muscles, often with paralysis. Bypass grafting or graft revisions are performed when thrombolysis reveals underlying disease that is not amenable to endovascular treatment.

Complications

Unfortunately, complications of thrombolysis are not rare and may be life-threatening. Complications increase with the age of the patient, the duration of treatment and the dose of the lytic agent. Stop the infusion if a complication develops.

- CVA, which can be thrombotic or haemorrhagic; overall incidence is 2–3%.
- Significant bleeding requiring transfusion or surgery occurs in 7%. If there is any sign of bleeding, stop the infusion, check the clotting, transfuse the patient with blood and FFP. Consult a haematologist for advice if bleeding persists. Surgical intervention is often necessary. Try to intervene early before the patient becomes unstable.
- Distal embolization of thrombus occurs in about 5% of patients; clinically, it is manifest as acute clinical deterioration with increased pain. Usually there are macroemboli, which will lyse spontaneously or can be aspirated. Microemboli are much more serious and may cause trash foot.

- Reperfusion syndrome is caused when there has been prolonged and severe ischaemia. Adult respiratory distress syndrome and renal failure are common sequelae, and there is a high mortality.

Thrombosuction

This is the endovascular equivalent of balloon embolectomy. Large-bore catheters can be used to aspirate thrombus from grafts and occluded vessels. Typically the technique is used as an adjunct to thrombolysis to accelerate reperfusion when there is a large volume of thrombus to clear. Thrombosuction is relatively safe in prosthetic grafts, which have a large smooth lumen and do not collapse when they thrombose (Fig. 14.4). The catheter can be safely manipulated without a guidewire. The situation is different in diseased native vessels, where repeated catheter passage is undesirable. The principal disadvantage of aspiration thrombectomy is the need for a large arterial puncture (7–8Fr) to permit passage of the catheter.

Equipment

- A sheath with a removable haemostatic valve is essential, or the thrombus will simply be stripped off by the valve during catheter removal.
- Large-lumen catheters: typically 7Fr straight guide-catheter (6Fr lumen) for prosthetic graft and native SFA; 5Fr catheter (4Fr lumen) for native popliteal and crural vessels.
- 50 mL syringe.

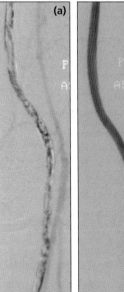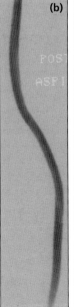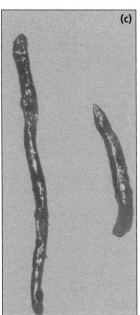

Fig. 14.4 ▓ (a) Thrombosed PTFE graft following (b) thromboaspiration with an 8Fr catheter. (c) Some of the thrombus removed.

Procedure

Access Ipsilateral arterial access is essential.

Catheterization The vessel is catheterized in the conventional manner, but a removable-hub sheath is used.

Technique The aspiration catheter is embedded into the proximal occlusion and then the 50 mL syringe is attached. Pull back the syringe plunger to create a vacuum and advance the catheter until it occludes with thrombus. Maintain suction and withdraw the catheter. When the catheter reaches the sheath, the hub is removed; this prevents thrombus trapping on the haemostatic valve as the catheter is taken out. Quickly put a finger over the sheath until the valve is replaced. Flush the contents of the catheter/syringe through a gauze cloth to allow examination. The procedure is repeated as often as necessary until the vessel is clear.

Troubleshooting

Thrombus cannot be aspirated; there are two main causes
- The thrombus is old: try again after a bolus of thrombolysis to soften the thrombus.
- The catheter/sheath is kinked at the arterial puncture site: replace the sheath and try again, keeping it under slight tension as the catheter is pulled back.

A central core of thrombus is removed but extensive thrombus remains
- This is common in artificial grafts and is a limitation of the technique; use adjunctive thrombolysis to clear residual thrombus.
- Some types of thrombectomy device, e.g. Trerotola, may remove a wider diameter of thrombus.

Thrombus embolizes distally   This is a pitfall of the technique; advancing a large catheter can 'bulldoze' thrombus distally and may even impact it in a distal vessel. Try thrombolysis to clear the block and consider surgical embolectomy if necessary.

Mechanical thrombectomy

Mechanical thrombectomy uses special catheters to macerate the thrombus. The residue is either small enough to pass through the distal circulation or is aspirated. The catheter must be an appropriate size for the vessel, and large sheaths may be necessary. These devices work best with fresh thrombus and small acute emboli.

Equipment

There are several commercially available devices but only a few basic modes of action:
- Impeller-type devices, typified by the Amplatz thrombectomy device (Fig. 14.5a). The impeller is driven by compressed air and rotates at up to 150 000 rpm. This creates a vortex that draws thrombus into the impeller, where it is fragmented into tiny particles that pass through the distal circulation. The catheter is activated by a footswitch and is cooled/lubricated by perfusion with saline. The catheter should not be run for more than 60 seconds at a time.

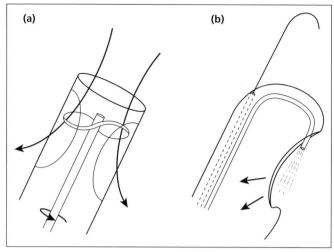

Fig. 14.5 ▨ Mechanical thrombectomy catheters. (a) The Amplatz thrombectomy device. The impeller draws in thrombus, which is macerated and expelled via the side ports. (b) A typical rheolytic catheter. A high-pressure jet creates a vortex, sucking in thrombus and removing the slurry via the exhaust port.

- Rheolytic catheters (Fig. 14.5). These devices utilize an injection pump to create a high-velocity saline jet, which produces a zone of low pressure at the catheter tip. Thrombus is sucked into the jet and is broken up. The resultant slurry is cleared through the catheter into a drainage bag.
- Fragmentation baskets, classically the Arrow–Trerotola device. These devices operate by retracting an outer sheath, which allows a constrained basket of wires to open. Thrombus fragmentation occurs by rapid mechanical rotation of the basket. The Trerotola device is available in both over-the-wire and unguided forms – the device is widely used for thrombectomy within prosthetic dialysis fistulae.

Some of these devices do not operate over a guidewire and hence cannot be steered except with a guide-catheter. The smallest of this type of catheter are 6Fr.

Procedure

Access Ipsilateral vascular puncture is necessary.

Catheterization A standard vascular sheath is used.

Technique Whichever type of device is used, it is switched on just proximal to the thrombus and then advanced slowly into the occlusion. It helps to advance the catheter only a few centimetres and then pull it back and repeat the procedure. This is continued until the vessel is clear. Some manufacturers advocate inflating a blood pressure cuff around the limb distal to an occlusion to prevent distal embolization.

Troubleshooting

The catheter will not pass down the vessel
- There is stenosis or occlusion blocking the way – treat with angioplasty.
- The vessel is tortuous – try directing the catheter with a guide-catheter.

The Amplatz thrombectomy device stops working

- The device will only function for about 15 minutes before it seizes. Use it intermittently and switch off when not advancing the catheter. Don't forget to turn on the saline 'coolant'.
- The catheter has been kinked and the drive shaft has fractured – keep the catheter as straight as possible because, once kinked, it is useless.

The catheter clears a central core but leaves residual thrombus   This is a limitation of the technique. Ensure that the catheter is correctly sized for the vessel – an 8Fr Amplatz thrombectomy device is necessary for the SFA and most grafts; the 6Fr device is suitable for the popliteal artery. Consider adjunctive thrombolysis to clear any remaining thrombus and distal emboli.

The device does not clear the thrombus   Unfortunately, this is not rare – check that the device is activated properly. If it is, then the thrombus is probably too organized to break down. Consider other techniques.

SUGGESTIONS FOR FURTHER READING

Thrombolysis

Consensus report on thrombolysis. J Intern Med 1996;240:343–355.

Belli A-M. Thrombolysis in the peripheral vascular system. Cardiovasc Intervent Radiol 1998;21:95–101.
The big picture of thrombolysis, how and when to do it.

Kessel DO, Berridge DC, Robertson I. Infusion techniques for peripheral arterial thrombolysis (Cochrane Review). Cochrane Library, 1, 2004. Chichester: John Wiley and Sons. CD000985.
Sexy as new techniques sound, there is no evidence that they improve the key outcome measures of amputation rates or mortality.

Percutaneous aspiration thrombectomy

Wagner HJ, Starck EE. Acute embolic occlusions of the infrainguinal arteries: percutaneous aspiration embolectomy in 102 patients. Radiology 1992;182:403–407.
Excellent results from the men who started it all. NB: Uses a selected group of patients without underlying peripheral vascular disease. Note also the high complication rate.

Mechanical thrombectomy

Gorich J, Rilinger N, Sokiranski R et al. Mechanical thrombolysis of acute occlusion of both the superficial and the deep femoral arteries using a thrombectomy device. AJR 1998;170:1177–1180.

Rilinger N, Gorich J, Scharrer-Pamler R et al. Short-term results with use of the Amplatz thrombectomy device in the treatment of acute lower limb occlusions. J Vasc Intervent Radiol 1997; 8:343–348.
Sends a clear message that best results are with emboli.

Rousseau H, Sapoval M, Ballini P et al. Percutaneous recanalization of acutely thrombosed vessels by hydrodynamic thrombectomy (Hydrolyser). Eur Radiol 1997;7:935–941.
Contains a mixture of dialysis access, peripheral grafts and native vessels, and concludes that best results are obtained in dialysis access.

Chapter Fifteen

Embolization

Embolotherapy is the deliberate blockage of blood vessels; it is usually performed to stop haemorrhage and may be life-saving. Embolization is sometimes used as an adjunct to surgery and in the treatment of some benign and malignant tumours. A variety of embolic agents are available to block vessels of different sizes, from arteries to capillaries. Some are temporary and others permanent. The choice of agent to be used depends on the individual circumstances of the case.

General principles

The aim of embolization is to block the target vessel or territory as selectively as possible to minimize 'collateral damage' to non-target structures. Good quality pre-embolization angiography is essential.

The target anatomy A thorough knowledge of the vascular anatomy is essential before embarking on a procedure. Arterial variants are common and must be considered during initial angiography. This is particularly important when there are anastomoses between arterial territories, in which case the outflow and inflow vessels must be blocked. This situation is typified in the case of a gastroduodenal artery aneurysm, which will receive supply from both the hepatic artery and the SMA via the pancreaticoduodenal arcade (Fig. 15.1).

What to block Decide at the outset whether you need to block a feeding vessel or an entire vascular bed, as this influences the choice of embolic agent. In general, to treat bleeding only the source vessel need be blocked, but to treat a tumour the entire tumour circulation should be occluded.

Consent issues Always consider the potential adverse consequences of blocking the target vessel(s) and of collateral damage, especially to end organs. Postembolization syndrome is common when embolizing tumour and solid organs. This should be discussed with the patient and referring clinician, and documented in the notes prior to attempting the procedure.

Which embolic agent The first question to ask is, Will temporary occlusion do the job? Most trauma cases can be satisfactorily treated with temporary occlusion using Gelfoam. Gelfoam occlusion lasts for between a few days and a few weeks and gives the vessel a chance to heal. Gelfoam is readily available, easy to use and prepare, and is fairly safe. If a permanent agent is needed, then determine the size of the target vessel; coils are used to occlude medium-to-small arteries; polyvinyl alcohol (PVA) particles are used to occlude multiple small arteries, arterioles and capillaries. Unless you are expert, avoid the use of liquid embolic agents.

Safety Use separate trolleys when dealing with particulate or liquid embolic agents to prevent contamination of the remaining equipment. Use either different-sized syringes or marked syringes to handle these agents. Discard any contrast, saline or syringes if there is any possibility that they might have mixed with the embolic agent.

Key steps for safe embolization

- Good-quality preliminary angiography.
- Think carefully about collateral pathways.

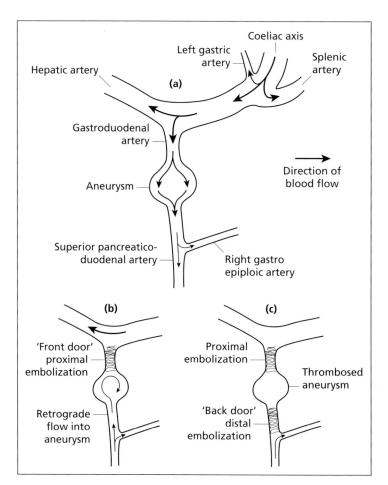

Fig. 15.1 ■ Embolization of a gastroduodenal aneurysm. (a) Aneurysm supplied from the hepatic artery via the gastroduodenal artery. (b) Proximal embolization only closes the 'front door'. The aneurysm is perfused retrogradely via the pancreaticoduodenal arcade. (c) Proximal and distal embolization closes the 'front and back doors'. The aneurysm is no longer perfused and will thrombose.

- Use the shortest, straightest approach, particularly if coils are involved.
- Always use endhole-only catheters.
- Get a stable catheter position and verify with the guidewire if using coils, or test injections of contrast if using particulate agents.
- Use non-heparinized saline to flush catheters and dilute contrast.
- Use continuous fluoroscopy during embolization.
- Perform intermittent runs to demonstrate the effect on flow.

EMBOLIC AGENTS

In broad terms, there are two types of embolic agent: those intended to occlude the target vessel permanently, and those that only induce temporary blockage. Embolic agents may be divided into:
- Mechanical occlusion devices: coils and balloons.
- Particulate agents: PVA, Gelfoam and autologous blood clot.
- Liquid agents: sclerosants and adhesives.

Coil embolization

Coils are permanent embolic agents and are used when you need to block a few feeding vessels or to pack small aneurysms. Coils have three effects:
- They damage the intima, leading to the release of thrombogenic agents.
- They provide a large thrombogenic surface.
- They cause mechanical occlusion of the lumen.

The first two factors are the most important: even the tightest packed coils will not effectively block a vessel without thrombus. There are many different types of coil; most are made of stainless steel or platinum and have fibres attached to promote thrombosis (Fig. 15.2). The coils resemble short segments of guidewire but do not have a central

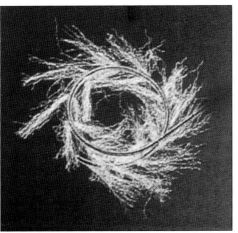

Fig. 15.2 ▨ A typical fibred embolization coil.

mandril. The coil is pushed through the catheter and extruded at its distal end. The rough surface of the coil tends to excoriate the lumen of the catheter, and this can cause considerable problems when multiple coils are required.

 Tip: Not all coils are MRI compatible. Stainless steel coils cause most problems. Check the manufacturer's guidelines if clinically relevant.

What size coil?

There are many types of coil available; all have three size parameters:

- **Diameter of the coil wire** This is equivalent to guidewire diameter and varies from 0.014 to 0.038 inch. Use a coil that is the correct diameter for your delivery catheter – too big and it will not fit; too small and it may jam with the pusher in the catheter.
- **Unconstrained length** This varies with the type of coil, but in general increases with the coiled diameter. Shorter coils are much easier to manage.
- **Diameter of the formed coil** Coils come in a large range of diameters, from 2 mm to over 20 mm. There are even 'straight' coils for blocking tiny vessels, e.g. in the colonic mesentery. Coils should be slightly oversized relative to the diameter of the target vessel, as this allows them to grip the vessel wall and to be closely packed (Fig. 15.3). Grossly oversized coils tend to behave like a guidewire and pass along the vessel rather than coiling up. Undersized coils do not lodge and may migrate. Some coils feature detachment mechanisms to allow them to be retrieved if they are incorrectly sized or misplaced.

 Tip: Coils that form perfect loops are undersized. Correctly sized coils are slightly compressed and have an irregular contour (Fig. 15.4).

For example, on Cook coils a coil labelled 35–5–10 will pass through a catheter that will accept a 0.035 inch guidewire; the total extended length of the coil will be 5 cm and the unconstrained coil diameter will be 10 mm.

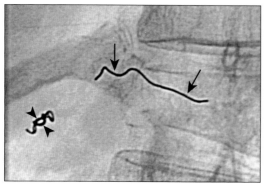

Fig. 15.3 ▇ Embolization of a vertebral artery for renal metastasis. The effect of coil size: 3 mm coils (arrowheads) have packed tightly but a 4 mm coil has remained straight (arrows).

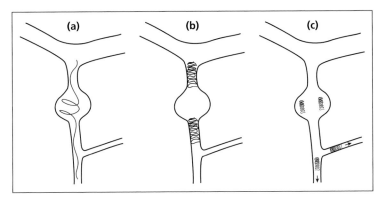

Fig. 15.4 ■ Importance of coil size. (a) Oversized – does not pack down and may not thrombose. (b) Correctly sized – packs tightly in the vessel. (c) Undersized – migrated distally, non-target embolization.

Using coils

Introducing coils into the catheter Coils are held straight in a short cartridge which is discarded after the coil has been pushed into the catheter. The tip of the cartridge is placed into the hub of the catheter and the coil is pushed into the catheter using the stiff end of a straight guidewire. Make sure that you hold the cartridge and the catheter tightly together if you do not want the coil to deploy in the catheter hub!

Tip: Many coils come in opaque cartridges. Dispose of these as soon as they are used to avoid sham deployment.

Coil pushers Once the coil is in the catheter, it is normal to use the reverse end of the guidewire to advance it 10–20 cm along the catheter. Coils can be pushed with conventional straight guidewires or using special pusher wires, two of which merit further consideration:

- Marsmann wires straighten out the coil and minimize catheter excoriation and are used with conventional 0.035–0.038 catheters. The Marsmann wire has a movable core that can be protruded beyond the end of the wire. The core is introduced into the middle of the straightened coil and the coil is pushed out of the cartridge (Fig. 15.5). The coil is introduced into the catheter and advanced to the catheter tip; the central core is then pulled back before the coil is extruded.

A variation on this theme is the Spirale coil (Balt). This is a very soft coil which can be packed very tightly. The Spirale comes in a range of lengths and diameters, both with and without fibres, and is available for microcatheters and conventional catheters. The coil comes on a straightening mandril rather than in a cartridge. The mandril is inserted into the delivery catheter, allowing the coil to be introduced. It is subsequently deployed like a conventional coil (Fig. 15.6).

Tip: The longest Spirale coils are 30 cm long. This is rather daunting even when packing a large aneurysm. It is possible to cut them with sharp scissors to form shorter coils.

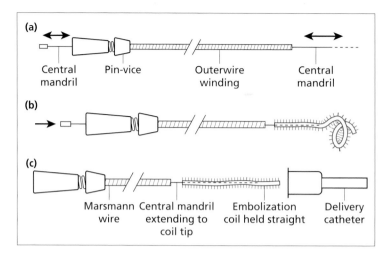

Fig. 15.5 ■ Marsmann-type coil-positioning wire. (a) Construction: the central mandril can be inserted or withdrawn. (b) The mandril is advanced into the coil cartridge and carefully into the central lumen of the coil. The cartridge may then be removed and the coil remains straight on the mandril. (c) The mandril is withdrawn when the coil has reached the end of the catheter and the coil will form normally.

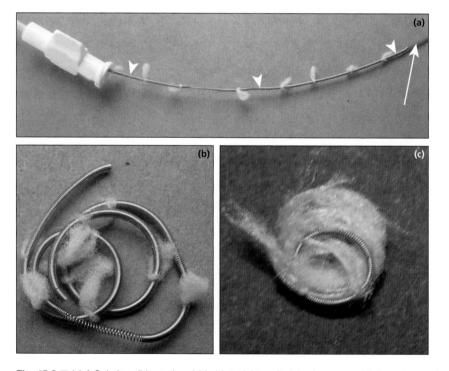

Fig. 15.6 ■ (a) A Spirale coil (arrowheads) held straight on its introducer mandril; there is a pusher (arrow), which is used to introduce the coil into the catheter. (b) Once deployed, the Spirale coil is 'floppy' and will conform to any shape; essentially it is a guidewire without a mandril. (c) A conventional embolization coil forms tight loops of a predetermined diameter.

- **Microcatheter coil pushers** The guidewires supplied with microcatheters cannot be used to deliver coils. Special microcoil pushers have a flexible plastic fibre tip on a stiff metal shaft. They are packaged separately and have to be requested! Use the back end of the wire until the coil is a least 30 cm into the catheter.

> **Tip:** Note how much of the pusher remains outside the catheter when the coil is about 15 cm from deployment. For subsequent coils, do not screen until you reach this stage.

Coil deployment

Position the catheter Before even opening the coil, check the catheter position is stable by passing the coil pusher/guidewire to its tip. If the catheter dislodges during this manoeuvre, it will definitely displace if you try to deploy a coil through it!

Extruding coils This is the stage when things are most likely to go wrong. Be careful to hold the catheter in position as the coil is pushed to its tip. Slowly start to push the coil out of the catheter; you may feel slight resistance as it starts to coil. Make sure that the catheter is not pushed back out of the target vessel. Continue slowly until the whole coil is out of the catheter. Problems are usually associated with incorrect sizing of the first coil, or the temptation to place 'just one last coil'. Avoid the chance of snatching defeat from the jaws of victory by stopping as soon as the vessel is occluded, and by using smaller, shorter coils towards the end of the procedure.

> **Tip:** If you cannot tell where the coil ends and the pusher starts, back the pusher off a few millimetres and look for the gap.

Packing coils To be effective, coils should be tightly packed together (Fig. 15.7). This can only be achieved if the catheter is in a stable position and the coils are correctly sized. Following placement of the first coil, the catheter may have to be pulled back a few millimetres to

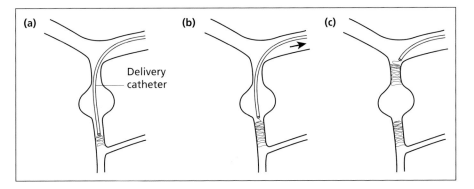

Fig. 15.7 ■ Coil packing. (a) Coils should be tightly packed together in 'nests', starting with the most distal. (b) The catheter should be withdrawn slightly with each coil. (c) Make sure that you leave enough space for the last coil to form in the target vessel.

allow subsequent coils to be deployed. After multiple coils have been deployed it can be difficult to be certain the last coil has been completely deployed and is clear of the catheter; always extrude the guidewire by a few millimetres before backing the catheter position off.

Completion angiography After a few coils have been deployed, perform an angiogram to assess flow. It is helpful to pull the catheter back a little and to inject gently in order not to dislodge newly formed clot. When the flow is very slow, wait for a couple of minutes to see if the vessel thromboses. If there is still brisk flow, then more coils are needed. If the flow has stopped you can usually stop too.

Troubleshooting

Unable to obtain selective catheter position Try using a hydrophilic catheter or a microcatheter. Guide-catheters can be useful in tortuous or aneurysmal vessels. If the optimal position is not obtainable, consider more proximal embolization, but remember that the collateral damage will increase.

Unable to obtain a stable catheter position There are several possible solutions; the basic principles of catheterization apply. Make sure that the catheter is the optimal shape for the vessel. Try a more supportive catheter (larger French size). Use a guide-catheter to support the catheter. Consider an alternative approach, e.g. from the arm rather than the leg.

The delivery catheter is pushed back during coil deployment Concentrate on holding the catheter in position. It is often helpful to get assistance from a colleague, particularly when using coaxial systems. A reasonably long coil that has had less than 25% extruded can sometimes be carefully withdrawn along with the catheter. This clearly risks coil misplacement and must be balanced against the risk of deploying the coil where it is.

A coil is misplaced This usually occurs when the catheter position is not stable, the coil is incorrectly sized, or when deployment is attempted in too short a vessel segment. The coil can either be left where it is or retrieved using a snare or endovascular forceps. Only attempt retrieval if the coil is likely to occlude a significant vessel, otherwise you will probably cause more harm than good!

A coil jams in the delivery catheter This occurs when the coil is the wrong size for the catheter, when there is a tight bend or kink in the catheter, or when the catheter has been damaged by previous coils or particulate agents. Fluoroscope to determine the position of the coil. First try to disimpact the coil by flushing with saline: use a 1 mL syringe, as this gives the highest pressure. If this fails try using the stiff end of the guidewire/pusher; unfortunately, this seldom works. If the coil is in the catheter outside the patient, then cut off the end of the catheter, including the coil. Put a guidewire into the catheter and exchange it for a new one. If the coil is in the catheter inside the patient, there is no option but to remove the catheter, with loss of the position.

Tip: Do not jeopardize a hard-won position: exchange the delivery catheter before it fails if you feel that there is increasing resistance to coil passage. Consider changing the delivery catheter if using coils after polyvinyl alcohol particles.

Detachable balloons

Detachable balloons are used to permanently occlude large vessels, particularly where coil occlusion might be hazardous, e.g. high-flow pulmonary arteriovenous malformations. They are rarely used outside specialist centres, as device preparation and deployment are complex and require an experienced operator.

Particulate embolic agents

Particulate embolic agents are used when blockage of small vessels is desired, e.g. tumour embolization. The smallest particles pass through to capillary level, and their use is likely to cause tissue infarction. There are three principal particulate agents:
- Autologous blood clot
- Gelfoam
- Polyvinyl alcohol particles (PVA).

Blood clot is rarely used and induces only temporary occlusion. Gelfoam pledgets cause thrombosis, which lasts for several days to weeks. PVA is a permanent embolic agent.

Exercise caution when there is arteriovenous shunting. To avoid pulmonary embolization, choose particles that will not pass through the shunt.

When using particulate material, stop embolization when there is virtually no flow in the vessel. If you continue until flow stops, you are left with a loaded catheter; any further injection or flushing will lead to reflux! When flushing the catheter, remember that it contains residual embolic material: careless flushing causes non-target embolization! Flush slowly and carefully with non-heparinized saline until no further contrast emerges; it is then safe to perform angiography.

Gelfoam

Gelfoam is a temporary embolic agent that dissolves after a few days to weeks and comes in two different forms with completely different uses:
- **Gelfoam powder** consists of small particles (40–60 mm in size); vessel occlusion occurs at the capillary level, hence tissue necrosis is likely.
- **Gelfoam sheet** is cut into pledgets 1–2 mm in size and blocks larger vessels; tissue infarction is rare. Gelfoam sheet comes in a variety of thicknesses: choose the thinnest available – some of the thicker sheets could more appropriately be used for loft insulation!

Preparing Gelfoam sheet This is simply prepared using sharp scissors to make parallel cuts about 1mm wide across the sheet until it resembles a comb (Fig. 15.8). This is then trimmed at right-angles to make 1 × 1 mm pieces. The pledgets are soaked in a gallipot of ~20 mL contrast for a few minutes to allow the Gelfoam to soften. Syringing the Gelfoam back and forwards in the gallipot will help soften the particles. When the pledgets become soft and slightly translucent, they are ready to use.

Using Gelfoam sheet Gelfoam pledgets prepared in this way can be injected through conventional angiographic catheters. It is best to suspend the pledgets in 20–40 mL of

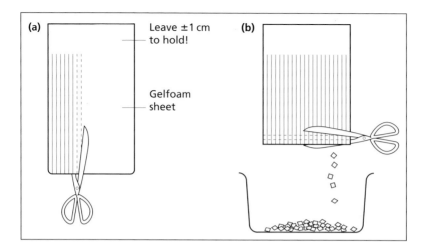

Fig. 15.8 ■ The Gelfoam comb. (a) Cut 1 mm longitudinal strips into the Gelfoam sheet. (b) Cut transversely across the Gelfoam comb. Do not forget to catch the pledgets in a gallipot.

contrast. The soft pledgets can be drawn up into a 5 mL syringe and are injected under continuous fluoroscopic guidance. Gelfoam floats in contrast, and therefore injection should be made with the syringe nozzle pointing upwards. Injection is continued until the flow in the target vessel is almost at a standstill.

Polyvinyl alcohol

PVA comes in a range of particle sizes 150–1000 μm. The particles wedge in vessels of the corresponding diameter, where they cause thrombosis and fibrosis. Particles in the range 300–500 μm are suitable for most purposes.

Preparing PVA One vial of PVA is suspended in 10–20 mL of full-strength contrast. The contrast allows the injection to be visualized on fluoroscopy. The suspension is mixed in a syringe.

Using PVA Aliquots of the suspension are injected slowly in small pulses under fluoroscopic control. Some PVA preparations tend to form clumps of particles; others rapidly 'float' to the top of the suspension. Frequent mixing is required in either case (Fig. 15.9). Check continually for reflux of the suspension. When there is slow flow, make a test injection with contrast to determine a safe rate of injection.

Tip: When using PVA use a 20 mL syringe as a reservoir connected via a three-way tap to a 5 mL syringe to inject the suspension (Fig. 15.9). This greatly simplifies mixing the PVA to avoid aggregation and separation of the suspension.

Microspheres There is an increasing variety of microspheres available, including calibrated PVA and novel compounds which are injected as particulate embolic agents. Do not assume

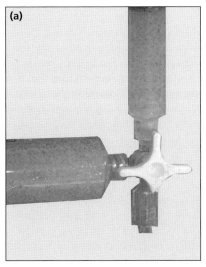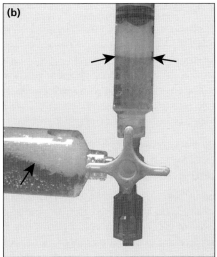

Fig. 15.9 ■ Mixing PVA. (a) Shows the PVA particles evenly suspended in the contrast; this suspension is ready to use. (9b) After about 30 seconds the PVA begins to float to the surface of the contrast (arrows). The suspension requires further mixing before it is used.

that these agents can be used interchangeably as conventional PVA. Early evidence suggests that they can produce adverse effects at particle sizes which would be considered safe with conventional PVA – take care when using these novel compounds.

Autologous blood clot

This is rarely used and is reserved for situations in which a short duration of occlusion is desirable. A sample of the patient's blood is withdrawn and allowed to clot. The clot is then aspirated into a syringe and injected into the target vessel. This is a relatively unpredictable procedure, and in practice is only applicable in high-flow priapism to occlude one of the cavernosal arteries.

Liquid embolic agents

Liquid agents divide into two categories: sclerosants and glues. The former include absolute alcohol and sodium tetradecyl sulphate (STD). The use of tissue adhesives, such as cyano-acrylate, ethibloc and onyx, has also been described, but these products are not readily available and are not licensed for intravascular use in many countries. Liquid agents are certainly the most difficult of the embolic agents to control and are the least forgiving. Their use is best restricted to expert hands, and therefore only a limited discussion is given here.

 Tip: Consider using an occlusion balloon catheter to prevent unwanted reflux of liquid agents during embolization.

Absolute alcohol

Absolute alcohol causes cell death by dehydration. It will damage any tissue it contacts. Extravasation will cause local tissue necrosis. Because alcohol is not visible fluoroscopically, safe injection rates, which do not cause reflux or extravasation, are determined by making test injections of contrast. Frequent check angiography is mandatory to ensure that the situation does not change as thrombosis occurs. As absolute alcohol injection is often very painful, suitable sedation and analgesia must be used. Alcohol is one of the ultimate permanent embolic agents and is used principally to treat vascular malformations and tumours.

Sodium tetradecyl sulphate

STD is commonly used as an adjunct to coil embolization during the treatment of varicocele. A few millilitres of STD are injected after the initial coils have been deployed. Take particular care to avoid spilling STD into the epididymal veins, as this will cause epididymitis. It is not as powerful a sclerosant as absolute ethanol, but should still be used with caution.

CLINICAL SCENARIOS

Varicocele

Embolization of varicocele is requested in symptomatic and subfertile patients. It is an elective procedure and very straightforward. It is therefore an ideal case on which to learn coil embolization.

Equipment
- Basic angiography set.
- Hydrophilic guidewire.
- Hydrophilic Cobra II and Sidewinder II catheters.
- Embolization coils and STD.

Procedure

Access The right CFV is often used, but the right IJV should be considered – the approach is inline and there is no need for bed rest post procedure.

Catheterization Most varicoceles are left-sided; the spermatic vein joins the midpoint of the left renal vein (Fig. 15.10). Catheterize the renal vein with a hydrophilic Cobra II catheter. It may be necessary to use a Sidewinder to catheterize the right spermatic vein, which joins the anterior IVC just below the right renal vein.

Runs Perform a venogram to demonstrate reflux down the spermatic vein. Use a hydrophilic guidewire and the catheter to cannulate the vein. If possible, the catheter should be taken down to the level of the inguinal canal. Deploy coils here and demonstrate blockage of the vein. The catheter is withdrawn to the midpoint of the vein. A further venogram

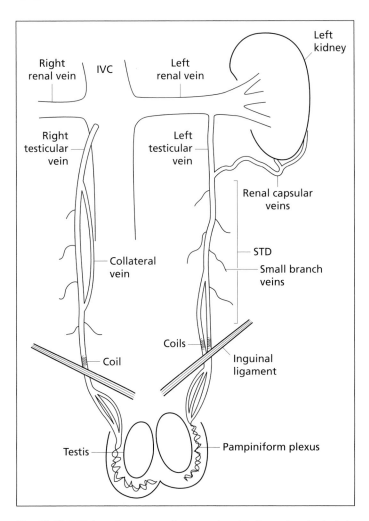

Fig. 15.10 ■ Varicocele anatomy. Coils are placed in the main veins just above the inguinal ligament. Sodium tetradecyl sulphate (STD) may be used to sclerose small branch veins/potential collaterals. IVC, inferior vena cava.

is performed to look for small collateral veins. These can be treated by further coil deployment, or some practitioners may use a liquid sclerosant such as STD. Use with caution, as the gonadal vein may communicate with important structures.

Make sure the coils are large enough to lodge in the spermatic vein or they will become effective pulmonary emboli.

Troubleshooting

The spermatic vein goes into spasm   Relax! Explain to the patient that this is not uncommon and always self-limiting. Give a small dose of GTN (100 mg), wait 1 minute, and then perform a gentle venogram. If the spasm has resolved, be gentle with the vein and this probably will not happen again. If spasm persists, give a further dose of GTN and then go and sit down for 5 minutes before looking again. The spasm will almost certainly have eased by now. If not, be patient. Give more GTN and go for a cup of tea before looking again. When the spasm does resolve, if you and the patient are feeling confident, continue as above.

Uterine Fibroid Embolization (UFE)

This is a relatively new technique that has shown encouraging results in the treatment of symptomatic fibroid disease. The procedure in itself is not particularly technically demanding; however, there is a lot of work in developing and implementing appropriate protocols for assessment, procedural pain relief and postprocedural management. It is essential that the service is delivered in conjunction with a gynaecologist, and in many countries there is a requirement that patients are included in a trial/registry.

Assessment

Patients should have both gynaecological and imaging assessment. The minimum is a pelvic ultrasound, but increasingly pelvic MR examination is used. Fibroid embolization should not be used if the fibroids are pedunculated.

Tip: GnRH analogues may be used in the medical treatment of fibroids. Delay embolization for 3 months after their use, as the uterine arteries are small and extremely difficult to catheterize during treatment.

Equipment
- Hydrophilic 4Fr catheter.
- Hydrophilic wire.
- Microcatheter.
- Particulate embolization, e.g. PVA or microspheres 500–1000 μm.

Technique

Fibroid embolization is a painful procedure and patients generally have severe cramping pain for 12–24 hours, with some milder discomfort lasting for weeks. Analgesia is more effective if given before the onset of pain and at regular intervals. Preprocedural analgesia normally includes a non-steroidal anti-inflammatory drug (NSAID) given by suppository, an intramuscular opiate and an antiemetic.

Bilateral uterine artery embolization is usually required for adequate treatment. The uterine arteries are branches of the anterior division of the internal iliac artery. The internal iliac artery is selectively catheterized with a Cobra catheter. If the uterine artery is suitably large the Cobra can often be advanced directly into the vessel. These vessels are prone to spasm, and a low threshold to using microcatheters should be practised. After selective catheterization has been achieved, embolization with permanent particles is performed, most typically PVA. The endpoint of embolization is to-and-fro flow within the uterine artery.

Intraprocedural analgesia should include an intravenous opiate. Midazolam is often also given to allieviate anxiety.

Alarm: The ovaries are very radiation sensitive, hence there are no figures in this section! Keep radiation to a minimum, use pulsed fluoroscopy if possible, and avoid performing angiographic runs.

Aftercare

Postoperative pain relief is best managed with a patient-controlled analgesia pump. NSAIDs should be continued, and an antiemetic is required. Most patients can be discharged 24–36 hours after the procedure on oral analgesia.

Complications

Fibroid embolization carries significant risks, but these should be balanced against the risks of a surgical procedure. It is essential that the patient receives both adequate information and an opportunity to discuss the potential complications (Table 15.1).

 Consent issue: Patients undergoing UFE are relatively young, and some are hoping to avoid hysterectomy in order to have children. They should be warned not only of the periprocedural risks, but also the possibility of premature menopause and infertility.

Trauma

Embolization is sometimes requested when there is persistent bleeding despite surgery, or when there is a contraindication to surgery. Only undertake this type of treatment if you are confident in your technical ability to perform selective embolization. Make sure that the patient is suitably resuscitated and is stable enough to survive the procedure. Initial angiograms to determine the source of the bleeding should always start with an overview of the target territory and proceed to selective catheterization as required. If a bleeding source is identified, ask the following questions:

- Is the amount of extravasation responsible for the patient's condition? It is possible to overlook another, more significant, source of blood loss. Make sure that this is the only site of bleeding.
- Is the bleeding vessel supplied from a single territory? This has implications for treatment, as both the 'front and back doors' may need to be 'closed'.

Table 15.1 Complications of fibroid embolization	
Premature menopause	2%
Fibroid expulsion	2%
Sepsis	1%
Hysterectomy	1%
Death	<0.01%

- What would be the consequences of occlusion of the vessel? This must always be considered, and is particularly important when dealing with end arteries.
- Is embolization or surgery the appropriate intervention? Embolization is appropriate if it is likely to lead to prompt cessation of bleeding without causing significant collateral damage. Discuss the situation with a senior surgical colleague.

If embolization is the appropriate therapy, perform it at the time of angiography. Gelfoam can be particularly useful where there are multiple bleeding points in one vascular territory, e.g. pelvic trauma. Use coils to embolize larger proximal arterial injuries as selectively as possible, and spare as much normal tissue as you can.

Consent issue: It is often impossible to obtain informed consent in the acute trauma patient, especially if they are ventilated and unconscious. Act in the patient's best interest, and if possible inform relatives what is planned and detail the pros and cons of the procedure.

Hepatic trauma   Blunt hepatic trauma more commonly causes venous injury than arterial injury, but PTC, biliary drainage and hepatic biopsy are all good sources of referral. The typical iatrogenic injury is a small pseudoaneurysm and often requires meticulous angiography for detection (Fig. 23.3). Hepatic arteries are not end arteries, and therefore it is essential to start coil deployment distal to the lesion to prevent collateral 'back-door' filling. Remember that the entire hepatic artery can be occluded if the portal vein is patent; if it is not, selective embolization is required, which should prevent hepatic infarction owing to the presence of intrahepatic collaterals.

Pelvic trauma   Major pelvic trauma is often accompanied by significant arterial and venous injury. Bleeding often stops when the fracture is stabilized. Patients with unstable fractures should have external pelvic fixation applied before angiography. If embolization is required, try not to occlude both internal iliac arteries as this increases the risk of pelvic ischaemia. Remember, even relatively minor pelvic fractures can cause major arterial haemorrhage (Fig. 15.11).

Renal trauma   This is often iatrogenic following biopsy and can usually be embolized highly selectively. Make sure that there are two kidneys before embolizing a large amount of renal tissue. Renal arteries are end arteries, therefore there is no need to worry about collaterals, just infarction.

Tip: Be pragmatic. If the patient is haemorrhaging and unstable, stop the bleeding and sacrifice the kidney. Don't waste precious time trying to perform highly selective embolization (Fig. 15.12).

Gastrointestinal bleeding   Embolotherapy has been described in the treatment of gastrointestinal bleeding in both the small and the large bowel. Duodenal bleeding can be safely treated because of the extensive collateral supply. Bleeding sites beyond the ligament of Treitz can be embolized, but the risk of infarction is much greater and embolization should only be undertaken if it can be performed highly selectively. The classic scenario is the gastroduodenal artery aneurysm caused by pancreatitis. This can be treated by embolization of the proximal and distal vessels (Fig. 15.13).

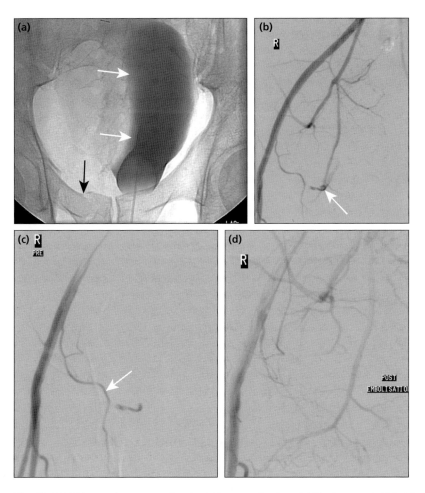

Fig. 15.11 ▧ Haemorrhage secondary to pubic ramus fracture. (a) Displacement of bladder by haematoma (white arrows), fracture (black arrow). (b) Initial angiogram suggesting extravasation (arrow) is from the internal iliac artery. (c) External iliac artery angiogram showing bleeding from the corona mortis branch of the external iliac artery (arrow). (d) Following embolization the patient stabilized.

Embolotherapy

Complications

Embolotherapy has a high potential for complications and catastrophes. Obviously, all the standard complications of diagnostic angiography are present, but the risks of vessel dissection are increased owing to the need to obtain selective catheter positions. Risks unique to embolization must be discussed with the patient before the procedure, and include:

- **Postembolization syndrome** Postembolization syndrome occurs as a consequence of tissue infarction, with the subsequent release of vasoactive substances and other inflammatory mediators. It is most common with solid organ embolization, e.g. the liver, and broadly related to the extent of tissue infarction. After embolization, patients typically develop severe pain within hours and over the next 24–72 hours have fever, nausea and

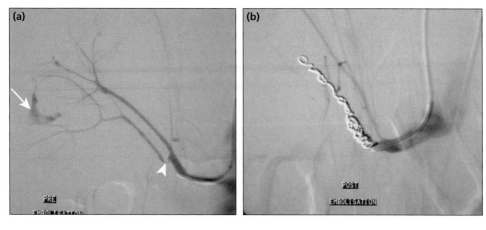

Fig. 15.12 ■ Postbiopsy haemorrhage. (a) Selective renal angiogram showing brisk extravasation (arrow) from a lower polar branch vessel with stenosis at its origin (arrowhead). The entire kidney is displaced upwards by the retroperitoneal haematoma. (b) Following non-selective embolization.

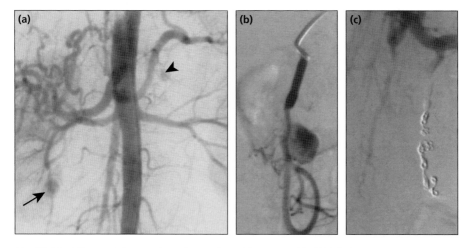

Fig. 15.13 ■ Recurrent haemorrhage in a patient with pancreatitis. (a) A flush aortogram shows false aneurysms of the gastroduodenal artery (GDA) (arrow) and left adrenal (arrowhead) arteries. (b) Selective catheterization of the GDA. (c) Completion angiography showing aneurysm exclusion. Note that the coils extend beyond the aneurysm to 'close the back door'.

vomiting, myalgia, arthralgia, and general debility. Affected patients need support with appropriate analgesia, intravenous fluids and nursing care. Symptoms tend to subside after ~72 hours, but it can be a worrying time for both the patient and the clinician.

- **Non-target embolization** As we explained earlier, with some skill and determination it is usually possible to retrieve a misplaced coil. Unfortunately, non-target embolization with permanent particulate or liquid agents is irretrievable. The consequences are dependent on the vascular bed affected, but may be life-threatening. Clearly, great care to avoid this complication is the aim, but for each case you must be aware of the potential innocent bystanders, and prompt recognition and appropriate treatment, surgical or otherwise, may be life-saving.

Abscess formation   Ischaemic and infarcted tissue makes a great culture medium, and prophylactic antibiotics are essential if a significant volume of tissue is embolized. If patients are persistently pyrexial after embolization, then blood cultures and appropriate imaging are needed.

Tissue necrosis   Necrosis occurs when a tissue has been completely devitalized, usually by occlusion of the capillary bed. This can occur with physical occlusion using very small-particle PVA, or with absolute alcohol, which also causes perivascular necrosis. The result will be tissue infarction in solid organs, or loss of overlying skin in more peripheral territories.

SUGGESTIONS FOR FURTHER READING

Embolic materials
Old articles, but then the technique is not recent!

Chow KJ. Transcatheter embolization with sodium tetradecyl sulfate: Experimental and clinical results. Radiology 1984;153:95–99.

Gianturco C, Anderson JH, Wallace S. Mechanical devices for arterial occlusion. AJR 1975; 124:428–435.
The original embolization coils.

Kunstlinger F, Brunelle F, Chaumont P et al. Vascular occlusive agents. AJR 1981;136:151–156.
All the original particulate embolic agents and glue.

Tadavarthy SM, Moller JH, Amplatz K. Polyvinyl alcohol foam (Ivalon): A new embolic material. AJR 1975;125:609–616.

Technique
There is no comprehensive review of embolotherapy, so here are a variety of articles covering some important areas.

Drooz AT, Lewis CS, Allen TA et al. Quality improvement guidelines for percutaneous transcatheter embolization. J Vasc Intervent Radiol 1997;8:889–895.
Standards for embolotherapy set by the SCVIR. Defines acceptable targets for success and failure.

Fenely MR, Pal MK, Nockler IB et al. Retrograde embolization and causes of failure in the primary treatment of varicocoele. Br J Urol 1997;80:642–646.

Fernando HC, Stein M, Benfield JR et al. Role of bronchial artery embolization in the management of hemoptysis. Arch Surg 1998;133:862–866.

Gomes AS. Embolization therapy of congenital arteriovenous malformations: Use of alternative approaches. Radiology 1994;190:191–198.

Katz MD, Teitelbaum GP, Pentecost MJ. Diagnostic arteriography and therapeutic embolization for post traumatic pelvic embolization. Semin Intervent Radiol 1992;9:4–12.
A clear overview.

Nicholson AA, Ettles DF, Hartley JE et al. Transcatheter coil embolotherapy: A safe and effective option for major colonic haemorrhage. Gut 1998;43:79–84.
Embolize distally and with caution.

Nicholson AA. Vascular radiology in trauma. Cardiovasc Intervent Radiol 2004;27:105–120.
A comprehensive overview of strategies for diagnosing and treating vascular trauma.

Pelage JP, Le Dref O, Mateo J et al. Life-threatening primary postpartum hemorrhage: Treatment with emergency selective arterial embolization. Radiology 1998;208:359–362.

Seppanen SK, Lepppanen MJ, Pimenoff G et al. Microcatheter embolization of hemorrhages. Cardiovasc Intervent Radiol 1997;20:174–179.
Selective coil and PVA embolization in haemorrhage.

Sonomura T, Yamada R, Kishi K et al. Dependency of tissue necrosis on gelatin sponge particle size after canine hepatic artery embolization. Cardiovasc Intervent Radiol 1997;20:50–53.
Size is important! Emphasizes the effect of particle size on target organ damage.

Worthington-Kirsch RL, Popky GL, Hutchins FL. Uterine arterial embolization for the management of leiomyomas: Quality of life assessment and clinical response. Radiology 1998;208:625–629.
Currently very topical.

Venous intervention

Percutaneous placement of IVC filters and treatment of superior vena cava obstruction (SVCO) are the cornerstones of venous intervention. Venous angioplasty, stenting and thrombolysis are sometimes performed, but remain controversial except in the management of haemodialysis access. The principles of negotiating and treating venous stenoses and occlusions are exactly the same as for the arterial system. This chapter covers some established indications for venous intervention and details aspects of intervention specific to the venous system.

IVC filters

IVC filters are placed to prevent pulmonary embolism from sources in the lower limbs, pelvis and IVC. Contemporary devices are readily placed percutaneously via the right IJV or femoral veins. Several permanent and some retrievable filters are commercially available. Temporary filters have largely been superseded by their removable counterparts.

Indications for IVC filtration

There are only two unquestionable indications for placement of a permanent IVC filter; several further indications may also be valid and should be considered on a case-by-case

Table 16.1 Indications for caval filtration and recommended filter type	
Indication	**Filter type**
Unequivocal	
Recurrent PE despite adequate anticoagulation	P
PE with contraindication to anticoagulation	P
Relative	
Free-floating ileofemoral/IVC thrombus with a high risk of embolization	P/R
Patients with PE and severely limited cardiorespiratory reserve	P
Spinal cord injury with paraplegia	P
Severe trauma	P/R
Prophylactic – before surgery on patients at high risk of DVT or PE, e.g. before hip surgery in the presence of ipsilateral femoral DVT	R
P, permanent; R, retrievable.	

basis (Table 16.1). Thrombosis rates vary between devices; overall, about 10% of permanent IVC filters will thrombose within 5 years. Permanent filters should be avoided whenever possible in patients with a long-life expectancy. Retrievable IVC filters can be removed a variable time after placement: the Gunther tulip filter should be removed within 2 weeks of insertion, as after this it will incorporate into the vein wall. Some of the latest devices on the market claim to be removable for 12 months or more (e.g. Recovery filter, Bard).

There are a few contraindications to caval filtration when there is a high risk of major pulmonary embolus. Introducer sheaths for IVC filters start at 7Fr and increase to 24Fr, and therefore coagulation must be checked. Coagulopathy should be corrected if possible, and if necessary venotomy can be performed. Insertion of large catheters into the femoral vein is itself a cause of DVT, hence the jugular approach has a distinct advantage!

Equipment

- Ultrasound for right IJV puncture.
- Basic angiography set.
- Cobra catheter.
- 3 mm J guidewire.
- An appropriate IVC filter set (see below).

IVC filters are supplied with different delivery systems designed for use from either the jugular or the femoral approach. Not all systems are interchangeable, so make sure that you have the correct device! Check also that you have an appropriately sized device for the IVC. The bird's nest filter is currently the only one that can be placed in a megacava.

Procedure

Access The right IJV is the 'universal gateway' and can be used for access even in the presence of ileofemoral DVT. Some filters have inflexible delivery systems and cannot be delivered from the left jugular or the left femoral vein.

Make sure that there is a contemporary ultrasound to document the site and extent of thrombus. Placing a catheter through a thrombosed vein is likely to result in iatrogenic PE!

Catheterization For the jugular route, use a Cobra catheter and 3 mm J guidewire to carefully negotiate through the right atrium to the IVC. For the femoral route, simply place a pigtail catheter at the iliac venous confluence.

Runs Angiography is required for three reasons:
- To demonstrate the patency of the IVC and assess its size.
- To document the position of the renal veins.
- Pulmonary angiography may be needed to confirm the diagnosis of PE, and sometimes also for pulmonary thrombectomy.

It is usually sufficient to perform a simple IVC injection through a pigtail catheter placed just above the confluence of the iliac veins. An initial gentle hand injection will ensure that there is no thrombus adjacent to the catheter; perform a more vigorous injection to demonstrate the entire IVC. The position of the renal veins is usually apparent because of streaming of unopacified blood (Fig. 16.1). If the renal veins cannot be identified, use a Cobra catheter to engage them and perform selective hand injections to demonstrate their position.

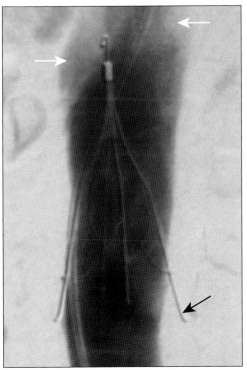

Fig. 16.1 ▨ IVC venogram performed prior to removal of IVC filter. Note the streaming effect of unopacified blood from the renal veins (white arrows). It is not uncommon to see a filter leg protruding through the IVC wall (black arrow): this does not preclude removal.

Tip: Use the patient's spine as a reference for the position of the renal veins and to measure the IVC. If your angiography equipment does not include measurement software it is helpful to place a radio-opaque ruler to the left of the spine.

Once the position of the renal veins has been established, do not move the table or the image intensifier. Do not forget to measure the diameter of the infrarenal IVC. Most IVC filters can only be used in a specified range of IVC diameters; if the filter is too small, the first place it will lodge is the tricuspid valve!

Positioning the filter There are two sites to place an IVC filter, and the position is determined from the cavogram.

- **Infrarenal** This is the optimal site; if the filter causes IVC thrombosis, the renal veins will be spared. Conical filters should be placed with the apex at the level of the renal veins; the high flow promotes dissolution of thrombus trapped or formed within the filter.
- **Suprarenal** In the presence of infrarenal thrombus a filter can be sited between the renal and hepatic veins. In this position, filter thrombosis can lead to renal vein thrombosis and renal infarction.

Deploying the filter Each type of filter is deployed differently, and there may even be differences for a single type of filter, depending on whether the jugular or the femoral route is used. Read the instructions carefully before use; if you do not understand them, seek help!

Alarm: If there is no contraindication, the patient should be anticoagulated while the filter is in situ to minimize the chance of filter thrombosis.

Bird's nest filter   The bird's nest filter comes with a long and very comprehensive set of instructions. The filter comprises two V-shaped anchoring struts and a very fine mesh of wire that sits between the struts, rather like an IVC Brillo pad! The deployment device consists of an outer sheath with an inner wire pusher, which is attached to the filter. The device is fairly complicated to use but has the advantage of being able to be placed in caval diameters up to 45 mm.

The deployment can be thought of in three stages (Fig. 16.2):
1. Deploy the first anchoring strut – the pusher is held in place and the sheath retracted.
2. Deploy the bird's nest wires – the pusher is held stationary and the sheath is retracted by 2–3 cm to give the nest space to form. While the sheath is held stationary, the filter wires are deployed by advancing the inner pusher until the junction point of the proximal hook wires is seen.
3. Deploy the second anchoring strut – the pusher and sheath are advanced to overlap the struts and the sheath is retracted to deploy the proximal anchoring strut. The filter is then released from the deployment mechanism using the push button at the end of the mechanism.

These instructions are essential and referred to during the procedure, even by experienced operators!

Gunther tulip removable filter   This is a simple conical filter which can be placed from either the jugular or the femoral approach. The filter has a small hook at the apex which

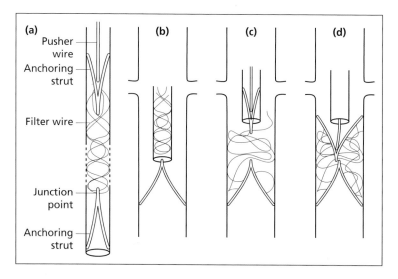

Fig. 16.2 ▪ Key steps in the deployment of the bird's nest filter (jugular deployment): (a) Filter in delivery catheter. (b) Deploy the proximal anchoring struts – the sheath is retracted. (c) Deploy the filter wires – the inner pusher wire is advanced. (d) Deploy the distal anchoring struts – the sheath is retracted.

allows retrieval using a snare and specialized retrieval kit. Separate femoral and jugular devices are required.

Filter removal Before attempting removal, perform a cavogram to see if there is any residual thrombus either in the filter (Fig. 16.3) or which would threaten significant PE. If there is less than 1 cm^3 of thrombus in the filter, it can be removed. The filter has a hook at its apex which can be snared from the jugular vein to allow it to be resheathed. It can be removed up to 2 weeks after placement, or left as a permanent filter. The snare must be placed at the top of the hook; the snare is held in place and the sheath advanced over it to close the filter (Fig. 16.3). The sheath and filter are removed together; even if the filter appeared completely clean there is always thrombus/tissue on the struts (Fig. 16.4).

 Tip: An alternative to exchanging the Gunther tulip after 2 weeks is to reposition it within the IVC. Ideally, if this needs to be performed more than once or twice the filter should be exchanged for an alternative design, such as the Bard Recovery Filter.

Complications

Significant procedure-related complications are rare and include:
- Access site thrombosis.
- Femoral vein thrombosis: this was particularly common with early devices, but with smaller contemporary devices is seen in only 2–3% of patients.

IVC perforation   Filter struts may perforate the caval wall; this is rarely clinically significant, but may make the filter irretrievable.

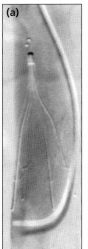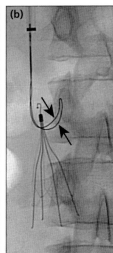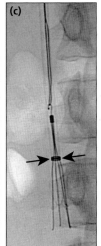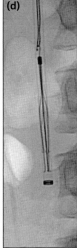

Fig. 16.3 ■ Removal of a Gunther tulip inferior vena cava (IVC) filter. (a) Initial IVC angiogram demonstrates that the filter is free of thrombus. (b) The snare (arrows) is passed over the filter and the apex of the hook is snared. (c) The filter closes as the sheath (arrows) is advanced over it. (d) When the filter is fully inside the sheath, they are removed together.

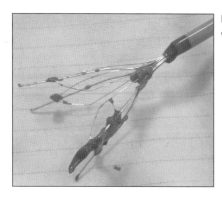

Fig. 16.4 ▦ Thrombus on filter struts despite normal venogram.

Incorrect deployment   There are four forms of incorrect deployment:
- Malposition in relation to the renal veins: if you have placed a permanent filter you are stuck, whereas a removable filter can be repositioned.
- Incorrect filter sizing: at worst, this will result in fatal embolization of the filter. More commonly it results in tilting or incorrect opening.
- Conical filters can be tilted: this may impair filter function.
- The filter may open incorrectly so that the struts are not evenly distributed. This is particularly common with the Greenfield filter, and it may also impair filter function.

If there is severe misalignment, a second filter may have to be placed above the first.

Late complications
- IVC thrombosis. This is seen in at least 10% of patients with Greenfield and bird's nest filters. Caval thrombosis is serious if suprarenal. Thrombosis of the infrarenal IVC is usually compensated by the development of ascending lumbar collaterals. Remember that until recently, surgical ligation of the IVC used to be the treatment for recurrent PE!
- Structural failure of the filter. This has led to several filter designs being withdrawn from the market.

The long-term structural integrity and patency of the newer designs of IVC filters remain to be established.

Superior vena cava obstruction

SVCO causes distressing symptoms including facial and upper limb oedema, headache and drowsiness. The majority of cases are secondary to intrathoracic malignancy, particularly central bronchogenic carcinoma. Patients with malignant SVCO usually have a poor life expectancy, and the aim of therapy is palliation of symptoms. Unless SVCO is treated promptly, extensive venous thrombosis often develops and greatly increases the complexity of intervention.

Alarm: SVCO is a palliative treatment; however, it is associated with a significant mortality and patients need to be aware that there is a procedure-related mortality rate of approximately 2–4%.

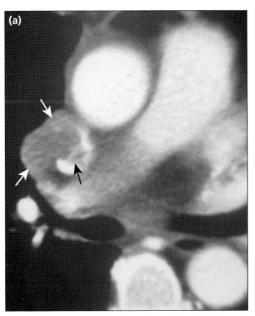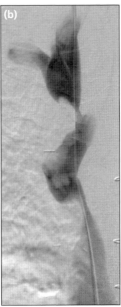

Fig. 16.5 ■ SVCO (a) Initial CT shows tumour adjacent to (white arrows) and invading the SVC (black arrow). (b) The venogram performed via a sheath in the RIJV confirms the findings.

SVCO is one of the most gratifying conditions for the interventional radiologist to treat: patients often feel a marked improvement immediately the stent is deployed.

Assessing SVCO

The aim of investigation is to delineate the extent of the venous obstruction and thrombosis and to plan the subsequent intervention. Many patients will have had chest CT, which will usually serve to delineate the cause and extent of the problem; it will also demonstrate complicating factors such as tumour invasion or thrombosis (Fig.16.5). Patients may have had bilateral upper limb venography to assess the peripheral and central veins. Remember, peripheral injection often fails to opacify the central veins (Fig. 16.6). If the jugular veins are patent, simply place a 4Fr dilator in the RIJV to perform venography; otherwise, central catheterization should be performed using 4Fr straight catheters placed via the basilic veins (Fig. 16.6).

 Tip: When assessing the central veins, ideally perform central injections (Fig.16.5) or perform simultaneous bilateral injection to minimize flow artefacts (Fig. 16.6).

Treatment of SVCO

There are two very different clinical scenarios:
- **Uncomplicated stenosis or occlusion** This is quick and easy to treat. Benign strictures may respond to angioplasty alone, but the majority of neoplastic lesions will be treated by primary stenting (Fig. 16.6c).

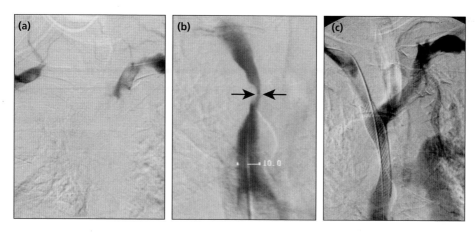

Fig. 16.6 ■ Superior vena cava obstruction. (a) Peripheral injection does not demonstrate the central veins. (b) Injection through a catheter in the innominate vein demonstrates a simple stenosis. Note measurement of the SVC diameter. (c) Following deployment of a single Wallstent, excellent bilateral drainage is restored.

- **SVCO complicated by thrombosis** The aim of treatment is to re-establish flow without causing pulmonary embolism. There are two distinct strategies: primary stenting, and stenting following thrombolysis and thrombectomy. The former is quick but may require additional stents. The thrombus is often organized and difficult to clear, making thrombolysis and thrombectomy a more complicated and time-consuming option.

Equipment

- Basic angiography set.
- Guidewires: curved hydrophilic wire, Amplatz superstiff wire 180 and 260 cm.
- Catheters: 4Fr straight, Cobra II, Berenstein, 80 cm, 8, 10, 12 and 15 mm angioplasty balloons.
- Sheaths: 5Fr, 7Fr and 10Fr.
- Stents: 8–16+ mm diameter.
- Vascular snares: 10 and 25 mm are sometimes required.

Procedure

Access The obstruction is often more readily traversed from the right internal jugular vein – the shortest, most stable route – and can readily accommodate large sheaths.

Catheterization Cross stenoses in a standard fashion using a shaped catheter and a hydrophilic wire. Exchange for an Amplatz wire before angioplasty/stenting. If necessary, cross the lesion from the arm and then exchange for a 260 cm guidewire, which can be snared and brought out of a femoral sheath. This 'bodyflossing' technique can be used to encourage catheters to pass around unfavourable angulations and through very tight stenoses.

Tip: When 'bodyflossing', a small catheter placed from the arm can be used to stabilize the position of an angioplasty balloon or stent by abutting the two catheters.

Runs Perform venography to delineate the obstruction and demonstrate the major collateral channels. Assess the extent and distribution of any thrombus.

Technique As a general rule, if there is not much thrombus it can be stented directly, but when there is extensive thrombosis an attempt should be made to debulk it by thrombolysis or mechanical thrombectomy. Most operators try to avoid thrombolysis; however, when performed it is usually using a low-dose infusion technique. It is essential that cerebral metastases be excluded by CT scanning, and that other potential bleeding sites such as the primary tumour are considered before starting thrombolysis. Thrombectomy with the Amplatz thrombectomy device can be very successful with fresh thrombus, but unfortunately the thrombus is often organized. Thrombectomy will not clear all the venous thrombus, but rather will create a central channel that will allow it to be stented over.

Choose the shortest stent that will completely cover the lesion. Choose a stent diameter that will be firmly anchored in the stricture: in practice, 12–16 mm. Do not leave the end of the stent in the right atrium, as it may cause emboli or even perforation. The stent will need to be balloon-dilated to an appropriate diameter. Following deployment, perform a venogram to demonstrate patency. If there is poor flow or extensive collateral filling, perform further angioplasty and consider further stent deployment.

Alarm: In the presence of thrombosis there is a risk of pulmonary embolus during stent placement, especially if the stent is placed from the femoral approach, as the stent opens from the jugular towards the SVC. Stents deployed from the jugular vein open from the SVC towards the jugular vein and so tend to trap the thrombus against the SVC wall as they are deployed.

Troubleshooting

Both brachiocephalic veins are involved   When there is bilateral obstruction, it is usually only necessary to treat one side.

There is a large discrepancy in size between the venous segments to be stented
This is an indication to use a Wallstent, which will taper to fit the narrower vessel. This will significantly increase its final length, so make sure that you allow for this.

The patient becomes hypoxic or hypotensive   Resuscitate them promptly and consider the possibility of pulmonary embolism or SVC perforation. Perform a venogram; if there is evidence of a leak then a covered stent should be deployed. SVC perforation can lead to rapid cardiac tamponade and death. If the venogram is negative then perform a pulmonary angiogram, and if there is a large embolism try to macerate it with a catheter.

Inferior vena cava obstruction

This is considerably less common than SVCO, but again mainly secondary to advanced tumour. Affected patients often have gross leg and lower body oedema. The basic principles are identical to those for SVCO, but particular care should be taken to avoid stenting over the renal or hepatic veins. The IVC is large calibre and there is a significant potential for stent migration, so choose a suitable stent diameter carefully.

Transjugular intrahepatic portosystemic shunt

The TIPS procedure involves forming a tract between the hepatic vein and the portal vein, thus shunting blood away from liver sinusoids and reducing portal venous pressure. The principal indication for TIPS is variceal haemorrhage not controlled by endoscopic banding or injection sclerotherapy. TIPS can also be used in the management of refractory ascites and in Budd–Chiari syndrome. It is a complex procedure with a limited durability which requires follow-up and, in a significant number of patients, reintervention. There is a 1% procedure-related mortality and a risk of new or worsening hepatic encephalopathy.

Anatomy for TIPS

TIPS tracts are formed between a hepatic vein and either the left or the right branch of the portal vein. Although any of the hepatic veins can be used, it is easiest and safest to pass from the right hepatic vein (RHV) into the right portal vein (Fig. 16.7). The RHV bears a reasonably constant position posterior and superior to the right portal vein (RPV). Bile ducts and hepatic artery branches frequently lie in between the RHV and the RPV and are often opacified during the procedure.

The middle hepatic vein may lie anterior to the RPV, and therefore punctures may need to be angled posteriorly. Anterior punctures from the middle hepatic vein risk capsular perforation. It can be difficult to differentiate the RHV from the middle hepatic vein in the AP projection, but this is easily done from a lateral projection.

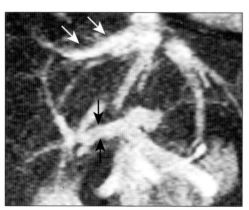

Fig. 16.7 ■ MRI showing the relationship of the hepatic veins to the portal bifurcation. The right hepatic vein (white arrows), which lies posterior and superior to the right portal vein (black arrows), is the optimal approach.

Guidance for TIPS procedure

The principal difficulty with the procedure is targeting the portal vein puncture. The position of the portal vein can be imaged in several ways. Wedged hepatic venography using conventional contrast or CO_2 can be used to fill the portal vein retrogradely (Fig. 16.8). An arterioportogram may be performed from an SMA injection and the position of the vein marked on the intensifier screen. Ultrasound allows real-time targeting, but relying on a colleague to direct the puncture with ultrasound will strain all but the best relationships. Percutaneous portal vein puncture can also allow targeting, but this increases the risk of the procedure.

 Tip: If you don't have CO_2 angiography and want to show the relative positions of the RHV and RPV, perform a hepatic venogram during the portal vein phase of an arterioportogram.

Equipment

- Basic angiography set.
- Guidewires: 3 mm J, curved hydrophilic wire (stiff), Amplatz wire.
- Cobra catheter, angioplasty balloons 8, 10 and 12 mm × 4 cm.
- 5Fr sheath.
- TIPS set (e.g. Cook UK Ltd)
  – 40 cm 10Fr sheath with endmarker
  – 51 cm curved guide-catheter with metal stiffener
  – 60 cm long sheathed needle.

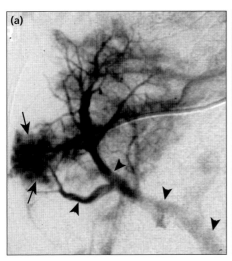 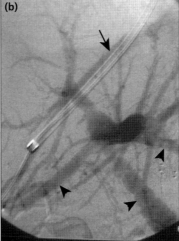

Fig. 16.8 ▦ Wedged hepatic venography. (a) Conventional contrast is forced into the sinusoids, causing a dense parenchymal blush (arrows), and then flows retrogradely into the portal vein (arrowheads). The portal bifurcation is clearly seen. (b) CO_2 wedged venogram showing the portal vein (arrowheads) and the hepatic vein (arrow). CO_2 opacifies the portal vein more reliably than conventional contrast.

- TIPS stents and stent-grafts 8, 10 and 12 mm.
- Vascular pressure transducer (to measure portosystemic pressure gradient).
- Ultrasound for right IJV puncture.

Procedure

TIPS is a painful procedure – sometimes for the operator as well as the patient – which will probably take you a long time to master. Leave yourself 3–4 hours for the case. Think of the patient and consider general anaesthesia; if you do not do this, the patient will require heavy sedation. This is easiest with anaesthetic assistance, as anaesthetic staff will also monitor the patient; variceal bleeders with hepatic encephalopathy are unstable.

Before starting, establish that the portal vein is patent using Doppler ultrasound. If there is portal vein thrombosis, then stop and seek expert advice.

Access Ultrasound-guided right IJV puncture.

Catheterization Introduce the TIPS sheath into the SVC. Pass the J wire and Cobra catheter into the IVC, taking particular care when steering through the right atrium. The RHV is the target vein. Rotate the catheter so that its tip points towards the patient's right, and slowly withdraw it until the tip engages the vein. Advance the hydrophilic wire and Cobra catheter into the vein.

Runs Perform a wedged hepatic venogram by advancing a 4Fr catheter into a distal and peripheral tributary of the hepatic vein. If the catheter is wedged there will usually be a satisfying sucking sound when the wire is removed. A gentle injection of contrast or CO_2 will demonstrate enhancement of the hepatic parenchyma, and may even show the portal vein. If the catheter is not wedged try a different position; if it is wedged, perform a run centred over the portal bifurcation (about 4 cm lateral to the spine, on the right!), including from the bottom of the right atrium down. This will show the relative positions of the portal vein confluence and the hepatic vein origin. If wedged venography fails, perform arterioportography with simultaneous hepatic venography. When you have obtained a good image, mark the positions of the portal veins and the hepatic vein on the screen with a chinagraph pencil, and lock the tabletop in position.

Further catheterization Place an Amplatz wire into the RHV and advance the TIPS sheath 4–5 cm into the vein. Exchange the Cobra catheter for the curved guide-catheter and advance this just beyond the tip of the sheath. The angled stiffener within the sheath gives excellent torque control but poor cornering ability, and will only negotiate suitably angled veins.

Puncturing the portal vein This is easy to describe but is one of those practical procedures that takes quite a lot of experience to really get the hang of. Remove the guidewire; remember that the RPV lies anterior to the RHV; and turn the guide-catheter so that the metal arrow points anteriorly and slightly to the right. Slowly pull the guide-catheter back until its tip is 2–3 cm into the RHV. Now advance the sheathed needle through the guide-catheter; aim to hit the RPV 1–3 cm from the portal bifurcation. Resistance is felt as the needle passes into the liver parenchyma; cirrhotic liver is particularly tough. The needle is passed out of the catheter in the direction of the RPV. Do not go beyond the projected portal vein position. It is common to feel increased resistance as the portal tract is reached, and a 'give' as the portal vein is entered. Withdraw the needle and attach a 5 mL syringe containing 2 mL of contrast to the catheter. Slowly pull the catheter back, aspirating as you go. As soon as you aspirate blood, stop and perform a short contrast run. There are three possibilities:

- Contrast flows towards the right atrium – you are still in the hepatic vein.
- Contrast flows towards the periphery of the liver – you are in either the portal vein or the hepatic artery. Portal vein branches are larger and are often visible to the periphery of the liver.
- Contrast flows towards the portal bifurcation and does not clear – you are in the bile duct.

If you are in the portal vein, congratulations! If not, continue pulling back until the catheter is in the guide-catheter. Put the needle back, redirect the guide-catheter and try again. Remember Robert the Bruce and his spider and, try, try and try again until the portal vein is entered.

Catheterizing the portal vein Once the vein has been punctured, introduce a hydrophilic wire well down into the main portal vein. Advance the catheter from the sheathed needle until it is in up to its hub. If there is any doubt about whether you are in the portal vein, check now with an injection of contrast. Gird your loins and advance the entire guide-catheter and sheath through into the portal vein; this is the defining moment of the procedure. Exchange the hydrophilic wire for the Amplatz wire and remove the catheter and guide-catheter over the wire. Put the Cobra catheter into the portal vein and pull the sheath back into the right atrium. Measure the portosystemic pressure gradient between the portal vein and right atrium. Keep the tip of the Amplatz wire under control: it will readily perforate the liver or the mesentery!

Forming the TIPS tract Once you are in the portal vein, make sure that you do not lose access! Dilate the tract with an 8 mm angioplasty balloon. If the patient is awake, now is the time for some heavy sedation and analgesia, as dilating the tract is very painful. The balloon will usually waist at the junctions of the liver parenchyma with the hepatic and portal veins.

Stenting the TIPS tract The tract must be stented if it is to stay open. Most operators prefer the Wallstent; the tract is usually about 4 cm long and a 12 × 60 mm stent is usually ideal. Obtain a high-quality venogram by injecting into the portal and hepatic veins simultaneously (Fig. 16.9a). The aim is to cover the tract, leaving some of the stent in the RHV and some in the RPV. Ideally, cover the entire hepatic vein. Do not leave stent protruding into the right atrium or dangling down the main portal vein! There is some evidence to suggest improved patency with the use of PTFE-covered stent-grafts. The Viatorr (Gore) has been designed specifically for TIPS and comprises bare stent, which extends into the portal vein, and a PTFE-covered portion intended to cover the intrahepatic tract and hepatic vein (Fig. 16.9b). This requires accurate sizing using a calibrated catheter (Fig. 16.9). The length of the covered part of the stent-graft is the distance from the portal vein end of the TIPS tract to the end of the hepatic vein; the diameter is that of the hepatic vein. The tract is dilated according to the pressure gradient. As neointimal hyperplasia does not narrow the stent-graft use smaller grafts: most operators would use a 10 mm stent-graft for bleeding and an 8 mm stent-graft for ascites.

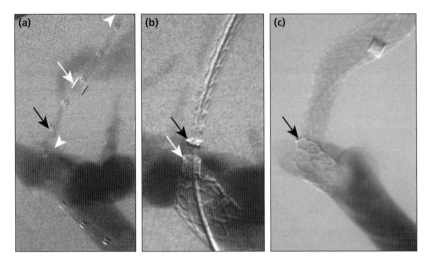

Fig. 16.9 ■ Using a Viator stent-graft. (a) Portal and hepatic venogram using a calibrated catheter (black arrow). The end of the TIPS sheath is in the hepatic vein (white arrow). Chevrons indicate the end of the hepatic vein and the portal end of the TIPS tract. (b) The sheath is placed in the portal vein and the stent is positioned so that the marker indicating the transition between the bare stent and the covered stent is at the distal end of the TIPS tract (black arrow). The sheath (white arrow) is then pulled back to deploy the bare stent. (c) Completion venogram showing correctly positioned stent graft.

Finishing off Dilate the tract to 8 mm and then measure the portosystemic gradient. If this is greater than 12 mmHg, dilate the tract to 10, then 12 mm until the gradient is abolished. If the gradient is less than 12 mmHg, perform a completion venogram. A satisfactory venogram shows almost all portal vein flow passing through the stent into the hepatic vein (Fig. 16.9c).

Troubleshooting

This section could potentially be as long as the procedure section.

Unable to catheterize the hepatic vein This is due to either an obstruction or unfavourable angulation. Review the previous imaging to ensure vein patency and perform a venogram to look for obstruction (Fig. 16.10). If there is a hepatic vein web, consider angioplasty rather than TIPS. If there is modest cranial angulation, consider shaping the introducer accordingly.

Unable to hit the portal vein Only practice helps here. Check that you are in the RHV and not the MHV. Try different points along the RHV and different degrees of torque on the metal stiffener. Consider bending the sheathed needle to alter the approach.

Hit an intrahepatic bile duct This is of little consequence per se. The cholangiogram will help indicate the position of the portal bifurcation. The main importance is that TIPS tracts contaminated by bile have an increased incidence of pseudointimal hyperplasia.

Hit the hepatic artery This is less common than biliary puncture but more likely to cause trouble. If intrahepatic, you are likely not to be in too much trouble – simply observe the

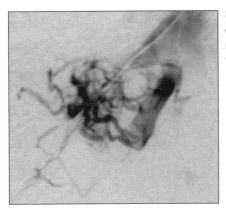

Fig. 16.10 ■ Budd–Chiari syndrome. The hepatic veins could not be catheterized. Injection into the stump of the right hepatic vein reveals the network of spidery veins typical of Budd–Chiari syndrome.

patient carefully during the remainder of the procedure. If extrahepatic, the potential to bleed is higher. Wait a few minutes and perform an angiogram. If necessary, embolize to stop the bleeding.

Hit peripheral portal vein You are unlikely to succeed unless the tract has a favourable course. If you are not too far peripheral and too angulated, proceed as normal. If not, start again.

Hit the main portal vein This is a dangerous thing to do, as there is a risk of massive bleeding if the vein tears, e.g. during angioplasty/stenting. Consider leaving a guidewire in situ to mark the position of the vein while you try again.

Unable to advance the TIPS catheter/sheath into portal vein Not uncommon in cirrhotic livers. Exchange the sheathed needle for an 80–100 cm 4Fr catheter and advance it into the portal vein, then exchange for the Amplatz wire. If it is still impossible, then carefully remove the curved guide-catheter, keeping the Amplatz wire in situ, and dilate the tract with a 4 mm angioplasty balloon. If this fails, exchange for a supportive 0.018 inch wire (e.g. platinum plus) and use a low-profile angioplasty balloon to dilate the tract.

The portal vein tears This is an emergency. Resuscitate the patient. The best advice is to stent or stent-graft the tract immediately. The drop in portal pressure will usually stop the bleeding. If this fails, surgery is the only solution.

Residual pressure gradient post TIPS If a >12 mmHg gradient persists following stenting and angioplasty, perform an angiogram to look for any obvious point of obstruction. Use further stents as necessary. If a gradient persists, a parallel TIPS may be necessary.

The patient is still bleeding Embolize the dominant varices through the TIPS tract. There is no need to routinely embolize varices.

TIPS follow-up

Make sure that the patient is followed up with Duplex ultrasound to confirm shunt patency and exclude stenosis. Intervention is frequently necessary, with only 50% primary patency at 1 year. Without intervention, virtually all TIPS have thrombosed by 2 years. At any sign of trouble, perform a venogram and measure pressures. If the gradient is >12 mmHg, then intervention is indicated. Stenoses tend to occur in the hepatic vein and within the TIPS tract. These are normally treated by stenting. These procedures can usually be performed as a day case via a 7Fr jugular puncture.

Tunnelled central lines

Tunnelled central lines are used when long-term central venous access is required for chemotherapy and total parental nutrition. All tunnelled lines are anchored by a subcutaneous cuff that induces fibrosis and prevents inadvertent removal.

The advantages of radiological placement are reliable venous access, accurate positioning and minimal procedural complications. Interventional techniques can also be used to gain vascular access in difficult cases, and also to salvage failing lines.

Learn your lines!

It is essential to understand what type of line you are dealing with, as this affects the sequence of tunnelling and line positioning. All tunnelled lines are variations on two designs:
- Lines that are cut to length, e.g. Hickman line. This type of line tunnelling is performed before positioning. Infiltrate local anaesthetic at the desired exit site on the anterior chest wall and make a small incision the width of a size 11 scalpel blade (~5 mm). The tunnel is fashioned back to the point of venous access using the blunt plastic tunneller provided. The catheter is attached to the tunnelling device and pulled through the tunnel until the cuff is ~2 cm into the tunnel. The line is placed on the skin to mimic the curve of the guidewire, and is then cut to the appropriate length to leave the tip in the right atrium.
- Lines that are fixed length, e.g. Groshong line. Tunnelling is performed after positioning. The line is inserted to optimum position and then laid on the skin to define the exit point 3 cm beyond the cuff. The tunnel is then made from the venous access site to the exit site using the steel tunneller provided.

Equipment
- Most proprietary devices come complete with the basic equipment necessary for placement. It is helpful to have some catheters and wires in reserve for difficult cases.
- Guidewires: angled hydrophilic, Amplatz superstiff.
- Catheters: Cobra II.
- Ultrasound machine: this is essential; a 5 or 7 MHz probe with a biopsy guide is ideal.

Procedure

There are three stages to the insertion of all tunnelled lines:
- Venous access – always the first stage
- Tunnelling
- Line positioning.

Access The right IJV provides the straightest route for central venous catheterization. The jugular vein seems less prone to thrombosis than other routes. Alternatives are the left IJV and the subclavian veins. Access may be limited by the presence of local disease, radiotherapy or stenosis/occlusion of the target vein. A 1 cm transverse skin incision is necessary to allow side-by-side placement of the line and the tunnelling device. Forceps can be used to perform subcutaneous blunt dissection, which will ease introduction of the catheter.

Use ultrasound to guide the venous puncture. Advance the guidewire into the right atrium/IVC under fluoroscopic guidance.

Tunnelling The aim is to tunnel in the subcutaneous plane; this is painless for both you and the patient. Introduce the tunneller and apply gentle forward pressure while rocking it from side to side. The exit site is usually on the anterior chest wall. Tunnelling over the clavicle from an internal jugular entry can be difficult; if using a metal tunneller, bending the shaft makes it considerably easier.

Think about the exit site, as a carelessly positioned line will cause discomfort by rubbing on clothing.

Line positioning The line is always introduced through a peel-away sheath (see Fig. 20.2). This is inserted just like a standard sheath. Remember the basic rules of vascular access: keep the guidewire under tension to avoid kinking. Tell the patient to stop breathing and take out the dilator and guidewire. Put your thumb over the end of the peel-away sheath and allow the patient to breathe normally.

Alarm: Air embolism can be fatal but is readily prevented. Instruct the patient to stop breathing while you remove the dilator. Keep your thumb securely over the end of the sheath after the dilator has been removed. Everyone can now breathe normally. Tell the patient to stop breathing again when you insert the catheter.

Ask the patient to stop breathing again and advance the catheter into the peel-away sheath until correctly sited. The tip should be advanced 2–3 cm into the right atrium. The line invariably ends in the SVC when the patient is erect and takes a full inspiration for the check X-ray. The sheath is then removed. Remember to keep your index finger on the catheter to hold it in position.

Final assembly A single suture is needed at the venous access site. Try not to kebab the line as you do this! Using a suture set with toothed forceps to hold the skin edge up will minimize the risk of a sharp stick injury to you and the line. If this worries even you with your level of coordination, do as some operators do and use a Steristrip, avoiding the risk altogether. Lines that are tunnelled towards the exit site need to have Luer lock fittings attached after tunnelling. The mechanism of attachment varies from system to system and is clearly described in the instructions. Test that blood can be aspirated and flush the line thoroughly. The line needs to be anchored by a suture for the first week until there is tissue ingrowth into the cuff. Cover both sites with a dressing.

Troubleshooting

Tip: The cuff should be 1–2 cm from the exit site. If it is further than this, line removal is difficult and requires a degree of dissection!

Arterial puncture Take the needle/dilator out and get the ultrasound machine while you obtain haemostasis!

Doubt about position
- Use fluoroscopy at the first sign of trouble.
- Put in a 4Fr dilator and inject contrast to confirm the anatomy.

Unable to advance the sheath
- Put in a 4Fr dilator to secure vascular access.
- If this fails, use serial dilators.
- Use the hydrophilic wire and Cobra catheter to access the IVC.
- Exchange for an Amplatz wire and use this to introduce the sheath.

Unable to introduce the line through the sheath
This can be tricky: the sheath is thin-walled and tends to kink at bends.
- Try to pull the sheath back while maintaining forward pressure on the catheter. Do not split the sheath yet. If this fails:
  - Replace the dilator and use a hydrophilic guidewire to try to negotiate the kink. Then reinsert the sheath fully: this may straighten the sheath sufficiently to use. If this fails:
  - Insert the catheter as far as it will go and peel away the sheath. Remember to apply forward pressure to keep the catheter in position. The catheter can usually be advanced once it is within the vein.

Unable to aspirate blood from the line
- Check the line position on fluoroscopy.
- Check for kinking at the venous puncture site.
- Sit the patient up and try other postural manoeuvres to alter line position.
- If all else fails, inject contrast through the line to delineate the problem.

Awkward venous access

Last-ditch venous access can literally be a lifeline for some patients – this is particularly true of haemodialysis patients. By the time a patient has had multiple tunnelled lines all of the central veins may be stenosed or occluded. At this stage the renal team usually resorts to temporary femoral access, but this is uncomfortable and usually results in infection. It is essential to re-establishing long-term central venous access. There are descriptions of using the hepatic veins and the IVC, but this is rarely necessary. The vast majority of patients can have access established via collateral veins using the same techniques to cross stenoses and occlusions that are described in the section on angioplasty and stenting. Remember that the aim is to establish venous access, not venous patency: if necessary, dilate stenoses or occlusions to allow introduction of the line. Only place a stent if there are symptoms of venous obstruction.

The first stage in the procedure is to perform an ultrasound scan of the neck veins. If an internal jugular vein is patent this is the optimal approach. There are always plenty of tortuous veins that cross the midline of the neck, but these are seldom useful. Look

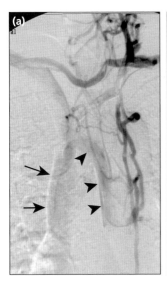 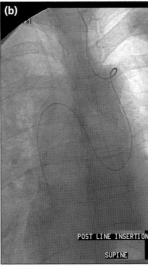

Fig. 16.11 ▨ Awkward access. (a) Injection into a vein in the left side of the neck shows collaterals communicating with the azygous vein (arrowheads) and into the SVC (arrows). (b) The Groshong line follows this tortuous path.

for the patent anterior and external jugular veins, or veins that lie more laterally in the neck.

Puncture the chosen vein under ultrasound guidance and insert a 4Fr dilator to perform venography. If there is a direct route to the central veins, then go for it. Dilate underlying stenoses as necessary in order to introduce the catheters. More often there is no direct route, but with knowledge of the likely course of the vein it is often possible to find a way through. Perseverance is the key: if the vein you have punctured is not 'the one' the venogram will often suggest an alternative (Fig. 16.11).

Remember, the aim for renal patients is not to re-establish venous patency but to simply get a line through the occluded segment to permit dialysis.

Impossible access – keys to success

- Good ultrasound.
- Plenty of time and determination.
- Use low-profile wires and balloons to cross tight strictures and occlusions.
- Once you have access into a central vein, don't lose it! Get a supportive wire (e.g. an Amplatz wire) in place, preferably through to the IVC.
- If dual catheters are required, e.g. for haemodialysis, resist the temptation to use the same puncture site for two wires. This only results in a venous tear and excessive bleeding. Instead, use ultrasound or fluoroscopy to perform a second puncture into the same vein about 1 cm from the first puncture.
- Use a long peel-away sheath – the sheath supplied with the catheter will not be long enough to support the catheter all the way through to the SVC/right atrium.

Maintenance of tunnelled central lines

All long-term central venous access is prone to four problems: infection, venous thrombosis, fibrin sheath and mechanical failure.

Infection limited to the exit site can be successfully treated with antiobiotic treatment; however, for tunnel infections and infected lines removal is usually required. Don't be tempted to place a new line until the patient has been clear of infection for 7 days, or you will be removing that line as well.

Line-related venous thrombosis is usually associated with symptomatic limb oedema, in which case the line is removed and the patient treated as for a DVT. If the thrombosis is asymptomatic, then anticoagulation alone is adequate.

Mechanical failure usually results in line fracture; extravasation then causes pain during injection, and sometimes leak of fluid from the skin entry site. Occasionally a line fractures or a totally implanted device such as a portacath separates from its hub, leading to migration of the line and requiring snaring (see Chapter 18, Retrieving foreign bodies).

Fibrin sheath formation In this condition fibrin deposits around the line to form a condom-like cover. This obstructs the line tips, prevents aspiration of blood, and may lead to extravasation. In dialysis lines it results in markedly reduced flow, which compromises dialysis.

When there is a problem with a line the first step is to establish the diagnosis with a lino-gram. This is simply an injection of contrast down the line under fluoroscopic control. Check the entire line from the skin to its tip. Look for:
- Extravasation: this most commonly occurs at points of flexion or compression.
- Free flow of contrast from the line lumen via the end- and sideholes. Sometimes it is necessary to perform a run to establish what is happening. Owing to cardiac motion this may be clearer on unsubtracted images.
- Reflux of contrast back around the line, often with a thin radiolucent 'membrane'; this indicates a fibrin sheath (Fig. 16.12).
- Line migration, typically into the pulmonary artery (see Chapter 18).

If there is a fibrin sheath the first approach is to flush the line vigorously. This may disrupt the sheath sufficiently to restore flow. The next step will usually be to try a low dose of thrombolysis. This is best given by infusion rather than as a bolus. The ward team can do this without your help. If this fails, then mechanically stripping the fibrin sheath with a Gooseneck snare is usually the answer. Warn the patient that even if this is successful the fibrin sheath may recur and require further treatment.

How to strip

The lines often abut the wall of the SVC, which makes them difficult to snare. In this case simply pass a guidewire through the line and into the IVC if it will go. If you are dealing with a Groshong line then only a hydrophilic wire will pass through it – it may take a little pushing to get it through the valve, but don't be deterred: it will go.

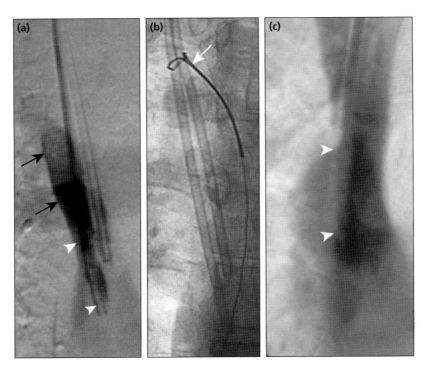

Fig. 16.12 ▪ Stripping a poorly functioning Tessio line. (a) Injection through the venous line. The line tip is occluded (arrowheads) and contrast outlines a fibrin sheath (arrows). (b) A Gooseneck snare has been placed around both lines. (c) Following stripping, the line fills to the tip (arrowheads) and contrast flows normally into the SVC. Normal function was restored.

Pass a Gooseneck snare from the femoral vein to catch the wire and then advance it over the line. If there are two lines, e.g. dialysis catheters, both can be snared at once. Take the snare as far up the line as it will go, and tighten it so that it grips the line fairly firmly (Fig. 16.12).

Pull the snare back: if it is gripped tightly enough it will tug the line down when you pull. It is best to warn the patient that they will feel as though someone is pulling on the line, because they are. You are aiming to get enough grip to remove the sheath but leave the line in situ. Repeat this once or twice, then repeat the linogram. If flow is restored and the lines aspirate freely, then stop. If not, try again.

Sometimes when there are two lines stuck together success is indicated by the line tips separating.

Tip: Leave the wire through the catheter while stripping: this allows the snare to be passed straight back up again. When performing the linogram you need to remove the wire, so park the snare high up the line so that you don't have to catch it again.

SUGGESTIONS FOR FURTHER READING

Venous intervention

Becker DM, Philbrick JT, Selby JB. Inferior vena cava filters: Indications, safety, effectiveness. Arch Intern Med 1992;152:1985–1994.

Linsenmaier U, Rieger J, Schenk F et al. Indications, management and complications of temporary inferior vena cava filters. Cardiovasc Intervent Radiol 1998;21:464–469.
A useful overview.

McFarland DR (ed) Interventional radiology in the venous system. Semin Intervent Radiol 1994;11.

Vesely TM. Technical problems and complications associated with inferior vena cava filters. Semin Intervent Radiol 1994;11:121–133.

SVCO

Nicholson AA, Ettles DF, Arnold A et al. Treatment of malignant superior vena caval obstruction: metal stents or radiation therapy. J Vasc Intervent Radiol 1997;8:563–567.
What can be achieved in good hands: the largest series to date.

TIPS

LaBerge JM. Anatomy relevant to the transjugular intrahepatic portosystemic shunt procedure. Semin Intervent Radiol 1995;12:337–346.
Why we try to use the right hepatic vein to approach the portal vein.

Saxon RR, Keller FS. Technical aspects of accessing the portal vein during the TIPS procedure. J Vasc Intervent Radiol 1997;8:733–744.
Guidance and practical TIPS tips.

Central lines

Hall K, Farr B. Diagnosis and management of long term central venous catheter infection. J Vasc Intervent Radiol 2004;15:327–334.

Mauro MA, Jaques PF. Radiologic placement of long-term central venous catheters: A review. J Vasc Intervent Radiol 1993;5:127–137.

Ramsden WH, Cohen AT, Blanshard KS. Central venous catheter fracture due to compression between the clavicle and first rib. Clin Radiol 1995;50:59–60.
A potential pitfall of the subclavian approach to central lines, which applies equally to stents and stent-grafts.

Trerotola SO, Johnson MS, Harris VJ et al. Outcome of tunneled hemodialysis catheters placed via the right internal jugular vein by interventional radiologists. Radiology 1997;203:489–495.
The RIJV is the approach to use with excellent patency and few complications.

Chapter Seventeen

Haemodialysis access – imaging and intervention

For patients on haemodialysis, their fistula or graft is a lifeline. Unfortunately, problems are not uncommon, and anyone working on a site with a dialysis unit will frequently see patients with problematic access. Stenoses lead to inadequate dialysis, prolonged bleeding, arm oedema and thrombosis. Large shunts may cause steal phenomena. The key to these procedures is to understand the anatomy and how to physically examine a fistula.

Fistula examination Feel the fistula for the 'thrill' at the anastomosis and in the draining vein. The vein adjacent to the anastomosis usually has a spongy feeling. If the fistula is underfilled there is a problem with the inflow. A tense distended vein indicates venous out-flow obstruction. A swollen arm indicates central venous obstruction (Fig. 17.1). Venous stenoses are often palpable as 'defects' in the draining vein associated with a change in the degree of venous filling and thrill.

Graft examination There is usually a thrill at the venous anastomosis, and examination is in essence the same as that for a fistula.

Diagnostic imaging

Arteriovenous fistulae The commonest fistula is the radiocephalic (Brescia–Cimino) fistula fashioned at the wrist of the non-dominant arm (Fig. 17.2). If this fails, it may be

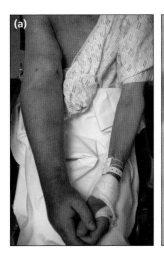
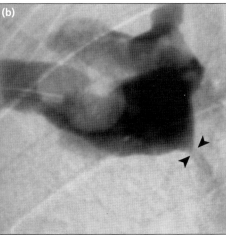

Fig. 17.1 ▦ Swollen fistula arm caused by high-grade stenosis in the subclavian vein (arrowheads).

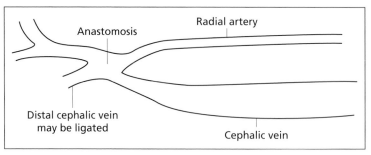

Fig. 17.2 ▒ Brescia–Cimino fistula (distal radial artery to cephalic vein).

revised or a more proximal fistula formed, usually between the brachial artery and the cephalic or basilic vein. Once the non-dominant arm sites are exhausted, the dominant arm is used; if this fails, a fistula may be formed at the groin.

Haemodialysis grafts These are an alternative to fistula formation and have the advantages of being ready to use immediately and allowing higher flow rates. The price for this is the frequency with which they develop stenoses and thrombose. Grafts often have a loop configuration. Typical sites are between the brachial artery and the cephalic or basilic vein, or between the femoral artery and vein.

Equipment

- Basic angiography set with a 3Fr straight catheter.
- Ultrasound.

Procedure

The same questions need to be answered for both fistulae and grafts, namely, the state of the inflow, the condition of any anastomoses, and the condition of the draining veins from the periphery to the central veins.

Access Retrograde arterial puncture of the ipsilateral brachial artery or the inflow limb of the loop graft is the ideal method. Performing the study via a 3Fr arterial puncture optimizes visualization of the inflow and allows complete assessment. The alternative, which seldom produces as satisfactory images, is to place a needle in the draining veins of the fistula and use a suprasystolic tourniquet to achieve retrograde flow through the arterial anastomosis. Remember that the patient will be heparinized during dialysis, so do not perform the study straight afterwards.

Catheterization Selective catheterization is only required for intervention.

Runs The principle is the same as in graft angiography: show the anastomosis in profile. Because of the high flow rates through fistulae, a high frame rate (4–6 fps) is used to study the anastomosis and the peripheral draining veins. As flow slows in the more central veins, the flow rate is decreased to 1–2 fps. For arm haemodialysis access sites, the venous return should be studied as far as the right atrium.

As always for arm angiography, it is necessary to rotate the angiography table to allow views down to the hand to be obtained. Start with the patient's arm in the anatomical position (palm up). Multiple oblique views are often necessary to sort out the anatomy.

Tip: To obtain oblique views, consider turning the patient's arm rather than rotating the C-arm.

Interpretation

- Significant stenoses are those causing greater than 50% diameter narrowing.
- There are often occluded venous segments with collaterals and retrograde flow. This may only be appreciated when the runs are reviewed frame by frame at the console.
- Filling of collateral veins around the central veins is always abnormal. If you cannot see a lesion, try another view.

Troubleshooting

Unable to puncture the fistula   Use ultrasound to target the puncture.

The arteries distal to the fistula do not fill   This is usually secondary to a steal phenomenon through the fistula. Apply a tourniquet to occlude the venous drainage. The arteries will normally now fill.

Angioplasty and stenting

There is controversy about whether to intervene on asymptomatic dialysis access stenoses, but symptomatic stenoses must be treated to improve dialysis, relieve swelling and prevent thrombosis. The commonest sites for stenoses are at the venous anastomosis and dialysis puncture sites. Central venous catheterization also predisposes to stenosis.

Before treating any stenosis or occlusion, make sure that everyone is aware of the objectives of the procedure, i.e. to preserve the function of the dialysis access site. Restenosis is frequent and repeat intervention is often necessary. Explain to the patient that treatment is a temporizing measure and not a miracle cure.

Access Choose the approach according to the location of the lesion and the condition of the adjacent vessels. For direct arteriovenous fistulae, the dominant draining vein is usually catheterized; this is almost always the vein that is used during dialysis. It is sometimes necessary to approach Brescia–Cimino fistulae via an antegrade brachial artery puncture. Haemodialysis grafts are directly punctured at a point that allows space to manoeuvre under the C-arm with respect to the lesion.

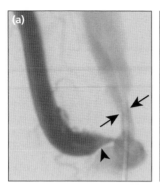
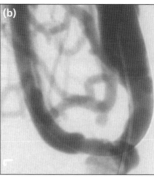

Fig. 17.3 ■ (a) Brescia–Cimino fistula with stenoses at the anastomosis (arrowhead) and in the draining vein (arrows). (b) Following angioplasty, excellent flow is restored.

Tip: The apex of some loop grafts is reinforced to prevent kinking. Check with the surgeon, or puncture away from the apex.

Angioplasty is performed in the conventional fashion (Fig. 17.3). Consider sending the patient for dialysis immediately after treatment. The sheath can be exchanged for a dialysis catheter, which is left in situ; discuss the best arrangement with the dialysis unit.

Stenting is reserved for those cases in which angioplasty alone is unsuccessful. Only stent if it will achieve good outflow; if not, the patient is better off with surgery. Take care when stenting the central veins as stent compression between the clavicle and the first rib is common. Try not to stent across other vessels that may be needed for central access in the future, especially the jugular veins. Make sure that the patient and clinician are aware of the position of the stent so that it is not inadvertently punctured. Long-term stent patency, particularly in peripheral veins, is poor.

Troubleshooting

Unable to puncture the draining vein   Use ultrasound guidance; colour flow is invaluable for this.

Unable to dilate a stenosis   It is often necessary to consider using a cutting balloon or prolonged high-pressure inflation to overcome fibrotic strictures (Fig. 17.4). Make sure that you have suitable angioplasty balloons before starting! Never use a stent when you cannot eliminate the waist on the angioplasty balloon – you are simply lining a stenosis with metal.

Rupture   Rupture is more common during venous intervention than during arterial angioplasty. It is probably more common when using cutting balloons (Fig. 17.5). Extravasation is managed in a similar fashion to arterial injury; remember that occlusion is often an acceptable outcome if the fistula was not functioning adequately.

Spasm   Spasm is common in the radial artery and in veins. Use vasodilators prophylactically and to treat spasm. Consider gentle dilation of areas of resistant spasm.

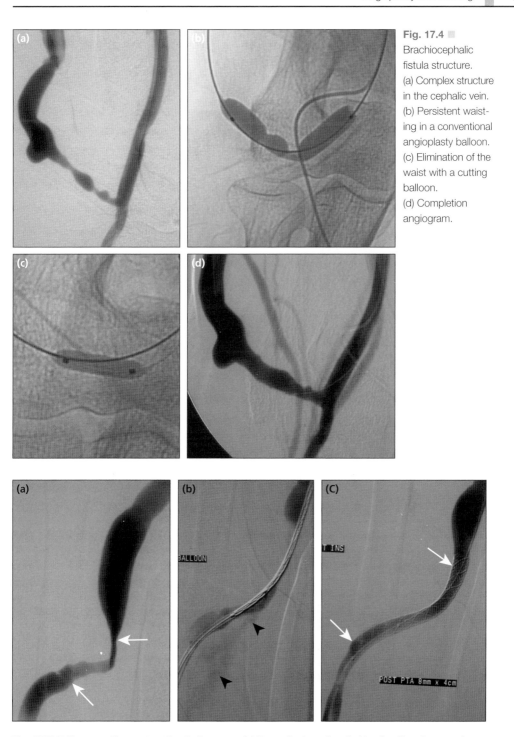

Fig. 17.4 ▦ Brachiocephalic fistula structure. (a) Complex structure in the cephalic vein. (b) Persistent waisting in a conventional angioplasty balloon. (c) Elimination of the waist with a cutting balloon. (d) Completion angiogram.

Fig. 17.5 ▦ Extravasation post cutting balloon use. (a) Preangioplasty flow-limiting basilic vein stenosis (arrows). (b) Brisk extravasation following cutting balloon angioplasty (arrowheads). (c) Completion angiogram following deployment of a covered stent.

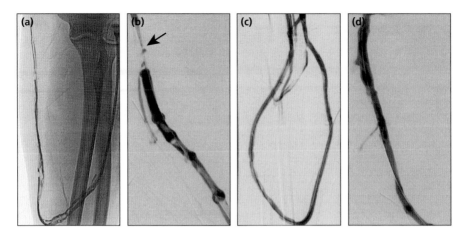

Fig. 17.6 ■ (a) Thrombosed forearm loop graft. (b) Stenosis in the draining vein. (c) Following mechanical thrombectomy, the graft is clear. (d) The cephalic vein is widely patent following angioplasty.

Thrombosis

Unfortunately, thrombosis is often the first sign of a problem. Radiological treatment options are thrombolysis and mechanical thrombectomy; the alternative is surgical embolectomy. Remember that there is almost always an underlying stenosis that must be treated when flow is restored. Ideally, treatment should be performed before the patient requires temporary venous access for dialysis, as this preserves central veins.

Remember the contraindications for thrombolysis. CVA during thrombolysis is probably less common in a young dialysis patient than in an elderly patient with peripheral vascular disease.

If the patient has a central line, check that there were no complications during placement that might compromise thrombolysis!

Direct AV fistulae Puncture the main draining vein about 10 cm away from and aiming towards the anastomosis. Perform gentle venography to confirm the anatomy. Position a 4Fr straight multi-sidehole catheter with its tip as close to the anastomosis as possible. Give a bolus dose of the thrombolytic agent (e.g. 5 mg rt-PA) and then start an infusion (see Thrombolysis, p. 184). Perform periodic check angiography to evaluate progress. When flow is re-established, perform check venography and treat any underlying stenoses.

Haemodialysis grafts The thrombus is usually confined to the graft, but may extend beyond it if there is a stenosis in the draining vein (Fig. 17.6). Occluded grafts can be treated by thrombolysis or thrombectomy using a crossed catheter technique (Fig. 17.7).

1. Punctures are made into the arterial and venous limbs and catheters manipulated round the graft. Puncture of the graft is usually straightforward, but if it is difficult to palpate use ultrasound.
2. Using a hydrophylic guidewire and a Cobra catheter, negotiate into the draining vein beyond the venous anastomosis and perform a venogram to demonstrate the venous

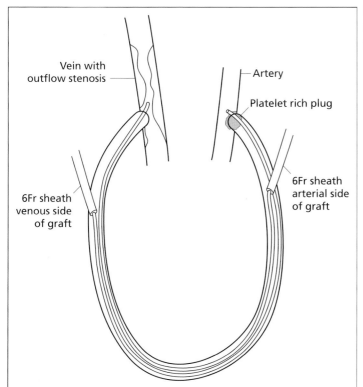

Fig. 17.7 ■ Crossed catheter technique for loop graft thrombolysis.

anatomy. If there is no direct venous drainage, stop now, as the graft needs to be surgically revised.

3. Perform either thrombolysis, usually with boluses of rt-PA, or thrombectomy using a mechanical thrombectomy device. Aim to treat the venous outflow first, then deal with the arterial limb. It is not essential to clear all the thrombus at this stage, but just enough to allow flow to occur.

4. There is usually a platelet-rich plug of thrombus at the arterial end of the graft which is resistant to thrombolysis. Use a hydrophilic guidewire to manipulate into the native artery and pass a small balloon catheter above the arterial anastomosis. Gently inflate it and pull it back into the graft (an over-the-wire Fogarty embolectomy catheter is ideal, though conventional angioplasty balloons will work). The platelet plug disimpacts and flow is restored.

5. Now is the time to tidy up the residual thrombus; often simple balloon angioplasty will macerate it.

6. Remember to look for the underlying lesion and treat it with angioplasty or stenting.

Mechanical thrombectomy

Particularly in loop grafts, thrombectomy is a good option as it can result in a single-stage procedure that allows immediate dialysis. A variety of devices are available, operating either as fragmentation baskets (e.g. Arrow, Trerotola) or on a rheolytic principle (e.g. Angiojet).

In reality, the most widely used system is the Trerotola device; this is a simple battery-operated fragmentation device that is available either with or without over-the-wire access. The device is cooled by a continuous flow of saline and is very effective at fragmenting thrombus.

Troubleshooting

Uncertain anatomy   Try hard to establish the type of fistula or graft before starting. Look for operation notes and speak to the surgical team in charge. Ultrasound will often clarify the anatomy. If not, adopt a 'suck it and see' approach.

Extravasation occurs during thrombolysis   This is almost inevitable when treating dialysis access grafts that have had frequent punctures. Warn the patient about this in advance. It is usually possible to complete treatment unless there is marked extravasation.

Intraprocedural thrombosis   Particularly with thrombectomy, it can be difficult to stop rethrombosis during the procedure. The key is avoiding delay between steps 4 and 5; it is essential to get flow through the fistula. Minor amounts of residual thrombus are easily resolved after flow has been established.

SUGGESTIONS FOR FURTHER READING

Beathard GA, Welch BR, Maidment HJ. Mechanical thrombectomy for the treatment of thrombosed hemodialysis access grafts. Radiology 1996;200:711–716.
An interesting paper on pulse-spray technique, with saline replacing the thrombolytic agent.

Beathard GA. Percutaneous transvenous angioplasty in the treatment of vascular access stenosis. Kidney Int 1992;42:1390–1397.

Lammer J, Vorwerk D. Hemodialyis fistulas and grafts. Semin Intervent Radiol 1997;14:1–110.
Everything you wanted to know …well, almost. The authors have not included thrombolytic therapy, but still a very good read.

Schuman E, Quinn S, Standage B et al. Thrombolysis versus thrombectomy for occluded hemodialysis grafts. Am J Surg 1994;167:473–476.
A thoughtful paper that reminds us of the established primary role of surgical thrombectomy, and that the principal advantage of radiology is to treat the underlying lesion.

Valji K, Bookstein JJ, Roberts AC, Davis GB. Pharmacomechanical thrombolysis and angioplasty in the management of clotted hemodialyisis grafts: early and late clinical results. Radiology 1991;178:243–247.
The strongest advocates of pulse-spray thrombolysis.

Valji K. Transcatheter treatment of thrombosed hemodialysis access grafts. AJR 1995;164:823–829.
An excellent overview with an extensive reference list.

Chapter Eighteen

Foreign body retrieval

Foreign body retrieval is usually for iatrogenic problems, most of which will have been of your own making. The techniques and equipment described can also be used for snaring guidewires for pull-through procedures, or to reposition misplaced central lines. The majority of foreign body retrieval is within the vascular system, though occasionally these techniques are required in the biliary or urinary systems. There are not many tools at your disposal, so a thorough knowledge of how they work and an inventive mind are the keys to success.

The toolkit

Amplatz Gooseneck snare (Figs 18.1, 18.2; see also Fig. 7.14)

This is the best-known and most popular snare. The snare loop comes in a range of sizes from 2 to 25 mm, and the chosen diameter should correspond to the target vessel. The snare is supplied with its own guide-catheter, which varies in size from 4 to 6Fr depending on the snare chosen. The guide-catheter has a radio-opaque tip marker and can be shaped if necessary to increase manoeuvrability.

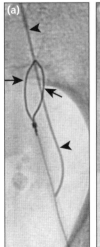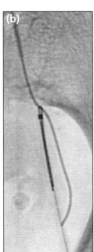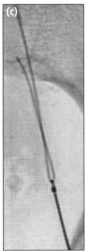

Fig. 18.1 Snaring a guidewire.
(a) The open snare (arrows) is positioned over the guidewire (arrowheads). (b) The snare is tightened to grip the wire. (c) The snare is pulled back into the sheath, bringing the guidewire with it.

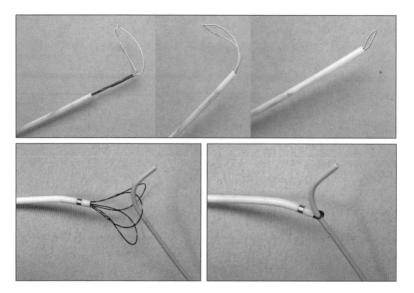

Fig. 18.2 ▢ Upper row: Amplatz Gooseneck snare fully open, partially open and closed. Lower row: EnSnare with catheter open and closed.

The EnSnare (MD Tech) (Fig. 18.2)

This snare is constructed with three loops and comes in different sizes. Each is designed to function in a range of vessel diameters, e.g. the mini snare will function from 4 to 8 mm and the large snare from 12 to 20 mm. This is a distinct advantage when working in a confined space, or when it is difficult to turn the snare.

Snares are simple to use; rather harder is deciding when a 'foreign body' will be relatively innocuous if left in situ, and when removing it is likely to cause more harm than good. A 'foreign body' which is free in the right atrium has the potential to be injurious, whereas an unexpanded stent in a minor branch vessel is not a big problem.

Using a snare in eight easy steps

1. First position a guidewire adjacent to the object to be removed. If you cannot manage this then you will not be able to remove it!
2. The guide-catheter is passed along the guidewire in the normal fashion and the guidewire is removed.
3. The snare is compressed within an introducer and then advanced into the catheter.
4. As the snare loop emerges from the catheter, it opens like a lasso (see Fig. 18.1).
5. Allow the snare loop to open so that occupies the entire vessel lumen. The snare loop can be rotated, advanced or withdrawn to position it over the target.

6. Once the target is in the loop it is kept still and the guide-catheter is advanced. This tightens the snare and grips the target (see Fig. 18.1).
7. The snare and its prey can now be pulled back to the access site.
8. The prey is either removed (Fig. 18.1c), parked somewhere safe or, in the case of a large object, held on to until the vascular surgeon can remove it safely.

Tip: Remember, many objects can be snared and retrieved but not all can be removed, and frequently a large sheath will be necessary, e.g. to remove a kinked catheter.

Endovascular forceps

The forceps are 3Fr in diameter and will pass down any catheter that will accept a 0.038 inch guidewire. This device is particularly useful when working in a confined space. Forceps are more traumatic than a snare and are usually reserved for circumstances where a snare has proved unsuccessful. The forceps have a shapeable guidewire tip and a side-opening jaw. The forceps are manoeuvred to lie in parallel with the target object, the jaw is opened and the target grasped and retrieved. Although the side-opening mechanism reduces the risks of intimal trauma, great care must be taken when using this device.

Stone-retrieval baskets

Dormier baskets are useful tools in the biliary and urinary systems but are too traumatic to endothelium to recommend for use in the vascular system.

Home-made snares

Snares can be made using a 0.018 inch guidewire and a 6Fr guide-catheter. The guidewire is simply doubled back through the guide-catheter to form a loop. Home-made snares do not function as well as the real thing, but are better than nothing in an emergency.

Clinical scenarios

It is essential to decide whether the foreign body needs to be removed. Stents, embolization coils and fragments of catheter and guidewire are likely to cause vessel thrombosis. Only if thrombosis is likely to be clinically relevant should retrieval be attempted; if not, leave the foreign body where it is. If something does need to be removed, it is a good idea to heparinize the patient to prevent thrombosis during the procedure.

Catheter and guidewire fragments Guidewire fragments are fairly straightforward. Find a free end and snare the fragment. Fortunately, wire fragments are small enough to be withdrawn through a 6Fr sheath even when doubled back. Catheter fragments and bits of central venous catheters are usually easy to capture, but will not come through a standard sheath. The first option is to increase the sheath size to approximately twice that of the target – this is often fairly large. Alternatively, bring the snared object back to the sheath, pull it snugly into the end of the sheath and withdraw fragment, snare and sheath simultaneously. In practice, this is the most frequently used option.

Embolization coils The ease of retrieval for coils is critically dependent on the size of the target vessel. If the coil has migrated into a small-calibre vessel, retrieval may require a microsnare. In many situations vessels of this calibre are not vital, and the safest option is to leave the coil alone. Particular care should be taken if the target coil is adjacent to a nest of coils, e.g. when the last coil of an embolization has extruded back into the main trunk. It is very easy to drag entangled coils back during the retrieval and make the situation much worse.

Stents Partially and even completely deployed stents have been successfully retrieved using snares. It is possible with a lot of patience to progressively crimp down stainless steel stents, but this is not a technique for stents that have undergone minor mispositioning. The stent must be in a site where it poses a significant threat to the patient, e.g. embolization to the heart or pulmonary circulation. Unfortunately, the majority of stents will not line up neatly and require a large sheath or an arteriotomy or venotomy for removal. Consider deploying the stent in a less harmful position, e.g. an iliac vessel. Remember that any of these options is a lot better than a thoracotomy. Self-expanding stents are even more difficult, as only a portion can be compressed; they almost always need to be 'parked' safely (Fig. 18.3). This is definitely an area for expert hands only.

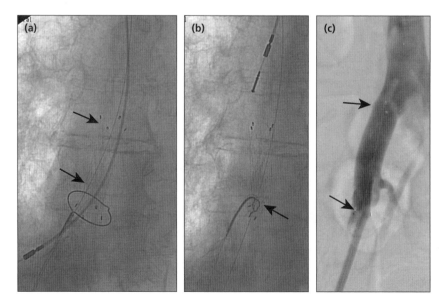

Fig. 18.3 ■ Retrieving a self-expanding stent from the right atrium. (a) An innominate vein stent (arrows) has been displaced during placement of a pacing wire. A 0.018 inch wire has been passed through the stent and a Gooseneck snare advanced over this. (b) The lower end of the stent is grasped and compressed (arrow); the upper end remains expanded. (c) The stent (arrows) has been pulled back and parked in the common iliac vein.

Repositioning central venous lines

The majority of these are subclavian central venous lines that either have passed from the subclavian vein into the internal jugular or have passed from the right subclavian into the left brachiocephalic vein. Non-tunnelled lines can often be readily exchanged by simply directing a guidewire through the original line into the SVC, then exchanging for a new line. Only in exceptional circumstances is it worth more elaborate manoeuvres for a non-tunnelled line. In addition, these lines are often made of stiff plastic that makes hooking the line down fairly difficult.

Tunnelled central lines deserve more effort. The tunnel means that it is less easy to simply exchange the catheter, and therefore more ingenious solutions are required. The first step is to attempt to hook the line down into the target vessel. Perform a femoral puncture and negotiate a pigtail catheter to the target line. Try to hook the line down using the pigtail; occasionally, it can be helpful to stiffen the pigtail by passing a guidewire partially round the loop. If this fails, it may be worth trying the same manoeuvre with a Sos Omni catheter (Fig. 18.4) or, if you can find one, a tip-deflecting wire.

If neither of these options is successful, then try using a Gooseneck snare. The difficulty with snaring is that the target object has to present a free end to capture. If the end of the misplaced line is in a decent-sized vessel, then it is possible to manipulate the snare and the guide-catheter into an appropriate position. If the line is in a small vessel, then access with a snare can be difficult. It is sometimes possible to move the end of the misplaced line into a more favourable position by simply performing a rapid hand injection of saline down the line.

Pull-through technique or 'bodyflossing'

This is a special form of guidewire retrieval and refers to putting a guidewire in at one site and bringing it out at another. This gives enormous strength and stability, as the wire can be held under tension and catheters can be placed end to end. It is typically used when it is simpler to traverse a lesion from one site while the other is the optimal route for intervention, e.g. large stents are best placed via femoral access rather than from the arm.

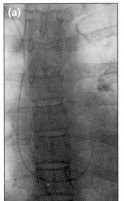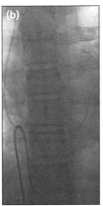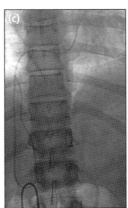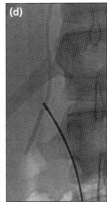

Fig. 18.4 ■ Retrieval of a broken catheter fragment. (a) The catheter tip has migrated into the right ventricle. (b and c) The catheter is hooked with a Sidewinder catheter and pulled down into the inferior vena cava. (d) The catheter is snared prior to being pulled out through the femoral vein sheath.

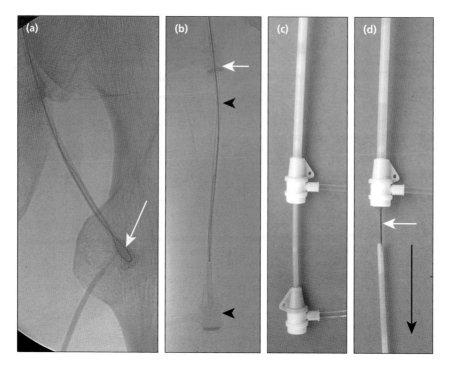

Fig. 18.5 ▪ Bringing a wire out through a sheath. (a) The hydrophilic wire (arrow) will not pass through the haemostatic valve. (b and c) Sheath in sheath. A smaller sheath (black arrowheads) has been inserted into the original sheath (white arrow) and the wire has been advanced into it. (d) The smaller sheath is pulled back (black arrow) to reveal the wire (white arrow).

In the first instance, an attempt should be made to steer a hydrophilic guidewire into the target sheath using a shaped catheter. Opacification of the target sheath with contrast will make it much easier to see. This will usually succeed, but may be quite fiddly. You will find that the wire will not pass through the haemostatic valve. In this case, pass a smaller sheath inside the larger one; the wire will pass into this; advance the wire as you retract this sheath (Fig. 18.5). The wire will come out of the valve.

If you cannot make this work, then use a Gooseneck snare to grasp the wire in the iliac artery or the aorta. This is quick, but much more expensive. The wire will usually be damaged during snaring, so do not use it again.

When applying tension to the wire to deliver devices, always place a catheter over the guidewire at any significant curves to prevent a cheesewire effect.

 Tip: It is surprisingly easy to steer a guidewire into a vascular sheath, but it is much harder to get it out through the haemostatic valve. The simplest way to solve this problem is to place a smaller sheath halfway into the larger one and push the wire into this up to the valve. Pull the sheath back out, and hey presto, there is the wire! (Fig. 18.5).

SUGGESTIONS FOR FURTHER READING

Brown PG, McBride KD, Gaines P. Technical report: Hickman catheter rescue. Clin Radiol 1994;49:891–894.

Egglin TPK, Dickey KW, Rosenblatt M et al. Retrieval of intravascular foreign bodies: experience in 32 cases. AJR 1995;164:1259–1264.
This is a large series of a variety of devices with a good reference section.

Hartnell GG, Gates J, Soujanen JN et al. Transfemoral repositioning of malpositioned central venous catheters. Cardiovasc Intervent Radiol 1996;19:329–331.

Hartnell GG. Techniques for intact removal of vascular foreign bodies. J Intervent Radiol 1996;11:29–37.
A 'How I do it' approach, with references.

Section Three

Non-vascular intervention

Chapter Nineteen

Imaging guidance for intervention

A wide range of interventional procedures can only be performed safely with accurate imaging guidance. The aim of this chapter is to outline the basic principles of imaging-directed intervention. Ultrasound, CT and fluoroscopy have complementary roles; individual circumstances dictate the optimal modality.

Ultrasound guidance

Ultrasound is ideal for many biopsy and drainage procedures and allows the procedure to be visualized in real time. Use ultrasound if it clearly demonstrates the target and a suitable approach. As a basic principle, use the highest-frequency probe that gives a good image from the skin to the target site. Use a 7.5 MHz probe for superficial structures and a 3.5–5 MHz probe for deeper structures. It is exceedingly helpful to have a probe with a small footprint, as this improves access.

Sterility   All invasive procedures should be performed using aseptic technique. Sterile ultrasound probe covers and ultrasound gel are readily available. Sterile ultrasound gel is used outside the ultrasound probe cover, but ordinary ultrasound gel can be used inside it. A clean drape should be used to cover the probe cable. Attach the cable to the drapes with a towel clip to save dropping an expensive probe.

Tip: If you do not possess a suitably sized probe cover, improvize with a sterile surgical glove. Cut the cuff off the second glove and use this as a 'rubber band' to attach the glove/drape to the probe.

Directing punctures   The ultrasound image represents a slice of tissue only 1 mm thick – much less than the width of the probe! For effective guidance the needle must pass along the scan plane, which runs directly along the midline of the probe; even a small degree of malalignment will mean that the needle is not in the scan plane. The importance of this relationship cannot be overemphasized: it is the single most important factor in successful ultrasound guidance.

Tip: If you cannot see the needle, look to check that the needle and probe are aligned correctly. Many probes come with a needle guide, which can be used for the majority of ultrasound-guided interventions; the alternative is to use the freehand technique.

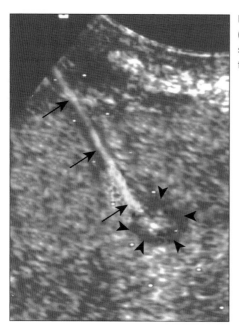

Fig. 19.1 ■ Biopsy of a small hepatic metastasis (arrowheads) using a needle guide. The white dots showing the projected needle path are clearly visible and the needle (arrows) can be seen entering the lesion.

A needle guide is so simple to use that no experience is needed to manage it. The guide attaches to the probe and constrains the needle to a predetermined path. The needle trajectory is displayed as two broken parallel lines superimposed on the image. The probe is positioned so that the projected needle path intersects the target. The needle is now advanced to the target (Fig. 19.1).

The freehand technique is required when there is no suitable path within the constraints of the needle guide. As the name suggests, the needle is advanced along the scan plane with one hand while the probe is fixed with the other. The most common problems are due to angulation or rotation of the probe relative to the path of the needle.

 Tip: When the needle tip is not clearly seen, then gently oscillating the needle backwards and forwards greatly enhances its visibility.

CT guidance

CT is used to guide biopsies and drainage of areas that cannot be seen on ultrasound, e.g. the lung, mediastinum, bone, and areas of the abdomen obscured by bowel gas. There are two chief disadvantages to using CT compared to ultrasound:

- Needle passage cannot be viewed in real time.
- The patient must be brought in and out of the scanner for each needle pass.

The principles of CT guidance are very simple, although the procedure can be technically challenging. When performing procedures in the chest and abdomen, it is important to explain to the patient the necessity to try to take the same size breath during each scan and needle pass.

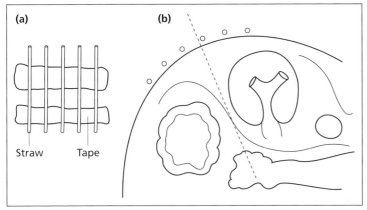

(a)

Straw   Tape

(b)

Fig. 19.2 (a) A CT grid can be readily made using plastic tubing and adhesive tape. (b) The optimal approach is determined by the markers.

Patient positioning   The diagnostic scans are reviewed and a suitable needle path is chosen. The patient is positioned either supine or prone, depending on the position of the target. Remember that although angled needle trajectories can be used, it is simplest to judge a vertical needle pass.

Tip: Sometimes it can be helpful to tilt the CT gantry, as this allows the needle to be angulated cranially or caudally while remaining in the scan plane.

The simplest way to mark the puncture site is to use a reference grid placed over the region of interest. Grids can be purchased or simply made from some thin plastic tubing (Fig. 19.2).

CT guidance: a step-by-step approach

1. The grid is positioned with the markers oriented perpendicular to the scan plane.
2. The patient is rescanned with the grid in place.
3. Select the slice that shows the optimal approach to the target and return the patient to this position.
4. Identify which of the grid lines corresponds to the best approach.
5. Turn on the light beam and simply mark where it intersects the chosen grid line.
6. Move the table to bring the patient out of the scanner gantry.
7. Cleanse, drape and anaesthetize the skin.
8. Advance the needle along the anticipated trajectory.
9. Rescan the patient.
10. Repeat steps 8 and 9 as necessary.

Tip: If you are uncertain about judging the approach, then use a 22G needle to verify the approach. A second needle is positioned alongside the first and its position again checked.

A common pitfall is for the needle to pass obliquely through the scan plane. This can be demonstrated by performing one or two cuts above and below the target plane. If the needle tip is still in a satisfactory position, proceed as normal; if not, reposition the needle, compensating for the incorrect angle.

Fluoroscopic guidance

Fluoroscopic guidance is used principally to biopsy pulmonary masses and for bone biopsy. Whenever possible, use an X-ray machine with a C-arm, and avoid machines with overcouch explorers. Remember the basic principle of radiology: two views are necessary for localization.

Position the patient for the procedure and fluoroscope to identify the target lesion. Centre the field on the lesion and mark the position with a pair of sponge forceps. It is nearly always possible to choose an approach that allows the needle to be advanced perpendicular to the skin. For pulmonary biopsy, ask the patient to suspend breathing. Advance the needle partway to the target and then fluoroscope to confirm that the tract is passing in the correct direction. Rotate the C-arm through 90° and fluoroscope again to determine the position of the needle tip relative to the target. Advance the needle until it reaches the target and reconfirm the position on the original projection.

The situation is slightly different during biliary drainage and nephrostomy, as an oblique approach is required for catheter and guidewire manipulation. When aiming at a specific duct or calyx, it is essential to know whether the needle is passing anterior or posterior to the target duct. This is resolved by rotating the C-arm (the patient can be rotated, but remember there is a long needle sticking in them) and observing the movement of the needle relative to the target. If the needle is posterior, when the C-arm is rotated the needle moves in the same direction as the C-arm rotation; if it moves in the opposite direction, it is anterior to the target. Remember that the reverse is true if you are turning the patient. When you think that you have grasped this concept, just wait until you try it in practice!

SUGGESTIONS FOR FURTHER READING

Matalon TAS, Silver B. US guidance of interventional procedures. Radiology 1990;174:43–47.
Essential ultrasound techniques; well illustrated.

Yeuh N, Halvorsen RA, Letourneau JG et al. Gantry tilt technique for CT-guided biopsy and drainage. J Comput Assist Tomogr 1989;13:182–184.
An invaluable technique for many lesions.

Chapter Twenty

Equipment for non-vascular intervention

The majority of catheters and guidewires used in the vascular system are also appropriate for non-vascular intervention. There are, however, several devices that are used mainly for non-vascular applications.

Mini-access set (Neff/Accustick)

A mini-access set converts a 22G puncture to 0.035 inch guidewire access (Fig. 20.1). The set is used mainly for PTC and more difficult nephrostomy insertion, e.g. in an undilated system. The set comes with a 22G needle for the initial puncture and a short 0.018 inch guidewire, which is inserted through the needle after successful puncture. An interlocked dilator system can then be inserted over the guidewire; essentially this consists of an inner 3Fr dilator with an outer 6Fr dilator. The inner dilator is then removed, leaving the 6Fr dilator, which will accept a standard 0.035 inch guidewire.

Torcon blue biliary manipulation catheter (Cook)

This is a short single-endhole steel braided polyethylene catheter which has excellent torque control and is invaluable for urinary and biliary work. Conventional angiographic catheters can be used, but tend to have poorer torque control.

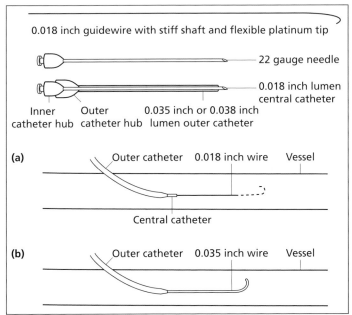

0.018 inch guidewire with stiff shaft and flexible platinum tip

22 gauge needle

0.018 inch lumen central catheter

Inner catheter hub   Outer catheter hub   0.035 inch or 0.038 inch lumen outer catheter

(a)   Outer catheter   0.018 inch wire   Vessel

Central catheter

(b)   Outer catheter   0.035 inch wire   Vessel

Fig. 20.1 ▦ Mini-access set. (a) Inner and outer catheters are inserted over 0.018 inch wire. (b) Inner catheter and 0.018 inch wire are removed and an 0.035 inch wire can be passed down the outer catheter.

Peel-away sheath

This is a non-haemostatic plastic sheath that has been bonded along its midline (Fig. 20.2). The peel-away sheath is inserted over a supplied inner dilator, which is then removed. Catheters and stents will readily pass down the sheath because of the reduction in friction and improvement in angles. The sheath is peeled apart by grasping the two proximal toggles. It is important to maintain some forward pressure on the device within the sheath to avoid inadvertently pulling it back while removing the sheath.

Ureteric stent systems

A variety of ureteric stent systems are available, but as always they operate on essentially similar principles (Fig. 20.3). The ureteric stent is usually a double-J configuration and straightened on the wire. A pusher is used to deliver the stent into position across a suitably stiff guidewire. The most common variation of design is the mechanism to pull back the stent if pushed in too far. In some systems an inner catheter is 'plugged' into

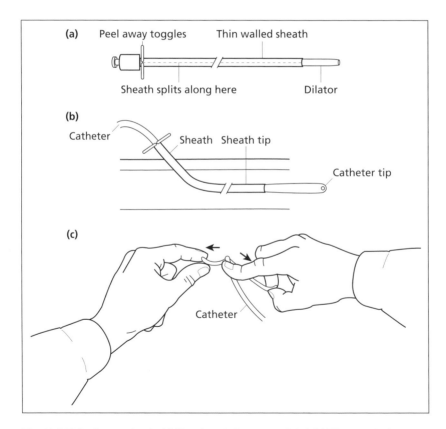

Fig. 20.2 ■ Peel-away sheath. (a) Sheath and dilator assembled. (b) Dilator and wire are removed to allow passage of the device. (c) Hold the catheter in place with a finger, then pull the hub to split and remove the sheath.

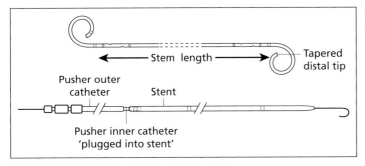

Fig. 20.3 ■ Double-J ureteric stent system.

the proximal end of the stent, which allows retraction of the stent. Alternatively, a suture loop may have been passed through the last two stent sideholes. After optimal stent positioning the inner catheter is withdrawn while maintaining the pusher in position to release the stent. In systems with a suture loop remember to cut the loop and remove it before withdrawing the stent pusher. An 8Fr 22 cm-long stent is appropriate for the majority of patients.

Chapter Twenty-One

Biopsy and drainage

This chapter is divided into three main sections:
- Fine needle aspiration cytology and biopsy
- Draining fluid collections and abscesses
- Biopsy and drainage of specific areas.

Complications of biopsy and drainage are discussed at the end of the chapter.

Biopsy and drainage procedures involve traversing normal tissue to reach an abnormal area. To do this requires a safe access route and accurate targeting. The principles of image guidance for intervention are discussed in the preceding chapter. The shortest, straightest route is usually the best, but there are important exceptions to this rule, e.g. peripheral liver lesion. Take time to plan an approach that avoids important structures, e.g. bowel, lung, major vessels and the gallbladder.

To minimize complications, the patient should be fasted for abdominal biopsy and coagulopathy should be excluded. Make sure that the patient has given consent and that all parties are aware of the potential risks (and their consequences) of the procedure.

 Consent issue: Explain the benefits of obtaining material for diagnosis/drainage. Problems tend to come from bleeding and traversing other structures, serious complications are rare.

FINE NEEDLE ASPIRATION CYTOLOGY AND BIOPSY

The aim of aspiration or biopsy is to obtain a satisfactory tissue specimen for cytology or histology. Ultrasound is used whenever possible, as it allows real-time guidance without exposing you or the patient to ionizing radiation.

The patient

The vast majority of biopsies are performed under local anaesthesia and patient cooperation is essential. Explain what the procedure entails; in particular, stress the importance of breath-holding during the needle pass. If the patient does not understand or cannot cooperate, then stop now! Most biopsies are not painful; emphasize that analgesia is available if needed. Make sure that the patient is aware that regular postbiopsy observations are normal and do not indicate a problem.

Contraindications

Abnormal clotting or platelets

- It is mandatory to know the platelet count and clotting status.
- No additional precautions are necessary when the INR is = 1.5 and the platelet count = 50 000.

When the clotting is more deranged, consider transfusion of FFP ± platelets.

Vascular lesion   Some tumours are highly vascular, e.g. renal cell tumour metastases. Switch on the colour Doppler if there is any doubt. If you need to biopsy a vascular lesion, make sure that the patient is adequately prepared. This may require large-bore IV access and cross-matched blood. Try to avoid the main tumoral vessels and be prepared to embolize the lesion if necessary.

Obstructed system   The target for biopsy is likely to be the point of obstruction, and fistula or intra-abdominal leakage can occur. It is best to drain the system before biopsy. Attempting drainage after a complication can be very difficult.

Uncooperative patient

- Consider sedation or general anaesthesia.
- Remember that a sedated patient will not be able to breath-hold.

Diagnosis irrelevant to management   Do not be persuaded to do the biopsy just because 'it would be nice to know'.

Which specimen – cytology or histology?

There are two sampling techniques: aspiration cytology and cutting needle biopsy. The local pathology service will guide you on the type of specimen they require. Usually only a few cells are needed to diagnose malignancy, but a core of tissue is needed to subtype tumours or assess diffuse liver/renal pathology.

Fine-needle aspiration cytology

Aspiration cytology, sometimes referred to as fine-needle aspiration cytology (FNAC), is performed with a 21G or 22G (Chiba) needle. The specimen only contains a few cells, but for many conditions this will establish the diagnosis. The risks involved are very small; FNAC is frequently possible even in hazardous areas.

The needle is placed into the lesion under imaging guidance and then attached to a 20 mL syringe. Draw a full vacuum on the syringe while the needle is passed back and forward through the lesion (Fig. 21.1). If you have an assistant, use a connecting tube or a 21G butterfly needle and get them to aspirate the syringe while you manipulate the needle under guidance.

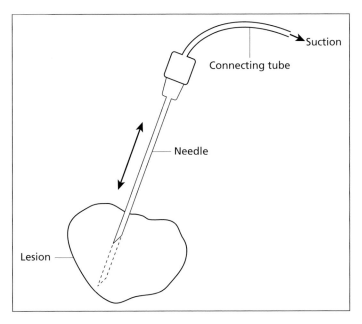

Fig. 21.1 ■ Aspiration technique. The needle is passed into the lesion under ultrasound control. A connecting tube and 20 mL syringe are attached to the needle. Draw a full vacuum on the syringe and then pass the needle backwards and forwards through the lesion. Slowly release the vacuum as the needle is withdrawn or the tiny sample will disappear into the syringe.

 Tip: Withdraw the needle under gentle suction, then remove the syringe. Vigorous suction results in the tiny sample being lost in the syringe; without suction, the sample stays in the patient.

Place the sampling needle on a slide and gently eject the contents on to the slide with an air-filled syringe. Also put any fluid in the sampling syringe on to a slide. Specimens may be simply air dried, but specimen preparation varies from centre to centre; check the preference of your cytologist. Specimens only contain a few cells, and therefore it is best to make at least two passes.

 Tip: It is helpful to have a cytologist to prepare the slide. The cytologist will make a better film, and also be able to make a preliminary inspection of the material to ensure that it is adequate.

Cutting needle biopsy

Cutting needle biopsy obtains a larger specimen, typically a 1 mm core 20 mm in length. The cutting needle consists of two parts: an outer cutting shaft and an inner stylet

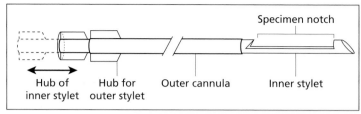

Fig. 21.2 ■ Construction of a cutting biopsy needle. Tissue prolapses into the specimen notch and is cut by advancement of the outer cutting needle shaft.

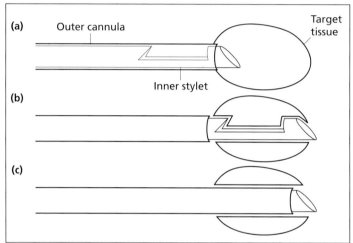

Fig. 21.3 ■ Mechanism of action of a cutting needle. (a) Needle is advanced to the edge of the target tissue. (b) Inner stylet is advanced into the target tissue. (c) Outer cutting shaft is advanced to resheath inner stylet and cut the specimen core.

(Fig. 21.2). Most centres use automated devices, but if you are using cutting needles manually it is essential to realize that the specimen is 'cut' when the outer shaft is advanced.

Manual biopsy needles   Many devices are available, but the most popular are automated versions of the traditional Trucut needle, as these reliably obtain a core of tissue for histology and can be used with an automated biopsy device (Fig. 21.3). The needle comes in various sizes from 14G to 18G, and with two different specimen lengths, 1 cm and 2 cm. In practice, the 18G 2 cm needle is suitable for the majority of biopsies.

Automated biopsy devices   The needles are always single use, but the mechanism may be disposable or reusable. There are two principal mechanisms, which differ in the way in which the central stylet is advanced.

The first is typified by the Temno needle. In this device, the inner stylet is advanced manually into the target. At this stage, resistance is felt and further pressure on the trigger mechanism fires the outer sleeve to cut the core. Important points to note are:

- The precise position of the core is ascertained before the biopsy is taken; this is particularly important in proximity to hazardous areas.
- It is an integral system. There is no handle to attach and detach, which means that it is smaller and lighter than the Biopty gun. This is an important consideration for CT biopsy, where the patient must be rescanned to confirm needle position.

The alternative system is fully automatic, and is typified by the Biopty Gun. Many radiologists use this, as it is simple, quick and reliable. The automated mechanism advances the device with a two-step action: first, the inner stylet is advanced 21 mm, exposing the specimen notch; then, almost instantaneously, the outer cutting shaft is advanced, thereby obtaining the specimen. The net effect is that the sample is obtained from the 20 mm immediately beyond the initial position of the needle tip – important if you want to avoid biopsy of adjacent vascular structures.

Tip: Some automated systems allow the operator to determine the length of the specimen, i.e. the forward throw of the needle – very useful if the biopsy is close to a vital structure.

Aftercare

There is no fixed regimen for postbiopsy care. The aftercare varies with the site of biopsy, the coagulation status and the general condition of the patient. Ensure that a written care plan is given to the staff who will care for the patient. If there is no established local protocol, the proforma in the box can be modified to suit most procedures.

Sample proforma for patient aftercare

Patient name   ID No.

Date   Time

Procedure

Anaesthesia/sedation

Needle size   No. of cores taken

Uneventful/complicated (specify)

Specimens   In formalin/saline/dry
                 Returned with patient/sent to

Aftercare
                 Flat bedrest for 2 hours
                 Pulse and BP   Every 15 minutes for 1 hour
                                                 Every 30 minutes for 1 hour
                                                 Every 60 minutes for 2 hours
                                                 Every 4 hours until discharge

                 Analgesia as necessary

Other, e.g. fluids only

Information for discharge

DRAINING FLUID COLLECTIONS AND ABSCESSES

Tapping fluid collections to drain them or to obtain fluid for laboratory investigation is an important and frequently requested procedure. The vast majority of collections can be managed with an appropriately sized and positioned catheter, but success depends on understanding a few key concepts.

Assessing abscesses

Use the preintervention imaging to identify:

- **The exact anatomical location of the collection** An understanding of the anatomical boundaries will dictate the ideal drain position and approach. Large collections will shrink, and to achieve complete drainage the drain should be placed in the most dependent portion.
- **The content of the collection** Ultrasound offers the most useful assessment of the viscosity of the collection and the presence of loculi and septa. Look for the following features, which will influence the type and number of drains required:

Anechoic collection	Probably clear fluid, e.g. urinoma
Few scattered echoes	Turbid fluid, e.g. thin pus
Extensive or swirling echoes	Thick fluid, e.g. viscous pus
Diffuse echoes with gas	Organized abscess or phlegmon
Simple collection	Single drain
Loculated collection – thin	Single drain – synechiae
Loculated collection – thick	Multiple drains – septae
Multiple collections	Multiple drains

 Tip: The ultrasound appearances are not an infallible guide and will occasionally be misleading – always try a diagnostic aspiration.

Which drain?

Drain size At the risk of stating the obvious, viscous fluid will not drain through a small-calibre drainage catheter. Use a 6–8Fr catheter for clear fluid, an 8–10Fr catheter for thin pus, a 10–12Fr catheter for thick pus, and a 12–22Fr drain for collections containing debris.

Drain type Virtually all drainage catheters are pigtail shaped. The pigtail in some catheters is locked in position to provide anchorage. The mechanism to lock the catheter usually involves tensioning threads between the catheter hub and the pigtail. As the locking mechanism varies between individual devices, familiarize yourself with the systems used in your hospital. Failure to unlock the catheter at removal will cause a large exit wound; intense screaming from the patient usually warns the alert operator.

Sump drainage catheters have a second lumen that allows air to pass to the distal tip of the catheter; this stops the cavity collapsing around the catheter tip. This is especially helpful during aspiration and drainage of very viscous collections, and when repeated irrigation is necessary.

Diagnostic aspiration

This is also the first step in any drainage procedure.

Equipment
- 21G needle (of appropriate length).
- 20 mL syringes.
- Specimen pots.

 Tip: Ensure that you know which samples are required and how they are to be handled en route to the laboratory. Some specimens must be examined urgently.

Procedure

Prepare and anaesthetize the skin at the desired puncture site. Aim the needle into the collection and aspirate the desired amount of fluid. If necessary, it is acceptable to traverse bowel with a 21G needle, but this tract cannot be used for drainage. If drainage is anticipated, only take a small sample as this leaves a larger target to aim at.

 Tip: Before plunging a needle into a collection, turn on the colour Doppler as this will prevent you from draining an aneurysm!

Troubleshooting
Fluid cannot be aspirated   Check that the needle tip is correctly sited within the collection and reposition as necessary. Sometimes the fluid is too thick to aspirate with a 22G needle; try again with an 18G needle. If this is unsuccessful, this is probably a solid mass; consider biopsy.

Therapeutic drainage

A selection of catheters and guidewires may be needed. A small amount of fluid is usually aspirated as a prelude to drainage; the nature of this specimen helps you decide which drain will function best.

Procedure

The precise technique depends on the type of catheter that has been chosen.

Prepare and anaesthetize the skin and the desired puncture site. Make a sufficiently large skin incision to allow passage of the drainage catheter. Pass a needle into the collection using imaging guidance.

In a **'one-step' procedure** the catheter is mounted on a central needle and stylet. A direct puncture technique is used. The central stylet is removed and fluid is aspirated to confirm that the tip is within the collection. The needle is held still and the catheter is simply advanced along the needle into the collection. This technique is only advisable for large collections which are easily accessed. Fluoroscopy is not required.

In a **'two-step' procedure** fluoroscopy is recommended. A guidewire is passed through the puncture needle into the collection. If a 21G needle was used to puncture the collection, either simply repuncture with an 18G needle or consider using a Neff set to convert to a 0.035 inch wire. The needle is removed over the wire and the track is dilated using fascial dilators to 1–2Fr larger than the drainage catheter.

Fix the wire securely to ensure that it does not kink and that you do not lose its position during catheter exchanges.

The catheter stiffener assembly is then passed over the wire into the collection. When you reach either a significant bend or the collection, detach the stiffener, hold it and the wire fixed in position, and slide the catheter forward over the guidewire (Fig. 21.4). The stiffener and guidewire are removed and the catheter is allowed to form. Most self-retaining catheters are introduced in this way.

 Tip: Always insert plenty of guidewire, as this allows a degree of latitude if you kink the wire.

Whichever technique is used, ensure that there is free drainage and that you have obtained adequate specimens for laboratory analysis. **When the collection contains pus, aspirate it as completely as possible!** In addition, consider gentle saline irrigation of the cavity, as this helps to clear thick pus and other semisolid debris. Make sure that you have a suitable drain bag to attach to the drainage catheter. Sometimes special adaptors are needed: do not wait until pus is running over your shoes to find this out!

Attach the catheter securely to the patient. There are several ways to do this:
• Suturing the catheter to the skin.
• Using adhesive anchor systems.
• Using adhesive tape – only secure with waterproof tape.

Make sure that the final position will be practical and as comfortable as possible for the patient.

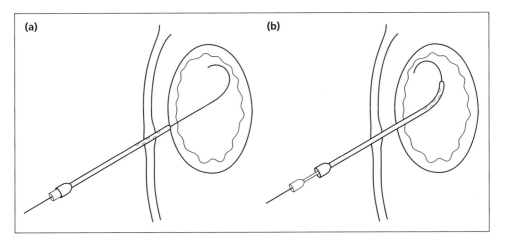

Fig. 21.4 Catheter stiffener assembly. (a) The entire assembly is advanced to the edge of the collection. (b) The Luer lock is loosened and the inner stiffener is held stationary with the wire and the drainage catheter pushed forwards.

Tip: It is always harder to puncture a partially drained collection. Avoid frustration and fix the catheter so that it stays put until you want to remove it!

Follow-up

The volume of fluid drained is charted. Febrile patients usually settle within 24–48 hours if there is adequate drainage. Most simple fluid collections drain quickly, with a steady decrease in the volume of fluid draining. Large inflammatory collections (e.g. pseudocyst, empyema) may take several weeks to resolve.

Thick viscous collections require irrigation and aspiration to ensure effective drainage. It is essential that the catheter is aspirated three times a day. Use a 50 mL syringe for maximum suction, and then irrigate with 5–10 mL of saline. The drain may need to be repositioned or replaced as the situation evolves.

The drain catheter can be removed when there is minimal drainage (<10 mL/day) and the collection has resolved as documented by CT or ultrasound. Catheters should be promptly removed when they have fulfilled their role if they are not to become a source of infection in their own right.

Troubleshooting

The drainage catheter will not advance into the collection

- Ensure that the skin incision is large enough.
- Use fluoroscopy to check for wire kinking. If it is kinked and there is sufficient wire, pull it until the kink is outside the skin, then insert a dilator and exchange for a stiffer wire.
- Large drains may need to be placed through a peel-away sheath positioned over a stiff guidewire.

The collection is loculated and does not drain freely

- Thin loculi can be disrupted by moving the catheter back and forth within the collection.
- If this is not successful, fibrinous bands can be broken down by instilling streptokinase into the collection. This is particularly useful for loculated empyema.
- Some collections require multiple drainage catheters.

The catheter drains initially but then stops

- Hopefully the collection is completely drained. Reimage the patient to assess the catheter position and the size of the collection.
- The drainage bag has been positioned above the collection, e.g. on the patient's locker. Place the bag in a dependent position.
- The catheter is correctly positioned but there is a kink in it or the drainage tubing. Kinks are almost always external and are often caused by fiddling with the catheter or dressings. Reattaching it appropriately can often salvage the catheter. If there is any doubt, replace the catheter/drainage tube.
- The catheter may need to be repositioned or replaced if the collection has changed size or shape, or if the catheter has been displaced.
- The catheter is blocked. Gentle flushing may clear it. If this fails, try using a guidewire to unblock it. An irreversibly blocked catheter must be exchanged. Catheters that have been in place for a week or more usually have a well-established tract. The catheter can be removed and a hydrophilic guidewire passed through the tract into the collection. A new drain is then simply positioned over the wire. An alternative option is to cut the hub off the catheter and then pass a sheath over the outside of it. The catheter is removed and a guidewire passed into the collection through the sheath; the sheath is removed and a new catheter positioned over the wire.

Fever does not settle after 48 hours Failure to improve implies incomplete drainage or another source of sepsis. If this occurs, the patient should be reimaged. Further drainage is often required. This scenario is common in patients with infected pancreatic pseudocysts.

There is a sudden increase in drainage or a change in the composition of the effluent
This implies that a fistula has developed; an injection of contrast into the drainage catheter will usually demonstrate the problem. Sometimes it is necessary to perform an alternative study if the fistula tract acts as a one-way valve. A fistula will usually resolve if there is an adequate alternative route of drainage, although prolonged drainage may be necessary. Where there is a connection with an obstructed system, this will also need to be drained if the fistula is to resolve.

BIOPSY AND DRAINAGE OF SPECIFIC AREAS

Liver

Liver biopsy is one of the most frequently requested interventional procedures and is usually one of the simplest to perform. Biopsies are targeted either to a focal lesion or to random cores in diffuse liver disease. Non-targeted biopsies are usually taken from the right lobe. When there are multiple lesions, choose the most accessible. To minimize the risk of

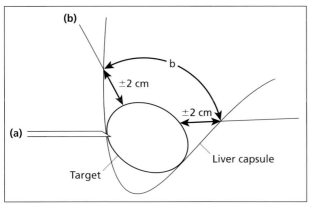

Fig. 21.5 ▪ Direct biopsy of peripheral liver lesions (a) increases the risk of extracapsular bleeding. Choose an approach (b) that passes through a cuff of normal liver tissue.

haemorrhage when taking a biopsy of peripheral lesions, always make a tract that passes through 2–3 cm of normal liver before hitting the target (Fig. 21.5).

When taking a biopsy of the right lobe of the liver, a lateral approach is usually chosen. The ribs can interfere with access; choose an approach that allows scanning parallel to the line of the ribs. Sometimes the needle has to be angled up or down to accommodate this.

Mild shoulder tip pain is not uncommon after liver biopsy, and the patient should be warned that this may occur. The risks of biopsy are increased in the presence of biliary obstruction and ascites, and so drainage is recommended before biopsy. In the presence of mildly deranged clotting, consider a plugged biopsy.

Plugged liver biopsy

The essence of this procedure is to prevent haemorrhage from the liver capsule by embolizing the needle tract using Gelfoam injected through a sheath in the needle tract. Using a sheath has the potential advantage of allowing more than one needle to pass through the same tract.

Equipment

- 18G biopsy needle.
- 18G sheathed needle.
- Gelfoam sheet.

Procedure

Prepare the Gelfoam in advance by cutting the sheet into 1 mm pledgets and soak them in contrast. Discard the needle from the 18G sheathed needle and fit the sheath over the biopsy needle. The needle and sheath are advanced into the liver as a single unit (Fig. 21.6). The biopsy is performed in the conventional fashion. The needle is withdrawn, leaving the sheath in situ, and the adequacy of the specimen is confirmed. The tract is now embolized

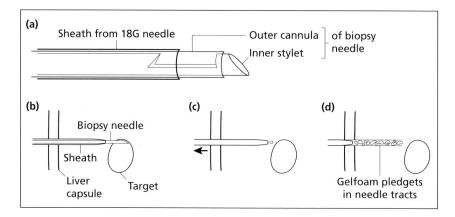

Fig. 21.6 ▓ Plugged liver biopsy technique. (a) The 18G biopsy needle is passed through the sheath of an 18G needle. (b) The needle and sheath are advanced into the liver and the biopsy is taken. (c) The biopsy needle is removed and Gelfoam pledgets are injected through the sheath as it is withdrawn. (d) The final result is a tract embolized with Gelfoam.

by injecting 1–2 mL of the Gelfoam pledgets as the sheath is withdrawn. Postbiopsy aftercare is the same as for a standard liver biopsy.

Transjugular liver biopsy

Transjugular liver biopsy (TJB) is a much more complicated and expensive procedure. It is reserved for patients with diffuse liver disease and deranged coagulation or ascites for whom plugged biopsy would still pose a significant risk. The rationale for TJB is that there is no puncture of the liver capsule, and therefore any bleeding from the needle tract will be contained within the liver or autotransfuse into the hepatic vein. TJB is not *carte blanche* to perform liver biopsy in any patient; as always, attempts should be made to correct the underlying coagulopathy before the procedure.

Anatomy

The hepatic veins join the IVC just below the right atrium. Biopsy is most safely performed from the right hepatic vein while angling the sheath anteriorly. This ensures that the biopsy is taken from the maximum volume of parenchyma and avoids inadvertent capsular perforation. Anterior biopsy from the middle hepatic vein should be avoided.

Differentiating the right from the middle hepatic vein can be difficult in the AP projection, but is easily done from a lateral.

Equipment

- Basic angiography set.
- 5Fr sheath.

- Cobra II catheter.
- Hydrophilic and Amplatz guidewires. A 1 cm floppy-tip Amplatz wire is very useful in small livers.
- Transjugular cutting needle liver biopsy set (Cook UK Ltd) which contains a 7Fr 49 cm long sheath, an angled metallic sheath stiffener, a 5Fr straight catheter, and a 60 cm long cutting biopsy needle. A metal arrow on the hub of the stiffener indicates the orientation of the curve.

Procedure

Access Ultrasound-guided right IJV puncture.

Catheterization Pass the J wire and the Cobra catheter into the IVC, taking particular care when steering through the right atrium. Rotate the catheter so that its tip points towards the patient's right; slowly withdraw it until the tip engages the RHV. Advance the hydrophilic wire and Cobra catheter into the vein.

Runs Hand-inject a few millilitres of contrast to ensure that the catheter is not wedged, then perform a hepatic venogram. The RHV is the target vein and typically has a suitably shallow angle that allows the sheath entry. The angled stiffener within the sheath gives excellent torque control but poor cornering ability, and will only negotiate suitably angled veins.

Biopsy An Amplatz extra-stiff wire is passed into the hepatic vein; take care not to puncture the liver capsule with the guidewire (Fig. 21.7)! Exchange the 5Fr sheath for the reinforced sheath, which is passed 3–4 cm into the hepatic vein. Use the directional indicator on the hub to direct the sheath anteriorly until it abuts the vein wall. The cutting needle is primed and advanced into the sheath until the tip is a few millimetres beyond the end of the sheath in the liver parenchyma. The patient is instructed to breath-hold and the inner stylet is depressed, taking the biopsy.

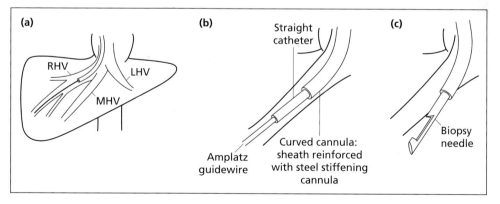

Fig. 21.7 ▦ Transjugular liver biopsy technique. (a) Catheterize the right hepatic vein using a Cobra II catheter. Then exchange for an Amplatz superstiff wire. (b) Advance the curved cannula into the right hepatic vein using a coaxial straight catheter and the Amplatz wire. Remove the catheter and wire to leave the curved cannula in place. (c) Turn the curved cannula anteriorly to abut the vein wall and advance the long biopsy needle into the liver parenchyma to take the biopsy.

Kidney

The kidney is the most vascular organ in the body and biopsy is associated with an increased risk of haemorrhage. Most renal biopsies in native and transplant kidneys are performed to investigate the aetiology of renal failure. These biopsies should be taken from either the upper or the lower pole of the kidney. Avoid biopsy adjacent to the renal pelvis, as this greatly increases the risks of urinary and vascular complications. Few biopsies are performed to investigate the nature of renal masses, as these are usually dealt with surgically.

Adrenal glands

The adrenal glands are usually approached posteriorly in the prone or lateral decubitus position; large lesions can be biopsied anteriorly. In most cases, CT is the best imaging guidance. Always measure the vanillylmandelic acid in patients who have an adrenal mass with no known primary tumour. When phaeochromocytoma is suspected α-adrenergic blockade is recommended to minimize the risk of hypertensive crisis.

Pancreas

Pancreatic biopsy is indicated in the investigation of a mass at the head of the pancreas. There is usually associated biliary and pancreatic duct obstruction. If obstructed, the biliary tree should be drained before starting. The pancreatic duct cannot be drained and there is a risk of pancreatitis and pseudocyst formation.

Pancreatic biopsy can usually be performed under ultrasound guidance. The biopsy track may be transgastric, but care should be taken to avoid inadvertent biopsy through the transverse colon (Fig. 21.8). Plastic biliary stents are readily seen on ultrasound and can be used to target pancreatic biopsy. As pancreatic biopsy is often painful, sedation and analgesia are recommended.

Peripancreatic abscesses, pseudocysts and phlegmons are common complications of pancreatitis. Infected collections often require drainage. The management of complex pancreatitis is best left to a specialist team, but the following guidelines are generally applicable. Collections in the lesser sac can usually be approached anteriorly through the transverse mesocolon between the stomach and the transverse colon. Collections in the left paracolic gutter are more difficult to approach and are best done with CT guidance to avoid colonic puncture. Loculated collections may require several drains. As always, frequent review is mandatory. This often entails serial CT scanning. Large pseudocysts that continue to drain can be treated by cyst gastrostomy.

 Alarm: If you cannot confidently identify the colon, opacify it with contrast. Do not risk a colonic kebab!

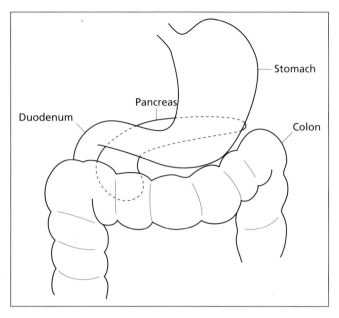

Fig. 21.8 ▦ Relationship between the stomach, pancreas and transverse colon. Transgastric biopsy is acceptable, but take great care to avoid the colon.

Retroperitoneum

Most retroperitoneal masses are best biopsied on CT unless they are very large. The retroperitoneum can be approached anteriorly if there is a window without bowel. The posterior approach is particularly useful for paraspinal masses.

Pelvis

The commonest difficulty in pelvic biopsy or drainage is identifying a route that does not traverse bowel or bladder. Gravity causes pus to collect in the prerectal space; this is difficult to access from an anterior approach. Alternative options include transrectal, transvaginal and transgluteal approaches.

The posterior transgluteal route traverses the sacrosciatic notch and uses CT guidance (Fig. 21.9). The patient is scanned in the prone position (Fig. 21.10) and the approach is planned in the conventional fashion. **Remember that the sciatic nerve and gluteal vessels pass through the anterior portion of the notch**. To avoid them, the tract should pass as close to the sacrum as possible. Burrowing through this much muscle can be difficult and may be uncomfortable for the patient, both during and after the procedure. Pericatheter inflammation can cause sciatica even when the catheter is appropriately placed.

Ultrasound-guided transrectal and transvaginal drainage and biopsy are readily performed and well tolerated. Although these approaches are unfamiliar, the basic principles of biopsy

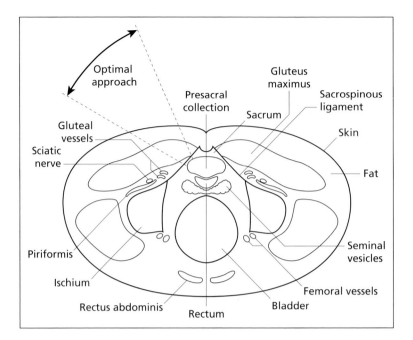

Fig. 21.9 ■ Approach for transgluteal drainage through the greater sciatic notch. The optimal path is posteromedial to avoid the gluteal vessels and sciatic nerve.

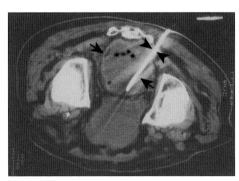

Fig. 21.10 ■ Transgluteal route for drainage of a presacral abscess (arrows). The catheter (arrowheads) passes close to the sacrum to avoid the sciatic nerve and gluteal vessels, which lie anteriorly.

and drainage apply. These routes offer a direct approach to posterior collections, with the advantage of draining well in the supine position. Most suitable probes have needle guides. Use sterile covers over the probe and guide. The collection is punctured under direct visualization. As always, aspirate some fluid; if it is purulent, formal drainage is performed; if not, the collection is aspirated to dryness. Catheter fixation is difficult and self-retaining catheters are preferred. The catheter can be taped to the patient's thigh and drained into a leg bag.

Transrectal procedures cause surprisingly little discomfort, but this is a 'dirty' route (Fig. 21.11). A cleansing enema is recommended to remove any faecal residue, and

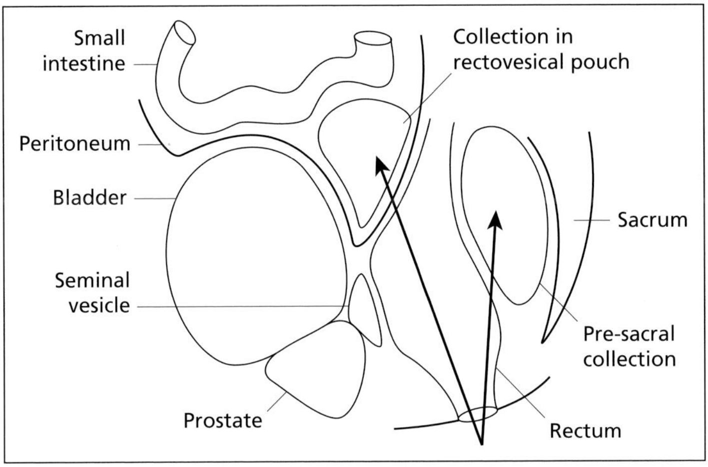

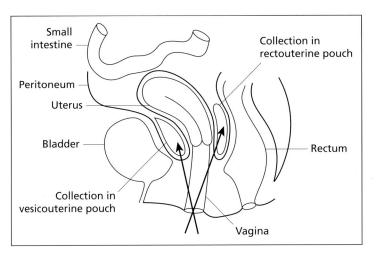

Fig. 21.11 ▦ Sagittal section through male pelvis showing routes for transrectal drainage.

Fig. 21.12 ▦ Sagittal section through the female pelvis to show transvaginal routes for abscess drainage.

antibiotic prophylaxis must be given. Contamination of the collection with faecal organisms is a potential pitfall, but is thought not to occur because of the positive intra-abdominal pressure during defecation. The patient is scanned in the lateral decubitus or lithotomy position. Drains up to 12Fr can be used. Catheter displacement during defaecation is common even with self-retaining catheters.

The transvaginal approach is performed with the patient in the lithotomy position (Fig. 21.12). Sedation is recommended, as the procedure tends to be uncomfortable and the vaginal wall can be difficult to traverse. The vagina and perineum are cleansed with povidone–iodine solution. Catheters up to 12Fr can be used but require the use of serial fascial dilators over a stiff guidewire.

Complications of biopsy and drainage

Fortunately, complications following biopsy are rare and the majority of complications are minor. The risks vary between individual patients and differing sites; this is discussed in the relevant sections. The most important complications are:

- **Bleeding** This may occur even in the best hands, particularly in the presence of a vascular lesion or organ. Ensure that the blood clotting and platelets are optimized before starting.

Alarm: The risk of haemorrhage is highest during:

- Biopsy of vascular organs (liver, spleen and kidneys) in the presence of abnormal clotting
- Biopsy adjacent to major blood vessels
- Biopsy of known vascular tumours, particularly when there is no surrounding normal tissue to tamponade bleeding.

In high-risk patients it is wise to group and save, or even cross-match blood for the procedure.

- **Perforation of a hollow viscus** Bowel can usually be avoided by using an appropriate approach. If the intestine must be traversed, use a fine needle (22G) rather than a cutting needle.
- **Pneumothorax** This is common following biopsy of lung or mediastinal masses. Pneumothorax can also occur when the pleural space is traversed during biopsy of upper abdominal lesions. Remember that the pleural space extends much further down posteriorly. This problem can be anticipated, and the patient should be warned that it might be necessary to have a chest drain following the procedure.
- **Fistula** May occur when performing biopsies in the presence of an obstructed system. For this reason, it is advisable to perform drainage before biopsy. This is particularly important in the presence of biliary obstruction.
- **Infection** This is rare if proper aseptic precautions are taken and the intestine is not traversed. When the bowel is traversed, e.g. transrectal biopsy, then prophylactic antibiotics should be given, e.g. gentamicin 80 mg and metronidazole 500 mg. If the colon is punctured, seek surgical advice. The patient will usually settle on conservative management, nil by mouth and antibiotics.
- **Tumour seeding of the biopsy tract** This is rare but can occur with any tumour. The risk can be minimized by passing through a 'normal' section of the target organ or the potential field of resection.
- **Death** This is usually due to haemorrhage and is very rare for routine biopsies.

SUGGESTIONS FOR FURTHER READING

General

Georgian-Smith D, Shiels WE. Freehand interventional sonography in the breast: basic principles and clinical applications. Radiographics 1996;16:149–161.

Gupta S. New techniques in image guided percutaneous biopsy. Cardiovasc Intervent Radiol 2004;27:91–104.
A comprehensive and contemporary overview with useful insights into newer modes of CT guidance, and also advanced biopsy techniques.

Livrahgi T, Lazzaroni S, Civelli L et al. Risk conditions and mortality rate of abdominal fine needle biopsy. J Intervent Radiol 1997;12:57–64.
Includes recommendations to minimize risks. A very worthwhile read.

Spies JB, Berlin L. Complications of percutaneous needle biopsy. AJR 1998;171:13–17.

Pelvic

Alexander AA, Eschelman DJ, Nazarian LN et al. Transrectal sonographically guided drainage of deep pelvic abscesses. AJR 1994;162:1227–1230.

Feld R, Eschelman DJ, Sagerman JE et al. Treatment of pelvic abscesses and other fluid collections: efficacy of transvaginal sonographically guided aspiration and drainage. AJR 1994;163:1141–1145.

Thoracic

Hubsch P, Bankier AA, Wilding R et al. Thoracic anatomy relevant to CT interventions. Semin Intervent Radiol 1994;12;211–217.

Moore EH. Technical aspects of needle aspiration lung biopsy: personal perspective. Radiology 1998;208:303–318.
Beautiful article with a wealth of practical information – a must-read.

Moulton JS, Moore TP. Coaxial percutaneous biopsy technique with automated biopsy devices: value in improving accuracy and negative predictive value. Radiology 1993;186:515–522.

Liver

Choh J, Dolmatch B, Safadi R et al. Transjugular core liver biopsy with a 19 gauge spring loaded cutting needle. Cardiovasc Intervent Radiol 1998; 21:88–90.

Smith TP, McDermott VG, Ayoub DM. Percutaneous transhepatic liver biopsy with tract embolization. Radiology 1996;198:769–774.
Good practical description of the technique.

Renal

Christensen J, Lindequist S, Knudsen DU et al. Ultrasound guided renal biopsy with biopsy gun technique – efficacy and complications. Acta Radiol 1995;36:276.

Adrenal

Hussain S. Gantry angulation in CT guided adrenal biopsy. AJR 1996;166:537–539.

Welch TJ, Sheedy PFr II, Stephens DH. Percutaneous adrenal biopsy; review of a 10 year experience. Radiology 1994;193:341–344.

Pancreas

Dodd LG, Mooney EE, Layfield LJ et al. Fine-needle aspiration of the pancreas: A cytology primer for radiologists. Radiology 1997;205:203–209.

VanSonnenberg E, Wittich GR, Chon KS et al. Percutaneous radiologic drainage of pancreatic abscesses. AJR 1997;168:979–984.
The best results achievable with a very aggressive radiological approach.

Chapter Twenty-Two

Percutaneous renal intervention

Percutaneous nephrostomy

Percutaneous nephrostomy is one of the most frequently performed interventional procedures and is a technique in which every radiologist should feel completely confident. The commonest indication is ureteric obstruction, which leads to gradual progressive renal loss, and nephrostomy is usually an elective procedure. In an infected obstructed system the resultant rapid renal loss and septicaemia are an indication for urgent drainage.

Equipment

- Undilated or minimally dilated system: 21G Accustick/Neff mini-access set.
- Dilated system: 19G sheathed needle.
- Heavy-duty 3 mm J guidewire.
- Fascial dilators to one size greater than the drain size.
- 6–8Fr pigtail nephrostomy drain.
- 5Fr Cobra catheter.
- Angled hydrophilic wire.

Procedure

The performance of a safe nephrostomy requires an understanding of renal anatomy, good ultrasound guidance and basic catheterization skills.

Target zone   The renal arteries and veins enter the kidney at the renal hilum and divide into larger anterior and smaller posterior divisions, passing around the renal collecting system. Much has been made of Brödel's avascular line, but in practice the least vascular zone, and therefore the safest area, lies within the arc shown (Fig. 22.1).

Interpolar posterior calyxes in the mid and lower poles are the best target and provide the most favourable approach for intervention. Direct puncture of the renal pelvis should be avoided, as this increases the risk of major vascular injury and persistent urine leak. Puncture of the upper pole calyces is only necessary for nephrolithotomy and is associated with a significant risk of pneumothorax (Fig. 22.2). Avoid anterior punctures: in addition to providing the least favourable access and causing renal haemorrhage, you may well traverse colon, liver or spleen.

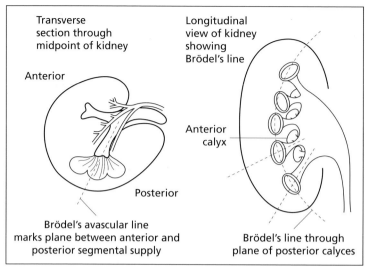

Transverse
section through
midpoint of kidney

Anterior

Posterior

Brödel's avascular line
marks plane between anterior and
posterior segmental supply

Longitudinal
view of kidney
showing
Brödel's line

Anterior
calyx

Brödel's line through
plane of posterior calyces

Fig. 22.1 ▨ Optimal approach for nephrostomy – posterior, lower or interpolar calyces along Brödel's avascular line.

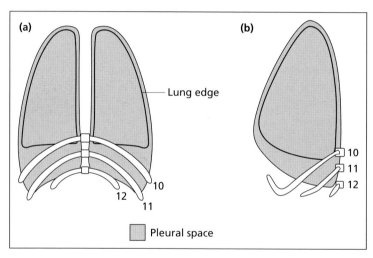

(a)

(b)

Lung edge

10
11
12

12   10
11

Pleural space

Fig. 22.2 ▨ Surface markings of the pleural spaces and the lungs relative to the lower ribs of (a) the posterior and (b) the lateral chest walls.

Ultrasound-guided puncture   Ultrasound guidance is by far the easiest and safest technique. It is easy to be anxious to get to the needle work, but take time at the start to get the ultrasound just right. If you have not read the section on ultrasound-guided punctures (p. 253), then read it now, if nothing else!

Scan the patient in either a prone or a prone/oblique position using a posterolateral approach to aim for a posterior interpolar calyx. Drape the patient, infiltrate local anaesthesia along the needle track, and make a 5 mm skin nick with a scalpel. Advance the puncture needle under continuous ultrasound guidance. When the needle tip reaches the calyx, advance it 5–10 mm with a darting motion. There may be a sudden 'give' as the calyx is entered. Apply gentle suction while slowly withdrawing the needle; aspiration of urine indicates entry to the system. Do not decompress the system completely, as this makes subsequent wire and catheter manipulation more difficult.

Achieving drainage   It seems nothing could be simpler now than to advance the nephrostomy drain into position, but many procedures go astray at this stage and frustrating hours can then be spent trying to puncture a now undilated system.

Using fluoroscopy, introduce a 0.035 inch J wire, which should advance without resistance. If you are lucky it will pass down the ureter, but often it will pass into an upper pole calyx or coil in the renal pelvis. Ideally, the guidewire should be passed into the ureter; it may be necessary to use a Cobra catheter to direct it. Advance dilators over the guidewire to 1Fr larger than the drain. Leave the dilator in place on the wire to tamponade the track.

In an uninfected system a 6Fr nephrostomy catheter is adequate, but pus requires at least an 8Fr drain for satisfactory drainage. Advance the nephrostomy drain until the tip is just within the ureter, then withdraw the wire to form the pigtail.

Never overdistend an obviously infected system with contrast. This is a sure way to give the patient septicaemia.

Inject a small amount of contrast to confirm your position, but generally, unless you have performed an immaculate puncture, a formal nephrostogram should be left for 24 hours as blood clot can simulate stones. Aspirate the drainage catheter:
- Pus: decompress the system completely.
- Blood – rosé coloured: connect to drainage bag.
- Blood – claret coloured: lavage with normal saline until it clears to rosé.

Finally, secure the catheter in position with either an adhesive dressing or a suture. Make sure that the catheter is firmly attached, or you will be replacing it later!

Troubleshooting

Difficult visualization
- Optimize the ultrasound; spend time looking for a good acoustic window before you start.
- Use a suitable probe: 3.5–5 MHz is best for nephrostomy.
- Use the best ultrasound machine available.

Aspiration of urine but cannot advance guidewire   The needle sheath is sitting against the wall of the calyx. Do not use force, as the calyx can be perforated. Very gently inject a little contrast to outline the position, carefully retract the needle sheath and advance the guidewire.

Unable to advance dilators/drainage catheter
- Check the skin nick. Is it large enough?
- Is the guidewire kinked? The wire most often kinks either at the skin surface or at the renal cortex. If you have inserted enough wire into ureter or renal pelvis, then it will be possible to withdraw the kink outside the skin. If there is insufficient wire to allow this, then it is usually possible to thread a 4Fr dilator over the most kinked wire into the renal pelvis. Insert a stronger wire, and this time do not let it ride forward during catheter insertion. Rarely, a stronger wire than the heavy-duty J is needed. Steer a 4Fr catheter into the ureter, then gently insert an Amplatz wire.

The pelvicalyceal system is undilated Exceptional for an emergency nephrostomy. Optimize your chances by using the best ultrasound machine. Consider giving 1 L normal saline and frusemide prior to nephrostomy to try to distend the system slightly. An Accustick system is best, as it is fairly unlikely you will access a suitable calyx first time round. Some operators will use contrast and puncture using fluroscopic guidance. For the more advanced, inject carbon dioxide after entering the pelvicalyceal system, and as this floats it allows the targetting of a suitable calyx.

> **Tip:** Do not try to jump too many French sizes but, as a general rule, go up in steps of two. Remember to dilate the tract to 1Fr larger than that of the drainage catheter.

Renal transplant nephrostomy

The good news about transplant nephrostomy is that the target is closer and hence ultrasound guidance easier. It is essential to avoid the temptation to perform a direct puncture of the renal pelvis. Ensure that the path of the nephrostomy catheter passes through parenchyma. Generally, transplant kidneys have an outer fibrotic capsule and it will require serial dilators to allow passage of the drainage catheter. Remember to insert plenty of wire; if necessary, use a catheter to steer down into the ureter. Finally, transplant kidneys do tend to be a bit more vascular, so do not be alarmed by bleeding during catheter changes as the nephrostomy drain will tamponade the tract.

Antegrade ureteric stent insertion

Antegrade stenting is performed when long-term ureteric drainage is required. It is more comfortable for the patient than having a nephrostomy, and has the obvious advantage of not needing any drainage bag. Ureteric stents can be placed retrogradely or antegradely. The antegrade approach is used when:
* There is a nephrostomy in situ.
* The retrograde approach has failed.

Indications
* Benign or malignant ureteric obstruction; malignant obstruction is by far the commonest indication.
* Ureteric injury, often in combination with nephrostomy drainage.
* Ureteric calculus undergoing lithotripsy.

Equipment
* Guidewires: 3 mm J, Amplatz, hydrophilic.
* Catheters: Cobra or Torcon blue.
* Peel-away sheath (usually 9Fr).

- Ureteric stent system (Boston Scientific, Cook UK Ltd).
- 8Fr nephrostomy catheter.

Procedure

1. A percutaneous nephrostomy may already be present. Alternatively, perform a nephrostomy aiming for a middle or lower pole calyx.
2. A shaped catheter, either a Cobra or a Torcon blue (Cook UK Ltd), is inserted using a J guidewire for access.
3. Contrast is introduced via the catheter to outline the ureter and the level of obstruction.
4. A hydrophilic wire (Terumo) is inserted into the catheter and directed down the ureter. The catheter is advanced down the ureter until it is just above the stricture.
5. The hydrophilic wire is gently advanced and rotated and will readily pass through the majority of strictures.
6. The catheter is advanced beyond the stricture and into the bladder.
7. The guidewire is now exchanged for an appropriately stiff wire such as an Amplatz or Flexfinder. Leave the catheter and wire in situ and prepare/assemble the ureteric stent system.
8. The tract should be dilated to 1Fr greater than the stent being inserted.
9. The ureteric stent system is inserted over the wire and, holding the wire perfectly still, advanced until the distal stent marker lies within bladder (Fig. 22.3).
10. Proximal end of stent is positioned within the renal pelvis and the guidewire is withdrawn.
11. The inner catheter is carefully withdrawn, releasing the stent, while keeping forward pressure on the pusher to maintain the stent in position.
12. A guidewire is inserted through the delivery system and a nephrostomy catheter placed in the renal pelvis. The nephrostomy catheter should be capped off, and if the stent functions adequately it can be removed in 24 hours.

Troubleshooting

Unable to negotiate the stricture with a guidewire   It is usually possible to negotiate strictures even if no route through can be seen on ureterograms. It takes skill and patience to negotiate these strictures, not force! Get a ureterogram and advance the catheter so that its tip is in the apex of the stricture. Use a hydrophilic wire and torque device to gently probe the stricture. This can take some time in the most difficult lesions. If this fails, then it is often worth leaving a nephrostomy in and allowing the system to decompress and ureteric oedema to settle over a few days. If after several attempts no route can be found, then it may be worth considering extra-anatomic stenting (see Further reading).

Unable to advance the catheter through stricture   Occasionally, the guidewire can traverse the stricture but the catheter will not follow. Try a 4Fr or hydrophilic catheter and try to rotate the catheter while advancing through the stricture. If this fails, take a deep breath and withdraw the guidewire and insert a 3 mm J guidewire down to the level of the stricture before advancing a 9Fr peel-away sheath into the distal ureter. The increased stability and reduction in friction means it is now often possible to advance a catheter. Exceptionally this may fail, and it is worth crossing the stricture with a 0.018 inch wire and using a low-profile small-vessel balloon to dilate the stricture.

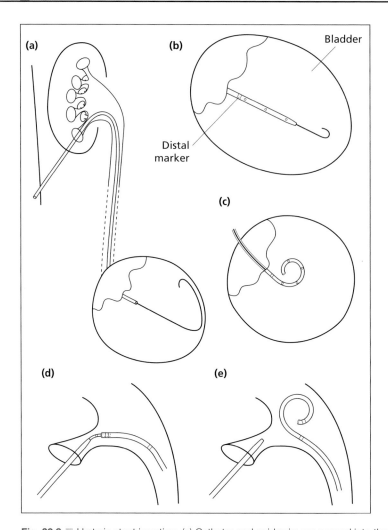

Fig. 22.3 ▉ Ureteric stent insertion. (a) Catheter and guidewire are passed into the bladder. (b) Stent is advanced until distal marker is in bladder. (c) Guidewire withdrawn until pigtail forms in bladder. (d) Proximal end of stent positioned so that pigtail will form in the renal pelvis. Guidewire pulled back. Final adjustment to stent position. (e) Central pusher catheter is withdrawn to release the stent.

Unable to advance the stent through the stricture   Advance a peel-away sheath across a stiff wire into the distal ureter or bladder. The reduction in friction means the stent usually passes readily. Remember to take care not to accidentally pull back the stent when peeling the sheath apart.

The pusher becomes impacted in the stent   With some stent systems the pusher can become impacted in the stent after the stent has been pushed through. This means that when the pusher is withdrawn the stent comes back with it. Always screen during withdrawal of the pusher, and if the stent seems to be coming back with it, rotating the pusher can often separate them.

The retraction sutures get entangled with the stent   Many systems have a suture loop through a sidehole of the trailing end of the ureteric stent to allow repositioning if the stent is inserted too far. After the stent has been positioned the loop is cut and the suture withdrawn. In practice, these sutures are often a cause of problems. Prevention is better than cure, and when advancing the stent always make sure the suture loop is not wrapped round it. If, after the loop has been cut, the suture is still pulling back the stent then don't just pull like fury – it is possible to remove the stent leaving an unsightly exit wound and a failed procedure. An elegant solution is to thread the longest part of the suture loop through a 5Fr dilator; then, using this as a buttress against the stent, it is usually possible to withdraw the suture.

Complications (of nephrostomy and antegrade ureteric stenting)

Disruption of the renal pelvis/extravasation of contrast   This will settle, provided the urinary system is adequately drained.

Bleeding   Some degree of haematuria is to be expected, particularly if multiple passes have taken place. Haematuria should clear within 48 hours. Blood clot in the pelvicaliceal system will lyse spontaneously because of the endogenous urokinase.

Renal angiography with or without embolization is occasionally required if there is persistent haematuria.

Inadvertent puncture of adjacent structures   Pneumothorax and colonic, liver and splenic puncture are all possible. These are much less likely under ultrasound guidance.

SUGGESTIONS FOR FURTHER READING

Barbaric ZL. Percutaneous nephrostomy for urinary tract obstruction. AJR 1984:143;803–809.
Cockburn JF, Borthwick-Clarke A, Hanaghan J et al. Radiologic insertion of subcutaneous nephrovesical stent for inoperable ureteral obstruction. AJR 1997;169:1588–1590.
An impressive technique, only to be performed with a responsible adult in the room.

Farrell TA, Hicks ME. A review of radiologically guided percutaneous nephrostomies in 303 patients. J Vasc Intervent Radiol 1997;8:769–774.

Ferral H, Stackhouse DJ, Bjarnason H et al. Complications of percutaneous nephrostomy tube placement. Semin Intervent Radiol 1994;11:198–206.
A contemporary update on an established technique.

Milty HA, Train JS, Dan SJ. Placement of ureteral stents by antegrade and retrograde techniques. Radiol Clin North Am 1986;24:587–600.
Zegel HG, Pollack HM, Banner MP et al. Percutaneous nephrostomy: comparison of sonographic and fluoroscopic guidance. AJR 1981;137:925–927.
Just in case you are in any doubt about the superiority of ultrasound guidance.

Chapter Twenty-Three

Biliary intervention

Biliary intervention involves mainly diagnostic cholangiography and biliary drainage. Until recently, percutaneous transhepatic cholangiography (PTC) and endoscopic retrograde cholangiopancreatography (ERCP) were the mainstays of biliary system investigation. Advances in non-invasive imaging, in particular CT and magnetic resonance cholangiography, have markedly decreased the need for percutaneous transhepatic cholangiography in the investigation of the jaundiced patient. In many centres, MR cholangiography is increasingly used to determine the site and nature of biliary obstruction. MR cholangiography can be invaluable in planning the approach for biliary drainage in patients with hilar lesions.

Percutaneous transhepatic cholangiography

Percutaneous transhepatic cholangiography is now rarely used as a primary technique to evaluate the biliary tree. In most patients the role of PTC has been downgraded to a component stage of biliary drainage. Before embarking on PTC, remember that patients with jaundice often have deranged liver function and abnormal clotting. Check platelets and coagulation before starting (see Patient preparation, Chapter 1, p. 3). Correct any underlying coagulation abnormality before proceeding; vitamin K is often all that is required, but needs to be given at least a day in advance; in urgent cases use FFP. Ensure that the patient is adequately hydrated prior to the procedure.

Equipment

- Chiba needle or Neff/Accustick access set.
- Connecting tube.
- C-arm fluoroscopy and a good ultrasound machine with a suitable probe and biopsy guide.
- IV access.
- Sedatives and analgesics.

Procedure

Planning your approach   As always, the shortest straightest route is usually best. It is helpful to review any cross-sectional imaging before starting to assess the size and shape of the liver, and to check for ascites. It almost always pays for you to have a quick look with the ultrasound before starting. Look for dilated ducts, and consider whether the ducts are uniformly dilated or there appears to be a segmental pattern of obstruction. Ultrasound guidance is always used for left lobe punctures, but is equally valuable to direct right-sided punctures. The patient should be prepared according to the planned approach to the right or left lobe, the procedure being much simpler if the hole in the drape is positioned over the puncture site.

Before starting:
- Take a control film of the right upper quadrant to look for calcification.
- Give intravenous antibiotics (check the local preference) to cover Gram-positive and Gram-negative bacteria.

Right-sided punctures   Blind puncture is traditionally made from the right flank below the 10th rib. The point of puncture is in the midaxillary line. Place sponge forceps at the proposed site of puncture, then fluoroscope to ensure it is over the liver and below the pleural reflection.

Tip: If you feel uncomfortable with this approach, use ultrasound to direct operations.

Infiltrate with local anaesthetic down as far as the peritoneum, but try to avoid puncturing the liver capsule. The intercostal vessels run along the inferior border of the ribs, and therefore it is best to puncture at the top edge of a rib. Make the initial pass with the needle, aiming just cranial to the hilum of the liver; angulate about 20° cranially and 20° ventrally (Fig. 23.1).

Left-sided punctures   The same principles apply; left-sided punctures are made from a substernal approach with ultrasound guidance (Fig. 23.2). The needle is advanced 10–15 cm into the liver, the central stylet is removed, and the connecting tube attached to the needle. Under fluoroscopy, gently inject full-strength contrast as the needle is slowly withdrawn.

Tip: You know you are injecting at the correct rate when the needle tract outlines as a thin line of contrast. Big splurges in the liver parenchyma indicate overinjection.

Look for filling of bile ducts and blood vessels. As the bile ducts fill contrast tends to flow towards the hilum; in obstructed ducts, the contrast often swirls as it dilutes. Portal vein and hepatic artery branches flow towards the periphery of the liver, whereas hepatic vein branches flow cranially towards the right atrium. Remember that the biliary radicals course together with portal vein and hepatic arterial branches in the portal triads, so that if you hit one, you are close to the others.

When you hit a bile duct, slowly inject contrast under continuous fluoroscopy. The dependent ducts tend to fill first, so the right lobe outlines before the left. The bile ducts have a

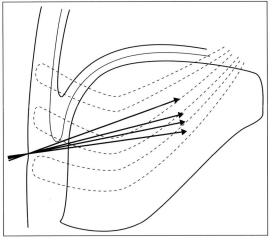

Fig. 23.1 ▓ Pattern of Chiba needle punctures at percutaneous transhepatic cholangiography. Note that the pleural reflection extends below the aerated lung.

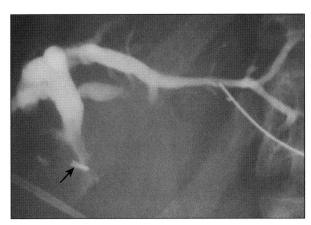

Fig. 23.2 ▓ Percutaneous transhepatic cholangiography from a left-sided approach showing a surgical clip occluding the common bile duct following laparoscopic cholecystectomy.

complex three-dimensional anatomy, and AP and both oblique views are required to analyse them. Take spot radiographs of any abnormal areas. Do not overdistend the bile ducts, as this is a sure-fire recipe for cholangitis.

At the end of the procedure, pull the needle out and put a plaster over the puncture site. You can press on it if you like, but it will not stop the liver from bleeding.

Interpretation

- **Filling defects** are caused by gallstones, tumour or blood. Gallstones appear as discrete, smooth intraluminal filling defects, sometimes visible on the plain film. Tumour may form mural nodules or strictures. Blood clot appears as extensive serpiginous intraluminal filling defects. Its appearance resembles the tramlining seen in DVT (Fig. 23.3).
- **Strictures** are caused by tumour or sclerosing cholangitis. The distribution of strictures should be noted and recorded.
- **Beading** is due to sclerosing cholangitis.

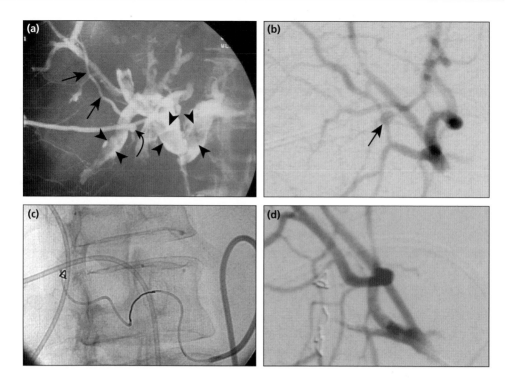

Fig. 23.3 ■ Haemorrhage following percutaneous transhepatic drainage. (a) Cholangiogram shows extensive blood clot (arrowheads) within the bile ducts. Note filling of a branch hepatic artery (arrows) and a false aneurysm (curved arrow) adjacent to the biliary drain. (b) Selective hepatic angiogram confirms the false aneurysm (arrow). (c) Coil embolization via a microcatheter. (d) Completion angiogram showing aneurysm exclusion. Adjacent hepatic artery branches are preserved.

- **Dilated ducts** are due to downstream blockage.
- **Displaced ducts** are due to an adjacent mass.
- **Distension of the gallbladder** is usually the result of downstream obstruction. This is typically caused by pancreatic carcinoma.

Troubleshooting

There is ascites This increases the risk of bleeding from the liver capsule. If there is extensive ascites, it should be drained before PTC. In the presence of a small amount of fluid, you can proceed if the liver abuts the peritoneum at the proposed puncture site. In the presence of small-volume ascites many operators would choose to perform an ultrasound-guided left lobe puncture. Make sure that you only make a single puncture of the liver capsule.

You do not hit a bile duct at the first attempt If you do not hit a bile duct on the first pass, angle the needle 5° caudal and dorsal to the initial pass and try again. Do not pull the needle right out of the liver. Stop before you cross the capsule, as fewer punctures equal less risk of bleeding. If the patient is not distressed, make up to five attempts and ask the radiographer to alert your boss that you may require assistance.

Contrast extravasates from the bile duct   Unfortunately, you have lost position or were in a small peripheral branch. This nearly always requires redirection of the puncture. If there is residual contrast in the biliary system you can aim for this.

The left ducts do not fill   The right-sided ducts are dependent and fill preferentially; sometimes the left ducts will only fill if the patient is turned right side up. Be careful not to dislodge the needle as you move the patient.

Extensive intraluminal filling defects are seen   This usually represents haemobilia and is an indication to stop. The patient should be closely monitored and resuscitated as necessary. The vast majority of cases of haemobilia will settle with conservative management; however, you should be prepared to perform a hepatic angiogram if bleeding continues (Fig. 23.3).

The patient has a rigor on the table   The patient has cholangitis and will rapidly deteriorate. Sepsis is more common in patients with benign strictures than in those with neoplastic disease. If the biliary system is obstructed, make sure to place a drain and contact the referring clinician. Aggressive resuscitation is often required.

Percutaneous biliary drainage

Percutaneous biliary drainage is performed in patients with obstructive jaundice in whom endoscopic drainage is unsuccessful or who have complex hilar lesions. The commonest indications are malignant disease of the bile ducts or pancreas.

 Tip: Patients with Roux-en-Y loops who develop biliary obstruction almost always require percutaneous drainage.

Equipment

As for cholangiography, plus:

- Neff/Accustick percutaneous access kit.
- Guidewires: stiff 0.018 inch platinum-tipped wire, heavy-duty 0.035 inch 3 mm J wire, curved hydrophilic wire, Amplatz wire.
- Catheters: dilators (at least 4–7Fr), 30 cm straight catheter, biliary manipulation catheter, Cobra II, Berenstein.
- Drains: there are many alternatives – pigtail, internal external drain, e.g. Ring catheter, Cope loop.
- Stents: most people use self-expanding metal stents if permanent drainage is required.
- Peel-away sheath.
- Sutures or catheter-retention device.

Procedure

It is useful to consider the Klatskin classification of hilar cholangiocarcinoma (Table 23.1).

In practice, it is only necessary to drain about a sixth of the liver to relieve the jaundice and the accompanying pruritus. This can usually be achieved with a single judiciously placed

Table 23.1 Number of stents required depending on tumour site

Klatskin type	Site completely	No. of stents to treat
Type I	Common hepatic duct	1
Type II	Confluence of left and right hepatic ducts	2
Type III	Confluence of hepatic ducts and first order branches	3+

drain or stent. The left hepatic duct has a longer course before it divides, and so a left-sided approach may offer more effective drainage for type II and type III tumours. For distal obstruction, the right-sided approach is usually chosen as it is technically simpler. Before starting, review the previous imaging to decide the most promising approach. Sometimes one lobe of the liver has atrophied and it is now too late to salvage function in it; use the other lobe!

Frequently with a right-sided approach to hilar tumours the initial duct entered is not appropriate for drainage: usually as it is too near the hilum. Use the first puncture to opacify the biliary system and fluoroscopically target a more suitable duct with a second Chiba needle.

Biliary drainage: a step-by-step guide

1. **Obtain IV access**: give antibiotics, sedation and analgesia.
2. **Perform a cholangiogram**: use a Neff set; this allows conversion to a 0.035 inch wire if you hit a suitable duct.
3. **Choose the optimal duct for drainage**: in practice, any duct draining a large part of the liver. Choose a duct with a straight approach to the site of obstruction that can be accessed from the conventional puncture sites.
4. **Puncture the duct**: aim for a point where the duct is large enough to accommodate the catheters and drains that you plan to use, but remember that there are fewer complications the more peripherally you puncture. Guide puncture with fluoroscopy and rotate the C-arm or the patient to demonstrate the position of the needle relative to the duct. When you are close to the duct, it will start to move when the needle is moved back and forth. When you reach the duct, it will indent as the needle tip contacts it. There is usually a 'give' when the duct is entered.
5. **Confirm intraduct position**: free backflow of bile indicates that you are in the duct. If this is not forthcoming, either inject a small amount of contrast or try to see if the guidewire will pass along the duct.
6. **Exchange the 0.018 inch wire for the 0.035 inch J wire**: use the mini-access set.
7. **Dilate a tract into the duct**: this is normally uncomfortable, so remember to give the patient adequate analgesia/sedation. Use 5Fr or 6Fr dilators, depending on the size of catheter you intend to use.
8. **Introduce the catheter you hope to use to cross the stricture**: most operators use either a Cobra or a biliary manipulation catheter.

9. **Take a sample of bile**: for microbiology and/or cytology.
10. **Cross the stricture**: this is often harder than it sounds. We usually start with the curved hydrophilic wire. The process is similar to crossing a stricture or occlusion in a blood vessel (see angioplasty, p. 144).
11. **Confirm intraluminal position**: always ensure that you are either back in the bile duct or through to the duodenum.
12. **Exchange for the heavy-duty J wire or the Amplatz superstiff**: an angled approach will need a stronger support wire.
13. **Position the drain catheter/stent**: internal external drains must have sideholes on each side of the obstruction, but not into the liver parenchyma. Stents must completely cover the lesion.
14. **Confirm free drainage**: make sure you do this before you attach the catheter!
15. **Fix the drain catheter to the skin**: there are many options for this; none is foolproof, so use either a suture or a proprietary skin fixation device.

Which drainage catheter?

There is a bewildering choice of drains available; the choice in biliary drainage depends on the anatomy.

Straight drain Only used as a last resort as a temporary measure when it is not possible to negotiate through a stricture into a large enough duct to form a pigtail. Straight catheters are easy to remove, often unintentionally. They should not be trusted and should be exchanged for a 'proper drain' as soon as possible.

Pigtail drain Use these when you cannot cross the obstruction but can access a sufficiently central duct. Even pigtail catheters can be inadvertently dislodged, so a self-retaining device, e.g. a Cope loop, is preferable. Pigtail catheters are usually used as a temporary measure until a definitive drainage procedure is performed.

Internal/external drain These drains are more secure than straight catheters or pigtails. They have multiple sideholes over a long length of the catheter (Fig. 23.4). When they are placed across the stricture, bile can be drained externally to a bag or internally to the duodenum. Additional sideholes should be punched along the proximal catheter to permit drainage from the intrahepatic biliary tree. Take care that no sideholes extend proximal to the liver parenchyma, as bile may then drain into the peritoneal cavity, particularly in patients with ascites. The position of the most proximal sidehole can be determined by this simple test. Before inserting the drain, put a green needle into the most proximal sidehole, then advance a guidewire into the drain. The guidewire will stop at the needle. Bend the guidewire at the hub of the drain. Insert the drain into the patient. Final positioning can be determined by using the previously bent wire to indicate the most proximal sidehole.

Rarely, internal/external drains may be used for long-term drainage. In this case, they should be allowed to drain externally for about a week before converting to internal drainage. The advantages of internal drainage are:
- Bile salts are not lost.
- It allows the patient to be ambulant without a bag.

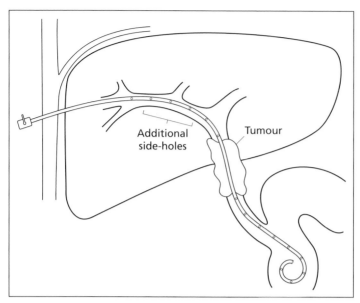

Fig. 23.4 ■ Internal/external biliary drainage catheter. Note that additional sideholes are often required to drain the proximal biliary tree.

- Skin excoriation is less common.
- The mature tract allows access for repeat procedures if the drain blocks.

Tip: When punching extra sideholes in drainage catheters, use a proper hole punch rather than a needle, as the results are much better. Do not punch holes directly opposite each other or in very close proximity, as this will weaken the catheter and may result in fracture.

Troubleshooting

Guidewire or catheter reluctant to advance   Bile is an effective lubricant and the passage of guidewires and catheters is usually easy. If you experience difficulty, this usually indicates a problem, e.g. you are not in the duct any more. Stop and confirm intraluminal position by aspiration ± contrast injection.

Initial cholangiogram fades   Inject more contrast, either through the initial puncture needle or through the catheter if you used the PTC tract to access the biliary tree.

Unable to cross the lesion with the guidewire   Do not be despondent: it is often very difficult to cross an occlusion in a very dilated system. Put in a pigtail drain (preferably self-retaining) and leave the catheter on free drainage for 2–3 days. When you try again, the system will be less capacious and less oedematous; frequently, it is now much simpler. If you still cannot succeed, seek an expert opinion. The adviser will help you decide whether to persist or to settle for permanent external drainage.

Unable to cross the lesion with the catheter   Try a 4Fr hydrophilic catheter or a tapered Van Andel catheter. If this is not successful, try to predilate the lesion with a low-profile angioplasty balloon. If the balloon will not cross the entire lesion, try to dilate it in stages. It is sometimes necessary to sacrifice the guidewire position and recross the lesion with a 0.018 inch guidewire to allow the use of a low-profile angioplasty balloon. These rarely fail to cross the lesion.

Unable to cross the lesion with the drain or stent   Consider balloon dilatation. If this fails, make sure that you have a stiff guidewire across the lesion and then insert a peel-away sheath. Cross the lesion with this if you can; if not, position it close to the obstruction and try again.

Biliary bleeding   Stop and put in a drain. Resuscitate the patient as necessary and monitor closely. Try again in 48 hours.

Drainage stops   Review the patient yourself. Often there is a benign cause, such as kinking or clamping of the drain tube. If this is not the cause, try flushing the drain with saline, as this may salvage a blocked catheter. If none of the above is successful, perform a cholangiogram through the drain to determine the problem; usually the catheter has been pulled out.

Biliary stenting

Both plastic and metal stents are available. Metal stents have a longer patency but cannot be removed; they should be avoided in benign disease or when the patient has a long life expectancy. Stents can be placed endoscopically, percutaneously or as part of a combined procedure.

Plastic stents

These are cheap, but are more likely to occlude than metal stents. Endoscopic stent placement is the first choice in most centres, with the other techniques reserved for those patients in whom endoscopic access has failed. The combined procedure, as its name suggests, involves both percutaneous and endoscopic techniques. The radiologist performs a percutaneous drainage and passes a catheter and a long (4.5 m!) guidewire into the duodenum. The endoscope is now positioned alongside the catheter and the guidewire snared. The wire is pulled out through the endoscope and then used to deliver the stent. The radiologist's job is to keep tension on the guidewire and to abut the percutaneous catheter against the stent. The stent and catheter can then be pulled through the stenosis. Plastic stents (Coons stents) can be placed percutaneously, but require at least a 10Fr tract compared to the 6/7Fr tract required for a metal stent, and are therefore rarely used nowadays.

Metal stents

Many units now deploy metal stents for malignant biliary obstruction. This is associated with extra capital costs, but these are offset by:
- Better patency, reducing the cost of reintervention as they will frequently stay patent for the remainder of the patient's lifetime.
- Ability to treat the patient in a single session in radiology because of the smaller tract size – usually 6 or 7Fr.

- The patient is spared the inconvenience of an external tube.
- Smaller tracts being required through the liver.

The Wallstent has been extensively used to palliate jaundice. It is flexible and comes in sufficiently long lengths to allow most lesions to be treated. The majority of biliary stent insertions occur in two stages, with initial decompression achieved preferably with an internal/external drain. Cholangiography is then performed and the pattern of disease assessed. Aim to cover the entire diseased segment with the stent. Hilar tumours often require stenting out to second-order ducts to achieve satisfactory drainage.

ROUX LOOP ACCESS

Many patients with benign biliary strictures will have choledochoenterostomy, usually to a proximal jejunal loop. Benign strictures tend to recur, and therefore an access loop of bowel is often apposed to the anterior abdominal wall. Roux loop access is preferable to percutaneous transhepatic access to the bile ducts when repeated intervention is required.

Equipment

As for percutaneous drainage.

Procedure

Access The Roux loop is punctured percutaneously. This sounds straightforward, but the bowel loop in question looks just like any other. Kind surgeons fix the Roux loop to the anterior abdominal wall and place radio-opaque marker clips to identify it. This greatly simplifies the procedure. It is more likely that there will be no markers, so either:

- Perform a limited abdominal CT to identify and mark the position of the loop that is anastomosed to the bile duct (see CT guidance, p. 254).
- Perform a percutaneous cholangiogram using a Chiba needle and then aim for the correct loop.
- Consider using ultrasound, but this is rarely helpful.

Catheterization Puncture the loop with a Neff set. Inject contrast to confirm intraluminal position, then introduce the guidewire. Dilate the tract and then place a heavy-duty J wire well into the lumen. You can now place a shaped catheter into the loop and use this to negotiate through the loop and into the bile duct. This approach can be used to perform diagnostic cholangiography, and intervention such as angioplasty can be performed through the loop.

Percutaneous gallbladder drainage (cholecystostomy)

This is generally indicated to drain an infected gallbladder in a critically ill patient or in unexplained sepsis, particularly in intensive-care patients. It also provides an alternative option for imaging the biliary tree in patients in whom ERCP and PTC have failed.

An acutely inflamed gallbladder will be thick walled and adherent to the peritoneum, and can be drained from an anterior transperitoneal approach. In theory, non-inflamed gall-bladders are better punctured transhepatically. In this way, any bile leakage will not cause peritoneal irritation. An additional advantage of transhepatic puncture is that the gallbladder shrinks towards the drainage catheter, whereas with transabdominal puncture the catheter may be displaced when the gallbladder decompresses.

Use ultrasound to guide gallbladder puncture and take particular care to maintain access and insert a self-retaining catheter. Vasovagal reactions are not infrequent, and atropine should be readily available. Drainage is normally performed for at least 2 weeks to allow a mature tract to form. Cholangiography should be performed to confirm cystic duct patency before the tube is removed. If there is obstruction, infection will recur or a biliary fistula will form. Clamp the tube for 48 hours prior to removal to confirm satisfactory internal drainage.

SUGGESTIONS FOR FURTHER READING

Adam A. Metallic biliary endoprostheses. Cardiovasc Intervent Radiol 1994;17:127–132. *Provides a good overview.*

Ferrucci JT, Mueller PR, Harbin WP. Percutaneous transhepatic biliary drainage: Technique, results and applications. Radiology 1980;135:1–13.

Hayashi N, Sakai T, Kitagawa et al. US guided left-sided biliary drainage: nine-year experience. Radiology 1997;204:119.

Lee MJ, Dawson SL, Mueller PR et al. Palliation of malignant bile duct obstruction with metallic biliary endoprostheses: Techniques, results, and complications. J Vasc Intervent Radiol 1992;3:665–671.

McPherson SJ, Gibson RN, Collier NA et al. Percutaneous transjejunal biliary intervention: 10 year experience with access via Roux-en-Y loops. Radiology 1998;206:665.

Rossi P, Bezzi M, Rossi M et al. Metallic stents in malignant biliary obstruction: Results of a multi-center European study of 240 patients. J Vasc Intervent Radiol 1994;5:279–284.

vanOverhagen H, Meyers H, Tilanus HW et al. Percutaneous cholecystotomy for patients with acute cholecystitis and an increased surgical risk. Cardiovasc Intervent Radiol 1996;19:72–76. *A mixture of transhepatic and transperitoneal drainages with a good discussion and references section.*

Wittich GR, vanSonnenberg E, Simeone JF. Results and complications of percutaneous biliary drainage. Semin Intervent Radiol 1985;2:39–49.

Chapter Twenty-Four

Percutaneous fluoroscopic gastrostomy

This straightforward procedure is used mainly to provide nutritional support for patients with swallowing disorders. There are two variants to the radiological technique: the traditional radiologically inserted gastrostomy (RIG) and the peroral image-guided gastrostomy (PIG). The traditional fluoroscopic gastrostomy (RIG) technique places a 12–14Fr tube, which can be prone to blockage. A newer variant, the PIG, delivers the gastrostomy via the oral route, allowing the placement of larger-calibre tubes (14–20Fr) that are often easier to manage in the long term.

Feeding via a percutaneous gastrostomy is associated with gastroesophageal reflux and aspiration in over one-third of patients. To prevent this, some practitioners choose to manipulate the tube around the duodenal loop into the jejunum, i.e. percutaneous gastrojejunostomy. The technique is similar for both procedures.

Equipment

Commercial kits are available for both PIG and RIG insertions, and in practice most departments will use a kit. Essentially this contains:

RIG Insertion
- 18G Seldinger needle.
- J guidewire 0.038 inch.
- Fascial dilators to 1Fr greater than the drain.
- A self-retaining catheter.

PIG Insertion
- 18G Seldinger needle.
- J guidewire 0.038 inch.
- Headhunter catheter.
- Superstiff wire.
- A 'push' gastrostomy tube and adapter.

If percutaneous gastrojejunostomy is necessary, a Cobra catheter, hydrophilic guidewire and gastrojejunostomy tube (e.g. CareyCoons catheter) are needed.

Technique: RIG

A nasogastric tube is inserted on the ward and any gastric content aspirated. The stomach is insufflated with air to bring it into apposition with the anterior abdominal wall. The target is a puncture at the mid/distal body of the stomach, equidistant from the lesser and greater

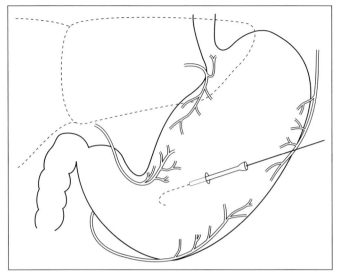

Fig. 24.1 ▪ Puncture site for percutaneous gastrostomy with puncture directed towards the pylorus.

curves to minimize the risk of arterial injury. Avoid puncture through the transverse colon and left lobe of the liver, which are adjacent innocent bystanders (Fig. 24.1).

Infiltrate local anaesthesia, go all the way in with the green needle and make a small scalpel incision. Puncture vertically downwards; avoid punctures directed towards the fundus, as these will be impossible to convert to gastrojejunostomy later. The final puncture through the gastric wall requires a short stabbing motion. It is usually possible to see the gastric wall tenting away from the needle when it is necessary to make that final thrust. Confirm entry into the stomach by injecting contrast through the needle, then insert the J guidewire.

T fasteners or anchors can be used to maintain the stomach in apposition with the anterior abdominal wall. Practice is variable, but most practitioners would not use T fasteners for a straightforward gastrostomy but may use them in the face of an uncooperative patient, ascites or a postoperative stomach.

How to use T fasteners　A T fastener, sometimes called a suture anchor, is a short metal bar attached to a suture/needle that is delivered through a puncture needle into the stomach (Fig. 24.2). An introducer needle is preloaded with the suture anchor and directed into the stomach. Contrast is injected to confirm position and a wire guide is then inserted into the needle, which pushes the anchor out into the stomach cavity. The introducer needle may then be removed and traction applied to the suture to bring the stomach into apposition with the anterior abdominal wall. While tension is maintained, the thread is sutured to the skin surface. The suture is cut after a period of approximately 2 weeks to permit tract formation.

The next step is tract dilation. You may have a distant memory of anatomy tutorials and the three muscular layers of the stomach. Practically, this means you need to push hard with the serial dilators. Finally, advance the self-retaining catheter into the stomach. There are a variety of different retention methods, including the usual pigtail loop catheters and balloons that tamponade against the gastric wall. Inject contrast to confirm satisfactory position, then secure the catheter to the skin.

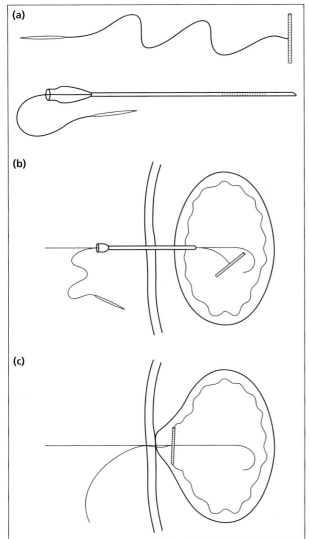

Fig. 24.2 ■ Suture anchors. (a) Basic design. (b) The suture anchor is pushed into the stomach using the guidewire. (c) Traction on the suture anchor brings the stomach against the abdominal wall.

If percutaneous gastrojejunostomy is required, the initial steps are identical but a Cobra catheter is used to negotiate around the duodenum; the gastrojejunostomy catheter may then be placed with its distal tip just beyond the ligament of Trietz.

Technique: PIG

Similar initial technique for percutaneous access to the stomach. Suture anchors are not required.

The gastrostomy tube for this technique is a completely different design and is pulled down through the orophaynx (Fig. 24.3). This technique can pull down oral flora to the gastrostomy site, and therefore a single dose of cefuroxime 750 mg is advised.

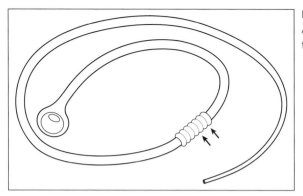

Fig. 24.3 ■ Peroral gastrostomy tube. Arrows indicate the point of separation of the long dilator from the gastrostomy tube.

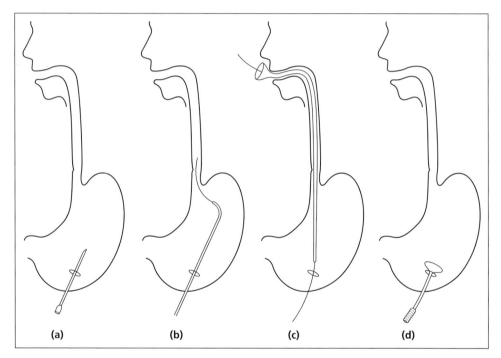

(a) (b) (c) (d)

Fig. 24.4 ■ Technique for PIG. (a) Percutaneous access to the stomach. (b) Retrograde catheterization of the oesophagus. (c) Push gastrostomy tube is advanced over the wire via the peroral route. (d) Gastrostomy tube is pulled down and the internal fixaton collar is pulled against the gastric mucosa.

A 4Fr sheath is placed through the gastrostomy tract and the oesophagus catheterized retrogradely with a Headhunter catheter and hydrophilic wire – this is more difficult than it sounds and can take 10–15 frustrating minutes. The catheter is advanced up the oesophagus and brought out through the mouth. The guidewire is exchanged for a 260 cm stiff wire. Working at the head end, the gastrostomy tube is then advanced over the wire until the distal extent exits the anterior abdominal wall. The catheter and wire are removed to avoid any risk of 'cheese-wiring', and the gastrostomy tube is pulled down into the stomach. It is a good idea to prepare the patient at this stage for the sensation of the tube crossing the oropharynx. The gastrostomy tube can then be fixed in place with the fixation disc supplied (Fig. 24.4).

Aftercare

Fast the patient for 6 hours post procedure, then if all is well start water for 6 hours at ~50 mL/h. If tolerated, commence enteral nutrition.

Results

Technical success rates are usually in excess of 95% for radiological gastrostomy. Complications occur in approximately 5% of patients and are principally peritonitis or puncture of adjacent viscera.

Troubleshooting

Unable to pass a nasogastric tube It is often possible to negotiate oesophageal strictures with an angiographic catheter and hydrophilic wire using the techniques described for oesophageal stenting.

Difficult access If it proves difficult to be certain that you have safe access avoiding other structures, the gastrostomy can often be safely performed under CT guidance.

Difficulty getting the catheter through the gastric wall A stiff guidewire and a peelaway sheath can be helpful, particularly if you are trying to negotiate the duodenum for a gastrojejunostomy.

Difficulty accessing the oesophagus retrogradely during a PIG procedure Pass a wire antegradely down the oesophagus via the nasogastric catheter. It is then usually straightforward to snare the wire using the gastric access.

The gastrostomy tube falls out after insertion If this occurs after less than 7 days, particularly if T fasteners have not been used, there is unlikely to be a track. Start again. If it is more than 7 days a track is likely to be present, and for long-term gastrostomies can be maintained by the attending clinical team passing a Foley catheter until a formal gastrostomy catheter can be replaced.

SUGGESTIONS FOR FURTHER READING

Cope C. Suture anchor for visceral drainage. AJR 1980;135:402–403.
Ho CS, Yeung EY. Percutaneous gastrostomy and transgastric jejunostomy. AJR 1992;158:251–257.
Laasch HU, Wilbraham L, Bullen K. Gastrostomy insertion comparing the options: PEG, RIG or PIG? Clin Radiol 2003;58:398–405.
An excellent description of the PIG technique.

Wollman BD, Agostino HB. Percutaneous radiologic and endoscopic gastrostomy: a 3-year institutional review. AJR 1997;169:1551–1553.

Chapter Twenty-Five

Gastrointestinal stent insertion

Stent insertion is being used with increasing frequency at either end of the gastrointestinal tract. In essence, the principles of GI stenting are not too different from those for stenting other systems. The stricture or occlusion is traversed with catheters and guidewires, and then a stent is deployed to restore 'flow'. The procedures are technically straightforward, provide excellent symptom relief and are well within the capabilities of most radiologists.

Oesophageal stent insertion

Oesophageal stenting is used to palliate dysphagia, particularly in malignant disease. Oesophageal carcinoma is a common condition, and 50% of patients are irresectable at the time of diagnosis. Traditional palliation of dysphagia with radiotherapy and plastic endoprostheses has a high complication rate and significant insertion-related mortality. Self-expanding metallic endoprostheses allow durable palliation of dysphagia in a single treatment session with minimal morbidity and mortality.

Oesophageal stents come in two main types, covered or bare. Covered stents have lower rates of occlusion secondary to tumour ingrowth, but initial designs had a high rate of migration. Improvements in design have reduced the migration rate to less than 10%, and many centres now use covered stents for all patients. A few stents are available that contain a one-way valve to prevent reflux and even have a suture loop to permit repositioning. These may be particularly useful in unusual applications, such as stent insertion for benign disease.

Accurate sizing is not important, but a device that is approximately appropriate in size should be used. In reality, few operators measure the true length of the lesion as the vast majority are covered by a single stent. As a guide, the length of the stent is usually around 2 cm longer than the lesion at either end. Large-diameter stents, i.e. around 30 mm, are best reserved for the dilated oesophagus, as they cause considerable pain in a normal-calibre oesophagus.

Equipment
- Oesophageal stent: 18–25 mm diameter.
- Hydrophilic guidewire: Amplatz superstiff, 260 cm.
- Berenstein catheter.
- Oesophageal dilation balloons: 10–20 mm.

Procedure

Perform an initial contrast swallow of the oesophagus with non-ionic contrast to identify the approximate level of the stricture. The throat is subsequently anaesthetized with xylocaine spray and the patient placed in the prone oblique position. IV sedation is administered and appropriate monitoring commenced.

Using fluoroscopic guidance, the oesophagus is catheterized with the Berenstein catheter via the oral route – it's tricky to get an oesophageal stent through the nose later in the procedure! The catheter is advanced to the approximate level of the lesion and a small amount of non-ionic contrast injected to outline the upper extent of the stricture. The catheter is then used to manipulate the hydrophilic guidewire through the stricture, using the techniques outlined in Chapter 12. The lower extent of the stricture can often be identified from the previous contrast injection, but if necessary the catheter can be pulled back while contrast is slowly injected to define the distal margin. The distal extent of lesions at the gastro-oesophageal junction can usually be outlined by air within the stomach. The position of the stricture can be indicated either by radio-opaque markers or by bony landmarks, but remember these are a considerable distance from the oesophagus, and even minor patient movement may be significant. The Amplatz guidewire is inserted into the stomach and, if an Ultraflex stent is to be used, predilation to 12 mm is performed. The stent is then carefully advanced over the Amplatz wire and deployed in position (Fig. 25.1). Deployment mechanisms vary between devices: the Ultraflex is held compressed by a long suture that is progressively withdrawn, deploying the stent; the Wallstent prosthesis, which has the advantage that repositioning is possible provided less than 50% of the device has been deployed, is released by progressive retraction of a sheath (see Chapter 13). Unless

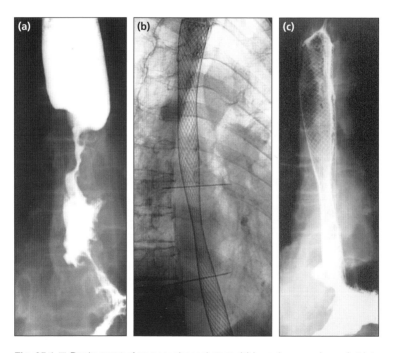

Fig. 25.1 ▓ Deployment of an oesophageal stent. (a) Irregular oesophageal stricture. (b) Immediately after deployment the stent is narrow but was not postdilated. (c) Stent fully open at 24 hours.

the stent is very narrow most operators will not postdilate, and prefer to wait for the stent to expand itself (Fig. 25.1).

Tip: If the markers move, or there is difficulty being sure of the length and position, use a long angiographic sheath over the wire to depict the proximal and distal extents of the stricture without losing wire position.

Aftercare

Clear fluids are permitted 4 hours after the procedure. If this proceeds uneventfully, a light diet may be commenced. It is not essential to perform a routine follow-up oesophageal study, but many centres will re-study at 24 hours. All patients should be advised to cut food into small pieces and encouraged to drink fizzy drinks, particularly cola, as they tend to prevent the stent from progressive sludging with food. If the stent extends over the cardia, the patient should be commenced on a proton-pump inhibitor to alleviate oesophageal reflux.

Results

Primary technical success is achieved in 95–100% of patients, with significant relief of dysphagia in most series. Complications consist of migration <10%, haemorrhage ~3% and fistula/perforation 2–3%.

Troubleshooting

The stent migrates through the cardia   Migration is more common with a stent that extends across the cardia, and *slightly* more common with covered stents. If this is partial at the time of insertion, then it may be possible to anchor the stent by inserting an over-lapping stent. More often, this occurs some time after the initial insertion and the stent is within the stomach. Most stents are left in situ within the stomach, but if the patient is symptomatic the stent can be retrieved (but not reused!) at endoscopy using an overtube.

The stent occludes   An acute occlusion usually indicates a food obstruction. Perform a contrast study of the oesophagus; if contrast is still percolating through, then try some cola! If this fails, the stent can usually be readily cleared at endoscopy.

More insidious onset of dysphagia indicates the stent has become occluded secondary to tumour overgrowth or ingrowth. If tumour overgrowth has occurred, then often a second stent will resolve this. If the problem is tumour ingrowth, then either a covered stent or laser therapy should be considered.

The lesion is high in the oesophagus   The majority of lesions are in the lower third, but high lesions in the upper third of the oesophagus need particularly critical positioning to avoid stenting open the vocal cords! Endoscopy during stent placement to identify the position of the cricopharyngeus muscle can be very useful. For the very brave, an alternative is a 1 mL submucosal injection of lipiodol at endoscopy to pinpoint the upper extent of the lesion. The Ultraflex oesophageal stent comes in a proximal release variant, and this permits more accurate proximal placement. It is generally better to use smaller devices in the upper oesophagus, and the Ultraflex stent, which has less radial force, may prove more comfortable for the patient.

The patient develops chest pain post deployment   This often occurs and is secondary to the expansile force of the stent. The sensation almost always resolves spontaneously.

Oesophageal fistulae and perforations

There is increasing experience in the use of covered stents to treat oesophageal perforations and fistulae. Malignant fistulae are readily treated by accurate placement of a covered oesophageal stent. Benign perforations are technically fairly straightforward, but long-term results may be less favourable because of the overgrowth of granulation tissue at the stent margins. It may be that placement of a temporary/retrievable covered oesophageal stent is appropriate in such cases. The only significant technical difference for this group of patients is to avoid predilation, as this will expand the oesophageal defect.

Duodenal stent placement

Gastric outlet obstruction secondary to either intrinsic or extrinsic tumour involvement can be readily treated by gastrointestinal stent placement. The technique is essentially the same as for oesophageal placement. Make sure the stomach has been emptied by a naso-gastric tube prior to intervention, as an empty stomach is a shorter and easier route. Even with this help it can be difficult to advance the stent round the greater curve of the stomach, and the use of a long sheath can be invaluable. In a few patients it is impossible to advance the stent via an oral route, and the procedure can be performed by creating a gastrostomy (see Chapter 24) to allow a much more direct route. It is usual to leave the gastrostomy in situ for a few weeks rather than immediate removal, as a leak may occur.

Colorectal stent placement

Acute left-sided colonic obstruction is a common surgical emergency. Frequently, the patient is dehydrated, frail, and has not had sufficient time for accurate staging of malignant disease. Emergency surgery and primary colonic anastomosis is associated with a high surgical morbidity and mortality, and colorectal stenting is an increasingly frequent treatment method for this group of patients.

Equipment
- Vertebral/Berenstein catheter.
- Stiff hydrophilic guidewire.
- Amplatz superstiff wire.
- Large-calibre sheath: 10–12Fr, 60 cm long.
- Colonic stents: an increasing variety of these devices is available. Most are simple to deploy, and we can only suggest that you familiarize yourself with those available in your own department. Typically, colorectal stents are between 20 and 30 mm in diameter and 70–100 mm long.

Tip: It's easy to find yourself with too short a wire in this procedure, particularly if you 'borrow' an endoscopic stent. Always think about the length of the stent deployment system.

Technique

Rectosigmoid lesions can be negotiated with fluoroscopic guidance alone; however, lesions higher in the colon usually need the presence of an endoscopist. Place the patient in the left lateral position and administer conscious sedation. Introduce a small amount of water-soluble contrast to outline the stricture. It is often best at this stage to turn the patient prone or prone oblique to profile the stricture. Advance the catheter and guidewire combination and carefully negotiate the stricture. This is often harder than it would appear, as the capacious colon offers little in the way of support for the catheter and it can be useful to insert a sheath to provide additional support. Once through the stricture, carefully insert the stiff guidewire. Advance the stent over the wire: this can be difficult if following a tortuous colon, and again a large-calibre sheath may be invaluable. Centre the stent over the lesion and deploy (Fig. 25.2). Regardless of how tight the stent looks, DON'T postdilate – this greatly increases the risks of perforation and misadventure. A successful placement is usually indicated by an escape of gas/faecal fluid – in most cases from the patient!

Finally, arrange for a plain film of the abdomen the next day to assess stent expansion, and check the stent position to make sure it has not migrated.

Results

Most stents are inserted for malignant obstruction and the overall success rate should be around 90%. Complications occur in 10% of patients and consist of perforation, migration

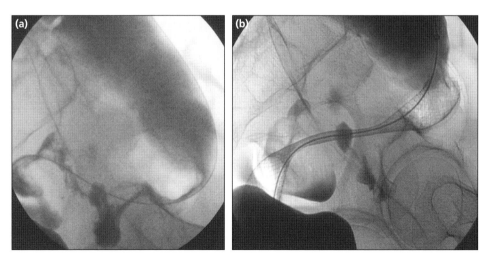

Fig. 25.2 ▓ (a) Gastrografin enema showing rectosigmoid tumour. Post deployment satisfactory position, but note stent remains narrowed.

and sepsis. Palliation is achieved in over 80% of patients and ~20% of patients will have recurrent symptoms secondary to either tumour ingrowth or overgrowth; most can be treated by additional stent insertion. Colorectal stents have been placed for a variety of benign indications, including diverticulitis, anastomotic stricture and colonic fistula, but tend to have a rather more complicated clinical course. Overall, they are best avoided in benign disease unless circumstances are exceptional.

Troubleshooting

Can't negotiate the stricture   Is the colon below the stricture empty? If it is full of faecal material, then arrange for a bowel washout. Generally, endoscopic assistance helps identify the stricture, and the use of a sheath to prevent the catheter 'flopping' about in the colon is helpful.

Oops, I've perforated the bowel   Catheter or guidewire perforation is usually without clinical consequence and it is appropriate to persevere and complete the procedure. Perforation secondary to either balloon dilatation or stent expansion is more serious and may lead to surgical intervention.

The stent has migrated   Management depends on the clinical situation. If the stent was placed for temporary relief of acute obstruction then often there is no need to replace the stent. If the case is palliative then the original stent can usually be readily retrieved and a further stent placed over the stricture.

SUGGESTIONS FOR FURTHER READING

Camurez F, Echenagusia A, Gonzalo S et al. Malignant colorectal obstruction treated by means of self expanding metallic stents: effectiveness before surgery and in palliation. Radiology 2000: 216;492–497.
Conio M, Caroli Bosc F, Demarquay JF et al. Self-expanding metal stents in the palliation of neoplasms of the cervical oesophagus. Hepato-Gastroenterology 1999;46:272–277.
A good series in a tricky area.

Morgan R, Adam A. Use of metallic stents and balloons in the esophagus and gastrointestinal tract. JVIR 2001;12:283–297.
If you have only time to read one article on GI then this is the one.

Morgan RA, Ellul JPM, Denton ERE et al. Malignant oesophageal fistulas and perforations: management with plastic-covered metallic endoprostheses. Radiology 1997;204:527–532.
O'Sullivan CJ, Grundy A. Palliation of malignant dysphagia with expanding metallic stents. J Vasc Intervent Radiol 1999;10:346–351.
Sabharwal T, Hamady MS, Chui S, Atkinson S, Mason R, Adam A. A randomised and prospective comparison of the Flamingo Wallstent and Ultraflex stent for the palliation of dysphagia associated with lower third oesophageal carcinoma. Gut 2003;52:922-926.
Well conducted study – turns out there's not much to choose between them.

Wojciech C, Tranberg K-C, Cwikiel et al. Malignant dysphagia: Palliation with oesophageal stents – long-term results in 100 patients. Radiology 1998;207:513–518.

Chapter Twenty-Six

Respiratory system

Biopsy of pulmonary and pleural masses

Most central endobronchial lesions are biopsied bronchoscopically. Inaccessible lesions are usually biopsied under CT guidance. Large parenchymal lesions can be biopsied under fluoroscopic guidance, which is certainly faster. Ultrasound is useful for lesions that abut the pleural surface.

Planning

Planning the procedure with review of previous imaging is essential. Plan a route that, if possible, does not transgress aerated lung, as this minimizes the risk of pneumothorax. Many parenchymal lesions will need a pleural puncture. The route chosen should puncture the pleural surface perpendicularly, and particularly avoid puncture of bullae and fissures, as these usually cause a substantial air leak. Always puncture just above the rib, as the neurovascular bundle travels along the inferior margin. Patient cooperation is essential and breathing instructions should be explained and practised. It is best to get the patient to breath-hold in early inspiration. The patient must be warned of the risks of pneumothorax (around 20%; about 2–5% require formal drainage), haemoptysis and air embolism. It is mandatory to have oxygen monitoring, and equipment for chest drainage should be immediately available.

Aspiration vs cutting biopsies

In suspected malignant disease, fine-needle aspiration biopsy will produce satisfactory results. Limiting the number of pleural punctures reduces the risk of pneumothorax, and if a number of passes are anticipated then the use of a coaxial needle technique is strongly recommended. Cutting needle biopsy is generally used where previous FNA has been negative, or when benign disease or lymphoma is suspected.

Postprocedural care

Most complications occur either immediately at biopsy or within a few hours. Immediately after biopsy the patient should be positioned puncture side down, as there is evidence that this minimizes the size of pneumothorax. Expiratory erect chest films should be obtained 1 hour and 3 hours after biopsy. The patient may be discharged if clinically stable and the 3-hour CXR is satisfactory. They should be given instructions to rest and avoid lifting, straining, or any other manoeuvres likely to cause a Valsalva. Minor blood streaking in the sputum is acceptable, but the patient must return to hospital if there is more significant blood loss.

Complications

Pneumothorax is the commonest complication and is more frequent if there is emphysema or obstructive airways disease. There are no absolute guidelines as to which patients require chest drainage. Symptomatic pneumothorax, a pneumothorax >30%, or a progressively expanding air leak are all likely candidates. Some patients can be simply managed by aspiration of the pneumothorax. Haemoptysis occurs in 5–10% of patients and is more likely with cutting needle biopsy. If there is a significant haemoptysis, withdraw the biopsy needle immediately and place the patient biopsy-side down to avoid aspiration into the other lung. If bleeding persists, consider bronchoscopic tamponade or pulmonary or bronchial artery embolization. Air embolism is a rare but potentially catastrophic complication that occurs when there is a bronchovenous communication. Needle withdrawal, 100% O_2 and Trendelenburg positioning to prevent cerebral air embolus are recommended.

Pleural effusions

Ultrasound guidance is ideal for diagnostic and therapeutic thoracocentesis. Diagnostic thoracocentesis can be performed with a 21G needle. Specimens are obtained for microbiology, biochemistry and, in appropriate patients, cytology.

Prompt drainage of complicated parapneumonic effusions (pH <7.0, glucose <40 mg/dL, LDH >1000 IU/L or positive Gram stain) will reduce the risk of empyema.

Thoracocentesis

The technique for thoracocentesis is straightforward:
- Position the patient seated leaning forward with his or her back facing the radiologist. Cross the patient's arms and support this position with pillows if necessary.
- A small diagnostic aspirate can be readily obtained with a 21G needle attached to a 50 mL syringe.
- Small effusions can be aspirated through a hypodermic needle. Larger collections are more effectively treated with a drain.
- Formal drainage of non-viscous pleural fluid requires only 6–8Fr drains; infected pleural collections can usually be managed with 16Fr catheters.
- Therapeutic thoracocentesis is performed either with a Seldinger technique or, for large effusions, with a one-step technique. Blunt dissection of the soft tissues with forceps will aid the passage of larger-calibre catheters through the chest wall.
- Connect the chest drain to a closed system or an underwater seal drain.
- Arrange a postprocedure erect chest X-ray.

Some infected effusions will not drain because of the presence of multiple loculi, and intrapleural fibrinolysis can be useful. Streptokinase is the most commonly used agent and is typically given as a 250 000 U dose in 100 mL normal saline once daily. The tube is clamped for 1–2 hours, then returned to suction. Several doses are usually required, success being judged by clinical and radiological resolution of the effusion. Complications are rare.

Bronchial artery embolizations

Bronchial artery embolization is a technically demanding but potentially life-saving intervention. Embolization is most frequently performed in patients with chronic inflammatory lung disease, such as cystic fibrosis, tuberculosis or bronchiectasis, who have developed hypertrophied, fragile bronchial arteries.

Embolization is usually reserved for patients who have sustained massive haemoptysis. The conventional definition is haemoptysis in excess of 300 mL in 24 hours. In reality, the operator will usually only get a vague approximation of the volume loss, but it is usually obvious the patient needs intervention. Continued haemoptysis usually leads to aspiration and hypoxia, and therefore prompt treatment is essential. Embolization does not cure the chronic lung disease, and therefore typically patients require repeated embolization sessions, with each treatment becoming more difficult as smaller vessels are involved.

Preintervention assessment must include chest radiography. Opinions on the value of fibre-optic bronchoscopy vary: occasionally it will lateralize the source of bleeding, but in many patients with massive haemoptysis blood will be present in both right and left bronchi. Contrast-enhanced CT can be valuable, as modern scanners will visualize bronchial and non-bronchial systemic feeder vessels and visualize abnormal parenchyma, allowing the embolization to be directed to the most appropriate area.

Anatomy The bronchial arteries usually arise from the descending aorta between T4 and T6; however, both the number of vessels and the exact site of origin are variable. The most frequent pattern is a common intercostobronchial trunk on the right and a single bronchial artery on the left, though there are many variations (Fig 26.1). Infrequently, bronchial

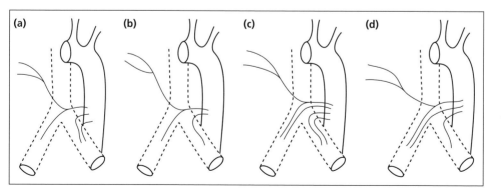

Fig. 26.1 ▪ Bronchial artery anatomy. (a) 41% – two bronchial arteries on the left and an intercostobronchial trunk on the right. (b) 21% – one bronchial artery on the left and one on the right. (c) 21% – two bronchial arteries on the left and two on the right. (d) 10% – one bronchial artery on the left and two on the right.

arteries can arise directly from an extra-aortic vessel such as the internal mammary, inferior phrenic or subclavian artery.

Patients with chronic lung disease, particularly if this involves pleural surfaces, may have a collateral bronchial supply from a variety of systemic arteries, including the subclavian vessels, inferior phrenic, internal mammary artery and thyrocervical trunk. The chest film will usually help identify which of these vessels is most likely to be a significant supply.

Technique Common femoral arterial access. Start with a descending thoracic aortogram using a pigtail catheter positioned just beyond the left subclavian artery. Give at least 30 mL at 15 mL/s, with a film rate of 3 fps. In most patients, particularly those with chronic lung disease, careful scrutiny of the run will reveal the origin of the bronchial arteries. If the origins are not visualized, choose a selective catheter and muster all your patience to start systematically hunting for the bronchial arteries between T4 and T6. Catheter choice is very much personal preference for this procedure, but a reasonable start is to use a Cobra or Headhunter. If you fail with these catheters, try again with a reverse-curve catheter such as a Sos Omni.

Tip: 90% of bronchial arteries are located within the lucency formed by the left main bronchus.

Interpretation

Hypertrophied bronchial arteries have a very characteristic appearance, with a tortuous course extending from the hila to areas of abnormal lung parenchyma (Fig. 26.2). Shunting to the pulmonary arteries or veins is fairly common. Extravasation is very rarely seen in

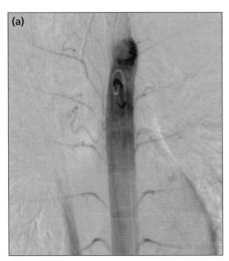

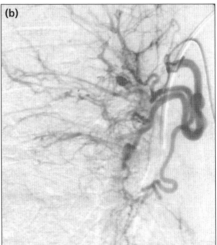

Fig. 26.2 ■ (a) Descending thoracic aortogram; the bronchial origins can be seen. (b) Selective right bronchial arteriogram showing marked hypertrophy of the bronchial artery.

bronchial arterial bleeding. Embolization is definitely indicated when hypertrophied bronchial arteries are seen, particularly when they clearly extend to areas of abnormal lung parenchyma. In the face of massive bleeding many operators will embolize morphologically normal bronchial arteries.

Embolization

Selective catheterization deep enough to permit embolization may require the use of microcatheters. Obtain good-quality angiograms to exclude an anastomosis with the artery of Adamkiewicz (anterior spinal artery supply), as embolization of this vessel could lead to tetraplegia. Polyvinyl alcohol particles (355–500 μm) are the most appropriate agent for embolization. Avoid the use of coils, as this simply makes subsequent embolization for patients with chronic lung disease more difficult.

Complications

There is a long list of potential complications related to bronchial embolization, but these should be balanced against the fairly dismal outcome of uncontrolled massive haemoptysis. The main complication is undoubtably paraplegia secondary to inadvertent embolization of the artery of Adamkiewicz, and very rarely can occur even with catheterization of the artery. Very careful scrutiny of the angiograms for the characteristic hairpin appearance of a spinal artery is mandatory. In addition, repeat angiograms during the embolization are advised, as the spinal artery may not be seen on the initial angiogram owing to preferential flow into the hypertrophied bronchial artery. Other rare complications include oesophageal necrosis, bronchial necrosis and pulmonary infarction.

Alarm: If you have catheterized both the bronchial arteries and the potential systemic collaterals and remain unconvinced that the source of bleeding has been identified, perform a pulmonary angiogram. Pulmonary artery pseudo-aneuryms, called Rasmussen aneurysms by the cognoscenti, occur in association with chronic infection and are treatable with embolization.

Tracheobronchial stenting

Tracheobronchial stenting is a useful, simple technique for the palliation of stridor secondary to airways compression by tumours within the upper mediastinum. The technique is usually restricted to the trachea and main bronchi, and best reserved for extrinsic tumours. Intrinsic tumours rapidly grow through the open stent mesh usually used in the airway. Generally self-expanding stents are used as they do not require occlusion of the airway by a balloon for deployment.

Preparation

These patients are usually breathless, with reduced oxygen saturations, and appropriate monitoring by skilled personnel is essential. With luck the patient will have recently had a CT scan to assess the mediastinum, and it is usually possible to measure the size of the affected airway from this examination. As a rough guide, 10 mm self-expanding stents are suitable for the main bronchi, and a minimum of 14 mm diameter for the trachea.

Technique

It is possible to perform this technique without the aid of a bronchoscopist, but why make life hard for yourself? The bronchoscopist will get through the cords easier and may even be able to get beyond the tumour. In addition, they will anaesthetize the airway more thoroughly than a radiologist can, and this may mean that you are not trying to deploy a stent during a coughing fit by the patient.

The throat should be thoroughly anaesthetized with lignocaine spray, and conscious sedation may be required. The bronchoscopist can usually identify the area of compression, and external radio-opaque markers can be used to indicate the target area. Pass a suitably long wire (260 cm) through the instrument channel of the scope. Take care manipulating the wire in the bronchi, as it is still possible to start a paroxysm of coughing. Carefully remove the bronchoscope. If you are already through the tumour and confident that you know the site of the stenosis, now is the time to load the stent. Occasionally it is necessary to inject contrast to outline the stenosis. It is nearly impossible to see non-ionic contrast, as it is coughed up so quickly, and it is better to use a few mLs of the more viscous lipiodol. Once you have markers applied to the target lesion it is usually straightforward to deploy the stent over the target. The only potential difficulty is the coughing. Be patient and wait for it to subside before deployment. The bronchoscopist can then go back down (carefully) and directly visualize the stent to admire your work. Often it is obvious from the oxygen saturation monitor that you have done the patient some good.

Index